TO HAVE AND TO HOLD

TO HAVE AND TO HOLD
The making of same-sex marriage in South Africa

edited by
Melanie Judge
Anthony Manion
Shaun de Waal

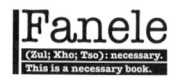 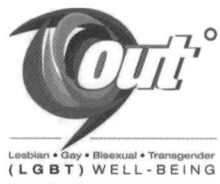 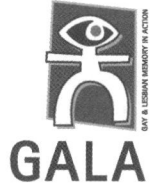 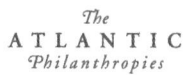

First published by Fanele – an imprint
of Jacana Media (Pty) Ltd – in 2008
Reprinted in 2008 and 2009

10 Orange Street
Sunnyside
Auckland Park 2092
South Africa
+2711 628 3200
www.jacana.co.za

© GALA and OUT LGBT Well-Being, 2008

All rights reserved.

ISBN 978-1-920196-05-9

Cover design by banana republic
Internal design by Shaun de Waal
Set in 10pt Sabon
Printed by Interpak
Job no. 000989

See a complete list of Jacana titles at www.jacana.co.za

Contents

Acknowledgements viii
Contributors ix

Introduction 1

1: AND WE WENT A-COURTING The legal steps to same-sex marriage

Getting to the Constitutional Court on time: A litigation history of same-sex marriage *Jonathan Berger* 17

Difference and belonging: The Constitutional Court and the adoption of the Civil Union Act *Pierre de Vos* 29

'A logical next step' *Interview with Beverly Palesa Ditsie* 42

'A space to challenge the norms' *Interview with Wendy Isaack* 44

'Reforming and renewing' *Interview with Dominee André Muller* 48

'It was a privilege to be involved in the case' *Interview with Sharon Cox and Diane Holdsworth* 52

Legal milestones for gay and lesbian rights in South Africa 55

Judgment days: The journey through the courts 58

2: TAKING IT TO THE PEOPLE The national debate

'This thing' and 'that idea': Traditionalist responses to homosexuality and same-sex marriage *Graeme Reid* 73

Lobbying for same-sex marriage: An activist's reflections *Fikile Vilakazi* 87

(Not) in my culture: Thoughts on same-sex marriage and African practices *Nonhlanhla Mkhize* 97

'Now we have reached consensus' *Interview with Andries Nel* 107

'Counting the gay faces' *Interview with Glenn de Swardt* 111

Putting it to Parliament: The hearings and debates 115

3: FOR BETTER OR FOR WORSE The Civil Union Act

The Civil Union Act: Messy compromise or giant leap forward?
  David Bilchitz with Melanie Judge 149

The achievement of equality and tolerance – how far have we travelled?
  Jody Kollapen and Judith Cohen 164

The Civil Union Act: More of the same *Elsje Bonthuys* 171

Marriage and murder *Tim Trengove-Jones* 182

On rupture and rhyme: Perspectives on the past, present, and future of
  same-sex marriage *Ruthann Robson* 193

A short guide to the Civil Union Act 202

4: DEARLY BELOVED … Religion and same-sex marriage

'Equality of the vineyard': Challenge and celebration for faith communities
  Keith Anthony Vermeulen 209

A way forward through *ijtihad*: A Muslim perspective on same-sex marriage
  Muhsin Hendricks 219

'It had such meaning' *Interview with Janine Preesman* 228

'A bright future for lesbian and gay Christians' *Interview with the Reverend
  Nokuthula Dhladhla* 232

'Justice for all is a core religious value' *Religious and spiritual responses to
  the Civil Union Act* 235

5: HAPPILY EVER AFTER? Reflections on marriage and the Civil Union Act

Blissful complexities: Black lesbians reflect on same-sex marriage and the Civil
  Union Act *Zethu Matebeni* 249

Lesbians and the Civil Union Act: A critical reflection *Mary Hames* 258

De-gendering unions: The Civil Union Act and the intersexed *Sally Gross* 268

Marriage, citizenship and contested meanings *Vasu Reddy and Zethu Cakata* 274

'Are our lives OK?' Reflections on 13 years of gay liberation in South Africa   *Gerald Kraak*   278

Queering marriage? The legal recognition of same-sex relationships around the world   *Craig Lind*   284

'We first need to be recognized ...'   *Activists reflect on same-sex marriage and LGBTI rights in Africa*   300

'The traditional model of marriage is oppressive'   *Feminist perspectives on marriage*   307

6: TYING THE KNOT   Marriage in action

'They knew we were serious'   *Interview with Charles Januarie and Hompi Januarie*   317

'Why is it okay when *they* hold hands, but not us?'   *Interview with Nozipho Ngcobo and Thulile Ngcobo*   321

'Saying to our children ... we are a unit'   *Interview with Lael Bethlehem and Emilia Potenza*   324

'The marriage ceremony was turned into a training session'   *Interview with William Stewart*   329

'Making the box bigger'   *Interview with Robert Hamblin and Sally-Jean Shackleton*   331

'I didn't marry the body, I married the person inside'   *Interview with Christelle Delport and Raven Delport*   335

'The guts to get married'   *Interview with Sadia Kruger and Zukayna Kruger*   338

'Rejoicing in merit'   *Interview with Wayne Sampson and Vajradhara*   341

'A living tradition'   *Interview with Margaret Auerbach and Liebe Kellen*   345

Index   349

Acknowledgements

This book could not have been accomplished without the assistance of many people and organizations. We wish to acknowledge and thank them.

The opportunity to develop and publish this book was provided by the generous financial support of The Atlantic Philanthropies. We owe a special debt of gratitude to the head of their South African office, Gerald Kraak, for his support. Our thanks also go to Gay and Lesbian Memory in Action (GALA) and OUT LGBT Well-being (OUT) for having the vision and courage to take on this project. We especially thank GALA director Ruth Morgan and OUT director Dawie Nel for their assistance and encouragement in bringing this book to completion.

Our publishers Caroline Smith and Russell Clarke of Jacana Media have been involved in shaping the book from the beginning. We thank them for the expertise and enthusiasm they brought to the project.

This book would also have been impossible without the hard work and commitment of the 21 essayists, and the interviewees who gave so generously of their insights and their time, and enriched the book immeasurably. Kerry Williams, Angelo Pantazis, Rehana Vally and Jonathan Berger read and commented on specific essays or sections of the book. Their input was invaluable. Adrienne Pretorius assisted in the standardization of our legal referencing. Karen Jeynes, Godfrey Phela, Phineas Riba and Graham Young provided transcriptions and translations for many of the interviews. Busi Kheswa and Paul Mokgethi of GALA provided important logistical support. Members of the Joint Working Group also provided assistance with the research and development of this book and special mention must be made of Behind the Mask in this regard.

David Bilchitz, Thuli Madi, Karen Martin and Graeme Reid shared with us their insights and perspectives in the initial stages of the project and helped us draw together a balanced and comprehensive book.

Many people assisted with the interviews: Joanne Bloch interviewed Sadia and Zukayna Kruger; Busisiwe Kheswa interviewed Nozipho and Thulile Ngcobo and assisted with interviews with Wendy Isaack and Dawn O'Reilly; Paul Mokgethi co-interviewed Charles and Hompi Januarie. The remaining interviews were conducted by the editors.

All royalties from this book will go to GALA and OUT and will be used to distribute the book to LGBTI organizations in South Africa, on the continent and elsewhere.

Finally, the editors wish to acknowledge the many people, deceased and alive, who have contributed to, and continue to fight for, the realization of LGBTI rights and justice in South Africa.

Contributors

Jonathan Berger is a senior researcher and policy, research and communications manager at the AIDS Law Project, and represents the law and human rights sector on the Programme Implementation Committee of the South African National AIDS Council. After serving as the legal education and advice officer at the National Coalition for Gay and Lesbian Equality, Jonathan clerked for Justice Kate O'Regan of the Constitutional Court. He holds degrees in architecture and law from the University of the Witwatersrand, Johannesburg, as well as a Master of Laws degree from the University of Toronto. Until recently, Jonathan served as a member of the board of the Lesbian and Gay Equality Project. He was integrally involved in the Constitutional Court challenge to the exclusion of same-sex couples from the marriage laws of South Africa. He also participated in lobbying and advocacy efforts leading up to the adoption of the Civil Union Act in 2006.

David Bilchitz has a BA (Hons) LLB *cum laude* from Wits University and an MPhil and a PhD from St John's College, University of Cambridge, in political philosophy and law. David is an admitted attorney and is also a sessional lecturer in jurisprudence at the University of the Witwatersrand Law School. He is currently a senior researcher at the South African Institute for Advanced Constitutional, Public, Human Rights and International Law. His main areas of writing interest involve socio-economic rights, lesbian and gay rights, and constitutional law in general. His publications include the book *Poverty and Fundamental Rights*. David was joint leader of the gay and lesbian student group at Wits University, Activate. He helped found and is presently the chairperson of Jewish OutLook, which caters for the needs of Jewish LGBTI people. In 2006, he played a key role in the campaign for civil marriage for same-sex couples in South Africa, and acted as legal adviser to OUT LGBT Well-being. In 2007, he helped lobby for the decision by the Progressive Jewish movement to conduct same-sex marriages and is now a religious marriage officer in terms of the Civil Union Act.

Elsje Bonthuys is an associate professor who joined the Wits Law School as a lecturer in 1999 and was appointed a professor of law in 2007. She teaches contract, family law and gender and the law. She previously held a lecturing post at the University of Stellenbosch and practised as a member of the Cape Bar. Scholarships from the Human Sciences Research Council (HSRC), the Cambridge Commonwealth Trust and the Association of Commonwealth Universities enabled her to read for a PhD at the University of Cambridge, which was conferred in March 2000. Her current research interests include family law, domestic violence and gender law.

Zethu Cakata is a senior researcher and a doctoral intern at the Gender and Development Unit of the Human Sciences Research Council (HSRC). She is a research psychologist whose interests include feminisms, gender, sexual politics, health, identity and marginal sexualities. She has a masters degree in research psychology. Her experience spans health research, gender and development (including sexualities) and citizenship and rights issues. She is currently working on her doctoral degree, entitled 'Knowledge, Attitude and Experience: Health Care Provision and Same-Sex Sexuality in South Africa'.

Pierre de Vos teaches constitutional law at the University of the Western Cape. He has published extensively on a wide variety of topics including sexual orientation and discrimination and the enforcement of social and economic rights. He also runs 'Constitutionally Speaking', a blog dealing with political and legal issues from a constitutional perspective. He was a member of the National Coalition for Gay and Lesbian Equality and was involved in the lobbying to secure the inclusion of the sexual-orientation clause in the 1996 Constitution. He was a founding member of Siyazenzela, an organization aimed at fighting racism and homophobia. He has been the chairperson of the Board of the Aids Legal Network for the past three years.

Shaun de Waal was literary editor of the *Mail & Guardian* from 1991 to 2006 and has been its chief film critic since 1998, as well as writing widely for the paper on books, the arts in general, and gay and lesbian issues since 1989. He has published fiction (*These Things Happen*, 1996; *Jackmarks*, 1998) and non-fiction (*Steven Cohen*, a monograph on the queer South African artist; with Robyn Sassen, 2003) and has edited several books, including *Pride: Protest and Celebration* (with Anthony Manion, 2006), and the booklet *Till the Time of Trial: The Prison Letters of Simon Nkoli* (with Karen Martin, 2007).

Sally Gross is an intersexed activist, founder of the Intersex Society of South Africa (ISOSA) and a member of the board of Engender from the time of its foundation. Born and bred in South Africa, she was actively involved in the struggle against apartheid and was in exile for many years as a result. Raised in a male role and trained rabbinically in her teens, she was a member of the English Province of Order of Preachers, serving as a priest of the Order and teaching both philosophy and theology. Her clerical and academic careers and connection with the Catholic Church ended in direct consequence of her being found to be intersexed. Since 1999, when she was able to return to South Africa, she has raised awareness concerning intersex and has secured amendments in law that ensure recognition of the intersexed and the strengthening of their rights.

Mary Hames is the director of the Gender Equity Unit at the University of the Western Cape. She holds an MPhil in Southern African political studies and is currently pursuing her doctorate in women and gender studies at the African Gender Institute, University of Cape Town. Her interests include women's human rights and sexual rights. She has made written and oral submissions to Parliament arguing for the legitimation and recognition of same-sex marriage. Mary has served on a range of boards, including the Development Education and Leadership Teams in Action (chairperson 2003–2007); Pride Shelter Trust (vice-chairperson 2006); Cape Town Pride (2007) and was a senator at the University of the Western Cape (2005).

Muhsin Hendricks studied Arabic and Islamic studies at the Islamic University of Karachi, Jamia Dirasat Al-Islamia, and returned four years later to South Africa to serve his community as an Islamic scholar, teacher and *imam*, until he was ostracized because of his sexuality. His personal life story bears testimony to the fact that queer Muslims experience trauma in reconciling their sexuality with their faith. His quest for the truth has led him to do research on Islam and homosexuality. Muhsin is the Director and co-founder of The Inner Circle, an NGO that provides services to queer Muslims and fights homophobia in the Muslim community through education, training, research and outreach.

Melanie Judge holds a masters degree in development studies from the University of the Western Cape and an honours degree in psychology from the University of Cape Town. She is a human-rights and feminist activist and has worked on policy, training, and service provision initiatives in the fields of HIV/AIDS, gender, and sexual rights in South Africa and Africa. Melanie has been actively engaged in LGBTI advocacy, and in the same-sex marriage campaign, both at OUT LGBT Well-being, where she works now, and at the Lesbian and Gay Equality Project. She was integrally involved in the lobbying and advocacy efforts leading up to the passing of the Civil Union Act. She is a board member of The Inner Circle, an NGO that provides services to and challenges homophobia in the Muslim community.

Jody Kollapen is the chairperson of the South African Human Rights Commission (SAHRC) and **Judith Cohen** is the head of programme: parliamentary liaison legislation and treaty body monitoring programme at the SAHRC. They are both lawyers by profession. The SAHRC is one of the independent institutions created to support democracy in terms of South Africa's Constitution. The Commission's parliamentary programme is actively involved in monitoring and advocacy work around new pieces of legislation, hence the Commission's participation in the public-hearing processes and advocacy around the Civil Union Bill.

Gerald Kraak is head of the South African office of The Atlantic Philanthropies, an international charitable organization. He is the author of the novel *Ice in the Lungs,* joint winner of the 2005 European Union Literary Award, and has published two other books on South African politics. He is also the director of the documentary film *Property of the State: Gay Men in the Apartheid Military*.

Craig Lind holds law degrees from the University of the Witwatersrand and the London School of Economics. Before taking up a post at the University of Sussex, he held full-time teaching posts at the University of the Witwatersrand and at the University of Wales in Aberystwyth. He has also taught at a number of other universities, including King's College, London, Brunel University of West London, City University and Birkbeck College, University of London.

Anthony Manion is the archives co-ordinator for Gay and Lesbian Memory in Action (GALA), Johannesburg. He is the co-editor with Shaun de Waal of the book *Pride: Protest and Celebration* (2006) and has been part of the development of a number of exhibitions, including *Balancing Act: South African Gay and Lesbian Youth Speak Out* (2006) and *Home Affairs* (2008; both in partnership with the Apartheid Museum). He was born in East London and educated at the University of Cape Town.

Zethu Matebeni is a doctoral fellow at the Wits Institute for Social Economic Research (WISER), Johannesburg. Her research proposes to understand and explore black lesbian identities and sexualities in post-apartheid Johannesburg. She has previously worked as a research manager for the South African government's national campaign on HIV and AIDS, TB and STIs, and has lectured at the University of Pretoria, Department of Sociology. Zethu is actively involved in various LGBTI organizations in the country.

Nonhlanhla 'MC' Mkhize is the director of the Durban Lesbian and Gay Community and Health Centre, which is a drop-in centre providing personal, legal and HIV/AIDS counselling, education and advocacy. She is a human-rights defender; an Amnesty International South Africa Durban Group Co-Chair; the 2006 GEM Awards Winner: Opinion and Commentary; and a final-year masters student in anthropology at the University of KwaZulu-Natal (Howard College). Her passion is research and advocacy work on human rights for children, women, youth and LGBTI people. She sits on the boards of Behind the Mask and the Lesbian and Gay Equality Project, and mentors and sits on the advisory committees of a number of youth, women, ethics and human-rights organizations and groups locally, nationally and internationally.

Vasu Reddy is a chief research specialist in the Gender and Development Unit, Human Sciences Research Council (Pretoria, South Africa). Before joining the HSRC he was head of gender studies at the University of KwaZulu-Natal (Howard College). He was previously a national executive committee member of the National Coalition for Gay and Lesbian Equality. He is also an honorary associate professor of gender studies in the School of Anthropology, Gender and Historical Studies at the University of KwaZulu-Natal. He is the co-founder of the Durban Lesbian and Gay Community and Health Centre and is currently board chairperson of OUT LGBT Well-being.

Graeme Reid is a lecturer at Yale University, teaching in LGBTI studies and anthropology. He is also a research associate at the Wits Institute for Social and Economic Research (WISER), where he was based from 2001 to 2006. In 1997 he established the Gay and Lesbian Archives (GALA, now known as Gay and Lesbian Memory in Action) at Wits University. His PhD, in anthropology, is from the University of Amsterdam. He has published extensively on same-sex sexualities, masculinities, and HIV/AIDS.

Ruthann Robson is professor of law and distinguished university professor at the City University of New York in the United States, where she teaches law and sexuality, as well as constitutional law. Her books include *Sappho Goes to Law School* and *Lesbian (Out)Law*, as well as the novels *a/k/a* and *Cecile*. In 2007, she was Bram Fischer Visiting Professor at the Oliver Schreiner School of Law, University of the Witwatersrand, Johannesburg.

Keith Anthony Vermeulen is the director of the Public Policy Liaison Unit – or parliamentary office – of the South African Council of Churches (SACC). Keith has been appointed to this position by the SACC, seconded by the Methodist Church of Southern Africa as one of their ordained clergy. Keith graduated from the University of Edinburgh with distinction in masters-degree studies in development and theology in 1991, studies that have contributed to his developmental focus. By virtue of his social location under apartheid as a 'second-class' and 'non-citizen', Keith is an activist for social equity. This orientation has placed him at the cutting edge of assisting the SACC member churches' response to the legal and constitutional challenges pertaining to freedom of religious belief. Keith's relationship with the Lesbian and Gay Equality Project, GALA and OUT LGBT Well-being developed and deepened after he was approached by these organizations to share in various workshops when the South African Law Reform Commission called for responses to their research on domestic and same-sex partnerships.

Tim Trengove-Jones lectures in English literature at the University of the Witwatersrand. He has written widely on gay politics and the politics of AIDS in both the mainstream media and academic publications. More popularly, he is known in a specifically gay context for his regular column appearing in the South African monthly gay publication *Exit*.

Fikile Vilakazi has an honours degree in Development Studies from the University of the Western Cape. She has been involved in development work since 1993 and has been actively involved in student politics, gender, feminism and women's-rights activism, lesbian, gay, bisexual, transgender and intersex activism in South Africa, Africa and Europe. She has a passion for grassroots development and believes in participatory development that works *with* people rather than *for* people. She is a growing and learning activist who aspires to make a difference in social and political reform for the rights of marginalized groups in society. She was born in Soweto.

Introduction

Melanie Judge, Anthony Manion and Shaun de Waal

> ... I think I should just pay tribute to gay and lesbian structures that actually helped wittingly and unwittingly in the development of equality jurisprudence in this country. All those struggles around rights of gay and lesbian people have in many ways allowed the [Constitutional] Court and allowed our Constitution and many other people to be able to express themselves around issues of equality, so we owe a lot of debt actually to gays and lesbians in this country, certainly around equality issues. – Deputy Chief Justice Dikgang Moseneke[1]

On 30 November 2006, South Africa became the first country in Africa to legalize marriage between people of the same sex. This book explores the processes that led to that historic moment, what the new legislation – the Civil Union Act – means, and what its impact has been on the lives of those now able to marry legally for the first time. Through the perspectives of a range of actors (activists, academics, commentators, organizations, and lesbian and gay individuals) we seek to tell the story of the making of same-sex marriage in South Africa.

There is no single story to be told, nor one interpretation of its meaning, as the contributions in this book show. Rather, we have attempted to assemble a range of understandings and reflections on the topic, and to place them alongside key information about and documentation of the legislative journey, the parliamentary process, and the Act itself. Our essayists offer a series of contour paths through this bumpy terrain, and we have interviewed various people who might be described as 'stakeholders', whether participants in advocacy or simply couples who share their experiences of marriage both before and after the inception of the Act. Every attempt has been made to be as inclusive as possible in the variety of voices presented, but we do not pretend this is the final word on the matter.

Was the passing of the Civil Union Act an outright victory or a compromise? What does the attainment of the right to marry mean for lesbian, gay, bisexual, transgender and intersex (LGBTI[2]) people, and what are its broader social and political implications? What does marriage say about sexuality, gender, power, and identities? Our contributors take differing positions on these issues, and their nuanced reflections and accounts of their personal experiences illuminate what marriage, same-sex or not, may mean in South Africa today. We provide documentation and argumentation that can be drawn on for the purpose of human-rights advocacy, critical engagement with the topic and historical record. We hope the book makes a contribution to continued activism in the struggle for lasting and meaningful social change.

The legal steps to same-sex marriage
In 2002 Marié Adriaana Fourie and Cecelia Johanna Bonthuys, a lesbian couple, approached the High Court wanting to marry. Their challenge to the common-law definition of marriage (then restricted to the union of a man and a woman) sought to attain the status, benefits and responsibilities that flow from marriage between heterosexual couples. The right to choose whether or not to enter into a marriage with another person of the same sex ('same-sex marriage'), had the potential to provide automatic legal recognition for all purposes where relationship status was at issue; and to accord equal social and legal status to both same- and opposite sex relationships.

At around the same time as what became known as the *Fourie* case commenced, the Lesbian and Gay Equality Project (the Equality Project) launched its first court application that sought to reform both the common law and the Marriage Act itself. Along with 16 other applicants (including Triangle Project, OUT LGBT Well-being, Forum for the Empowerment of Women, the Durban Gay and Lesbian Community and Health Centre and six same-sex couples), the Equality Project approached the courts for relief.[3] An increasingly visible, vocal and mobilized LGBTI sector drove what became the same-sex marriage campaign. Targeted litigation, supported by direct lobbying and advocacy on the part of LGBTI individuals, activists and organizations, was central to the process.

When the *Fourie* case reached the Supreme Court of Appeal (SCA) in 2004, Justice Edwin Cameron ruled that the common-law definition of marriage discriminated unfairly against same-sex couples and ordered that the law be developed immediately to include them. (See excerpts from this judgment in 'Judgment days' in part one of this book.) But this finding was to be appealed and cross-appealed by the applicants and the state, taking the matter all the way to the Constitutional Court.[4]

On 17 May 2005 both the *Fourie* case and the Equality Project's application for direct access to the Constitutional Court, was heard in that court. The resulting judgment would be the culmination of a process begun against the backdrop of the interim Constitution of South Africa in 1994. The birth of democracy was the beginning of a new era for all South Africans, including LGBTI people. The historic equality clause[5] in the final Constitution (ratified in 1996) set the stage for the development of precedent-setting jurisprudence around rights for sexual minorities, as one by one discriminatory laws were challenged. The strategic litigation efforts of the National Coalition for

Gay and Lesbian Equality (NCGLE), and its successor, the Lesbian and Gay Equality Project, along with a number of brave individual citizens who took to the courts to challenge various pieces of discriminatory legislation, paved the way for a series of landmark cases that would usher in a new post-apartheid legal dispensation for LGBTI people. During the period from 1996 onwards we witnessed legislative and jurisprudential developments that demonstrated a growing recognition in law of same-sex relationships and families. Moreover our courts had consistently acknowledged that there are multiple family forms that are evolving over time; recognized the historical and ongoing discrimination faced by lesbian and gay people; and identified a lack of comprehensive family law rights for lesbian and gay people. (The key cases in this process are listed in 'Legal milestones for gay and lesbian rights in South Africa' in part one of this book.)

Finally, on 1 December 2005, amid a buzz of anticipation – trepidation for some, excitement for others – Justice Albie Sachs delivered his momentous judgment. (See 'Judgment days' for excerpts; the judgment is extensively discussed throughout this book.) The Constitutional Court found that the failure of the common law and the Marriage Act to provide the means whereby same-sex couples could enjoy the same status, entitlements and responsibilities as heterosexuals do in marriage constituted an unjustifiable violation of their rights to equality and dignity.

Yet same-sex couples were not to have justice on that day. Marié and Cecelia would have to wait another year before they would be able to exercise their choice to marry. The Court had suspended the order of invalidity and given Parliament a year to enact legislation to correct the constitutional defect in the marriage laws. If Parliament failed to do so, the Court would automatically order that Section 30 (1) of the Marriage Act be read as including the words 'or spouse' after the words 'or husband' as they appear in the marriage formula, thus allowing same-sex couples to marry. (Justice Kate O'Regan, in her dissenting judgment, argued that the order of constitutionality should not be suspended and that, in line with the SCA finding, the applicants should be granted immediate relief. See 'Judgment days'.) Sadly, as a result of this delay, Marié and Cecelia were never to make it down the rainbow aisle. Marié passed away before the legislature acted to give effect to the Constitutional Court ruling.

Part one of this book, 'And we went a-courting: The legal steps to same-sex marriage', examines the route from the equality clause in the Constitution to the Constitutional Court judgment that eventually gave rise to the Civil Union Act. **Jonathan Berger**'s essay traces the litigation history that led to same-sex marriage in South Africa, beginning with the case for the decriminalization of the common-law crime of sodomy. (See also Mary Hames's piece on lesbian activism around equality law in part five.) **Pierre de Vos** examines Justice Sachs's emphasis on the importance of an acknowledgement of 'difference' in post-apartheid South Africa, as well as the need of marginalized minorities to 'belong', and how that challenges heteronormativity. He discusses how the key principle of difference informed the ultimate Constitutional Court decision on same-sex marriage, and what message that communicates to South Africa today.

Also in part one, interviews with activists engaged in the struggle for the equality and recognition of LGBTI people help trace the thinking that shaped the same-sex marriage campaign. **Beverly Palesa Ditsie** was a founding member of the Gay and Lesbian Organization of the Witwatersrand (GLOW), which became the public – and, importantly, largely black – face of lesbian and gay activism in the early 1990s. She talks about how the desire for equality of marriage rights was embedded in such activism even at that time. **Wendy Isaack** discusses the development of the campaign for same-sex marriage, and its consequences, from the perspective of the Equality Project at the time. Dominee **André Muller** talks about the Reforming Church he founded, its drive to perform life-commitment ceremonies, and his support to Marié and Cecelia. **Sharon Cox and Diane Holdsworth** were among the couples who joined the court cases to declare the heterosexual limits on marriage unconstitutional; they talk about the process and what meaning it had for them.

The section concludes with a timeline of the important court cases that secured gay and lesbian formal equality in South Africa, in the lead-up to *Fourie*, and provides a series of extracts from the SCA and Constitutional Court judgments in response to the legal challenges to discriminatory marriage laws.

The national debate on same-sex marriage

The Constitutional Court judgment in *Fourie* gave Parliament the responsibility of addressing the discriminatory aspects of the 1961 Marriage Act. In August 2006, the Department of Home Affairs released the first draft of the Civil Union Bill, which sought to establish a new, 'separate but equal', civil-partnership institution, for same-sex couples only. The Bill was then subjected to an extensive process of public engagement and deliberation. The National Assembly's Portfolio Committee on Home Affairs held a series of hearings in all provinces, in September and October 2007, and then in Parliament.

The public debate on the Bill unleashed a range of responses from all sides of the political spectrum. LGBTI organizations, including the Joint Working Group (JWG),[6] along with other human-rights activists and civil-society actors, argued that the Bill fell short of constitutional requirements: it sought to establish a 'separate but equal' institution for same-sex couples only. The proposed 'separate but equal' (which is never equal) regime was reminiscent of apartheid, and it relegated LGBTI people and their relationships to second-class status. The first draft of the Bill did not allow for the designation 'marriage' in the legal classification of same-sex relationships. The solution favoured by LGBTI organizations and many other human-rights activists was simply for Parliament to amend the Marriage Act to render it gender-neutral. On the other side of the political spectrum, religious conservatives and traditional leadership argued vehemently against the Bill, suggesting that it had gone too far in its recognition of same-sex relationships, and that granting same-sex unions the same legal status as 'marriage' would destroy the traditional concept of marriage as exclusively heterosexual.

Around the period of the public hearings, religious reactionaries arranged country-wide marches protesting against same-sex marriage. (See picture pages.) There were calls for a constitutional amendment to protect the 'sanctity' of (heterosexual) marriage. Radio talk shows and TV debates were filled with argument on the issue. The public discourse, inside and outside Parliament, was often characterized by flagrant expressions of hate speech, demonizing LGBTI people and their relationships. Same-sex marriage was the first LGBTI rights issue to enter the public arena for orchestrated, nation-wide debate. All previous LGBTI-related legal reforms had passed without much of a fuss. In a sense, the same-sex marriage debate became far broader than the question of whether same-sex couples should have the right to marry: it went to the heart of beliefs about and attitudes to gender, sexuality, power, democracy, religion, culture and the like.

As Nozizwe Madlala-Routledge, the former deputy minister of health, put it, 'The nature of the debate around the Civil Union Bill illustrated the importance of promoting the Constitution and the rights it protects. Although the rights of gays and lesbians are embroidered into the fabric of our Constitution and the Bill of Rights, some of the arguments used against the bill were very worrying. They displayed ignorance and intolerance on the part of various sections of our society, in the faith-based sector and structures of traditional leadership. It takes all pervasive leadership to build a culture of accountability and openness and ensure that these rights and freedoms are not undermined or lost.'[7]

Part two of this book, 'Taking it to the people: The national debate', outlines the public positions taken around the issue of same-sex marriage. Before the Constitutional Court had made its finding in *Fourie* and the Equality Project case, and with the buzz about same-sex marriage in the air as a result of the SCA judgment, the National House of Traditional Leaders (NHTL) conducted its own roadshow of public hearings. This process focused on the 'traditionalist' response to homosexuality and same-sex marriage, producing a stark opposition between such responses and the human-rights ethos of the Constitution. In the essay kicking off part two, **Graeme Reid** examines the views expressed during the NHTL hearings, and contrasts them with the construction of sexual identities in rural South African communities, where traditional gender roles are inflected in intriguing and innovative ways.

As the campaign for same-sex marriage moved through Parliament, LGBTI organizations engaged in joint advocacy strategies to garner support, lobbying key sectors and decision-makers towards their goal: 'Equal marriage for all: nothing less'. **Fikile Vilakazi,** one of the activists centrally involved in lobbying around the Bill, tracks the advocacy approach of the marriage campaign during the Bill's journey through the legislature. In the context of the traditionalist resistance to same-sex marriage, **Nonhlanhla Mkhize** conducts an investigation into the opinions and feelings of individuals and couples in her reflective exploration of what same-sex marriage may mean in the context of 'African culture' and how culture may accommodate divergent sexualities, or not.

The interviews in this section take the story further. The ruling party's deputy chief whip, **Andries Nel,** describes the process from within the African National Congress (ANC) and from within Parliament. From without Parliament, as it were, **Glenn de Swardt** of Cape Town's Triangle Project talks about the involvement of LGBTI people in the campaign for same-sex marriage, the experience of the public hearings, protest activities, and dealing with the media.

'Putting it to Parliament: the hearings and debates', which concludes part two of this book, presents excerpts from the parliamentary submissions, revealing the core arguments for, against, and somewhere in between. As these extracts show, voices opposed to equality for LGBTI people dominated, informed as they were by conservative, religious and traditionalist views, and staged in an often apocalyptic manner. But other important voices to the contrary were heard as well, and in the end it was the duty of Parliament to respond to the Constitutional Court's judgment.

The Civil Union Act

As the interview with Nel in part two (partly) indicates, there were divisions within the ruling party about extending marriage to include same-sex couples. The ANC executive had to assert its authority and remind members of Parliament, both in caucuses and in the National Assembly (NA) debate, of the party's policy commitment to equality for all South Africans, as underscored by both the Freedom Charter and the Constitution. As the extracts in part two show, the debates in the NA and the National Council of Provinces (NCOP) reflected some of the ideological contestations the Bill evoked. The final vote on the Bill was a result of a three-line whip, in terms of which ANC members of Parliament were obliged to be present in the NA and vote in favour of the Bill. On 14 November 2006, the Bill was passed by the NA, and on 28 November it was confirmed by the NCOP.

Despite that victory, the Civil Union Act is flawed: among other defects, it did not repeal the Marriage Act of 1961, which is still exclusively for heterosexual couples, and it allows civil marriage officers to "conscientiously object" to solemnizing same-sex unions. In their essay, which introduces part three of this book, 'For better or for worse: The Civil Union Act', **David Bilchitz and Melanie Judge** explore the shifting content of the Civil Union Bill during the legislative process, and ask where it came out: messy compromise or giant leap forward, with a transformative potential for South African family law?

In her response to the Act, **Elsje Bonthuys** sees it as premised on a particular form of 'globalized' gay and lesbian identity. (See also Zethu Matebeni's essay in part five.) Bonthuys argues that the Act fails to acknowledge the long history of same-sex relationships in African societies, or to reflect the complex practices and beliefs surrounding such relationships. She suggests that, as a result, the Civil Union Act did not grasp the opportunity to imagine the richer concepts and forms of legislation that customary law could have inspired.

Tim Trengove-Jones's essay situates itself in the space between the Sachs judgment and the murder of two black lesbian women that occurred in July 2007. Why, he asks, are we so surprised and outraged when our lives (and deaths) show how far our society has fallen short of its constitutional ideals? His detailed examination of the Sachs judgment, in the light of the '*Bildungsroman*' that is the progressive jurisprudence around LGBTI rights, offers some thoughts on this complex issue. **Ruthann Robson,** by contrast, offers a personal perspective on the Act, from the viewpoint of an American (where same-sex marriage has been a battleground for decades, and the battle is ongoing), and playfully imagines a future Constitutional Court challenge to the constraints and dangers that potentially come with the very marriage regime many fought so hard to attain.

Part three concludes with a quick, practical guide on the Act, what it means and how to gain access to its provisions. For those of our readers eager to 'tie the knot', this is the place to start.

Religion and same-sex marriage

As the parliamentary hearings showed, the issue of religion was central to social and moral engagements with the notion of marriage between people of the same-sex. Since the passage of the Civil Union Act, 35 religious denominations or organizations have been granted the designation to solemnize same-sex marriages and civil partnerships under the Act; unsurprisingly, none of the mainstream Christian denominations are among them. In part four, 'Dearly beloved ... Religion and same-sex marriage', a range of voices from across the religious and spiritual spectrum discuss the often uncomfortable intersection of traditional religious moralities and LGBTI sexualities and rights. **Keith Vermeulen,** from the South African Council of Churches, presents a Christian viewpoint at odds with the conservative perspectives that so dominated the parliamentary hearings, as shown by the excerpts in part two. His reasoning throws up a bold challenge to Christians who see the Word of God as limited in interpretation and who have defined themselves in relation to the achievement of institutionalized power, rather than drawing from scripture a fundamental message about love, trust and care – particularly for the oppressed and marginalized. Writing from the perspective of a Muslim imam, **Muhsin Hendricks** is one of the few people prepared to engage publicly with homosexuality and same-sex marriage from an informed Islamic perspective. His essay explores the promise of *ijtihad*, the 'independent reasoning' licensed by the Quran, in grappling with the stifling effects of orthodoxy on Muslim constructions of sexuality and marriage.

In the interviews in part four, Pastor **Janine Preesman** shares her personal reflections of conducting the first legally sanctioned religious same-sex marriage on the continent, and the Reverend **Nokuthula Dhladhla** discusses the hopes for a reconciliation of Christianity and the sexual minorities it has historically despised. Rounding off part four is a group discussion coordinated by the editors, in which people working within various faith-based organizations or groups (including Buddhist, Hindu, Pagan, Jewish and African traditional-religious perspectives) grapple with the challenges of religious doctrine, sexuality and the social sanction of relationships through marriage. In order to provide a contrast with the immovable prejudices expressed by so many religious groups at the parliamentary hearings, the editors solicited contributions from those whose faith communities are positively and constructively engaging with these issues.

Reflections on same-sex marriage and the Civil Union Act
For all the triumphalism expressed by many LGBTI individuals, couples and activists following the promulgation of the Civil Union Act on 30 November 2006, a range of contributors reveal the myriad contradictions in the struggle for the realization of the right to marry. Against the backdrop of continuing homophobia and hate motivated crimes in South Africa (never mind the rest of the continent), the question of whether we have emerged victorious is a vexed one. There is an insidious incongruence between social mores and constitutional values, and the battle around same-sex marriage highlights the contradictions inherent in the dual projects of social transformation and intimate exchange.

The extracts from the parliamentary submission of the Congress of Traditional Leaders of South Africa (Contralesa) in part two show that the accusation that homosexuality in any form, let alone same-sex marriage, is 'unAfrican' is pervasive. Reid and Mkhize explore this in their essays in part two and other contributors touch on this sensitive topic as well. South Africa is undoubtedly emerging from the ravages of colonialism and apartheid, when indigenous identities and cultures were systematically denied and fractured by colonial masters. Coming after centuries in which African identities meant relegation to an underclass, redefining what it means to be African is a critical part of an ongoing engagement in post-colonial reconstruction. African identities are, rightly so, a site of major contestation, and legitimate questions must be raised about the interface of so-called traditional cultures and the reclamation of human rights in a pluralistic constitutional democracy. In this regard homosexuality and same-sex marriage often seem to be acting as lightning rods, and may be the site upon which these identity contestations play themselves out. As such, same-sex sexuality and marriage, within our current socio-political context, is more than simply a constitutional 'litmus test' because it speaks to the consolidation of democracy and the aspiration to 'unity in diversity'.[8]

What is clear is that same-sex sexuality and relationships existed in a variety of places and periods in Africa. How people understood such relationships has also varied greatly over time and in different regions, and continues to be the subject of debate. Frequently cited examples of pre-colonial same-sex practices stand in contrast to claims by African opponents of same-sex marriage that such practices are 'unAfrican' and a Western import. In *Hungochani: The History of a Dissident Sexuality in Southern Africa*, Marc Epprecht suggests, instead, that same-sex sexuality in pre-colonial Africa was often accepted as long as it did not preclude marriage and children and was enacted discreetly. He has uncovered little evidence to suggest that Africa had an extensive pre-colonial history of persecuting people for same-sex relations. Epprecht argues that it is in fact homophobia that is the Western import, introduced into the region by European colonialists and preachers.[9]

Similarly, the essay by **Zethu Matebeni** in part five of this book draws on some of the rich anthropological and archival material on same-sex relationship forms in Africa, exploring the history of woman-marriages in South Africa to show that such relationships can take different forms and mean different things to the people involved, offering a mobility of relationship forms that 'tradition' would seem to deny. In the light of this, she engages with the perspectives of four black lesbian women on marriage and the Civil Union Act, suggesting that the Act has extended the traditional parameters of woman-marriages in that it offers a Western-style pact that juxtaposes the desires of the individuals concerned with the structural needs of family and clan affiliation. In the same section, **Mary Hames** puts a lesbian-feminist mirror to the institution of marriage and traces the key contributions of lesbian women to the development of the jurisprudence around LGBTI rights. She interrogates what marriage may mean for black lesbian women, as it is inflected by dynamics of race, class and citizenship.

Sally Gross addresses the impact of same-sex marriage on the intersexed, showing how it offers liberation from the entrenched gendering that is formalized through the Marriage Act. She considers the significance of a de-gendered marriage regime in the light of the divergent accounts of the primal union of Adam and Eve in the book of Genesis, echoing and extending the discussion of religion and same-sex marriage in the previous section. **Vasu Reddy and Zethu Cakata** interrogate the meanings of citizenship as thrown up by the same-sex marriage question. While marriage is now a condition conferred or denied by the state, they argue, our very bodies and their pleasures represent deep political conflicts over identity and morality. Activism must continue, they argue ... and we know that funding helps. **Gerald Kraak**'s essay discusses the advancement of LGBTI rights in South Africa over the past 13 years from the perspective of a key donor, and talks about how the same-sex marriage campaign was one that crossed boundaries of gender, class and race. He also asks what the way forward for LGBTI activism might be.

In some ways, South Africa now stands as a model of progressive legislation for LGBTI rights. **Craig Lind** provides a comprehensive global overview of the achievement of, or movement towards, the kinds of rights represented by the Civil Union Act, and asks whether such initiatives are on their way to 'queering' family law. Given South Africa's approach to human rights and our transition to democracy, and given the contestations around African identity mentioned above, the editors of this book go on to ask a range of LGBTI activists from across Africa what the impact of legal same-sex marriage in South Africa has had or might have in their countries. Coming as they do from places where any form of same-sex sexuality is usually criminalized, their responses are a poignant but hopeful reminder of the fact that the battle for freedom in Africa does not cease because formal colonialism has ended.

Closing part five, there is a colloquium of women who reflect on the implications of marriage as a key site of women's oppression from feminist perspectives. They ask whether this institution can be reformed – or whether the desire for the legalization of same-sex marriage barters freedom for approval in a socially regressive order.

Marriage in action
At the time of going to print, 1 070 couples had registered their relationships under the Civil Union Act.[10] On 1 December 2006, Tony Hall and Vernon Gibbs became the first same-sex couple to marry under the Civil Union Act, at a Home Affairs office in George, Western Cape. (See picture pages.) The following day, on 2 December 2006, Janine Preesman, the first religious marriage officer to be designated under the Act, officiated at the first religious marriage ceremony to be conducted under the Act, as described in part four.

The sixth and final part of this book is devoted to interviews with couples – the first wave of pioneers to take advantage of this new marriage regime. Questions of identity, race, social positioning and same-sex marriage in a religious context are taken up once more, but given expression through these accounts of lived experience. The couples interviewed here give personal testimony to the very real ways in which such issues inflect their daily lives – these are not simply abstract matters of law and rights, but have a deep impact on the most intimate core of people's existence. What does marriage mean for those who have done it? What issues does it raise for gender, sexuality and relationality? These stories reflect the diverse ways in which couples chose to create meaning through marriage.

Hompi and Charles Januarie describe their old and new weddings, the first a commitment ceremony that expressed their drive to be united 'before God', and the second a powerful endorsement of that union under the law. They talk about what it means to them to finally be 'legal' as a couple. Like the Januaries, **Nozipho and Thulile Ngcobo** discuss the family issues that arose when they solemnized their union legally and religiously – and the implications for them as they move towards a traditional African marriage too. They also talk about the hate crime they suffered soon after their wedding, highlighting the ongoing systemic discrimination and violence experienced by LGBTI people in South Africa, a discrimination potentially intensified by the 'coming out' of same-sex marriage. **Emilia Potenza and Lael Bethlehem**, too, had a commitment ceremony as well as a marriage under the Act, some time later. They talk about what this signified to them, as parents, and what the impetus was that brought them to a unique space within the Home Affairs offices in Edenvale. The reality of the Civil Union Act – in action – has not always been positive. **William Stewart** tells of marrying his partner Richard Holden and how a lack of understanding at the relevant Home Affairs office threw the ceremony into disarray.

While entranced by 'romance' and working out the politics of the engagement party, as they plan their wedding, **Robert Hamblin and Sally-Jean Shackleton** are highly aware of the sexual complexities at play: Robert is a transman and Sally-Jean a lesbian activist. They have to deal not only with a sometimes disapproving family but with how to craft new sexual and social identities outside of the gender box. In this interview, questions about gender itself are up for grabs. By contrast, **Christelle Delport** is a transwoman who was previously married (as a man) under the Marriage Act, and had to divorce her partner **Raven Delport** in terms of that Act. Now, negotiating new gender identities, they plan to remarry under the Civil Union Act.

The theme of religion and same-sex marriage is picked up once more in the last three interviews in part six of this book. **Sadia and Zukayna Kruger** defied the opprobrium of their Muslim community to marry, at last. **Wayne Sampson and Vajradhara** describe having not a Buddhist wedding but a wedding 'in a Buddhist context', while **Margaret Auerbach and Liebe Kellen** talk about how they reworked the Jewish marriage ceremony to give them a wedding that answered to their needs as feminists while invoking the power of an ancient tradition.

Beyond the honeymoon
Some argue that the right to marry has the potential to enhance the integration of sexual minorities within mainstream society, and to mitigate prejudicial social attitudes in the long run. Same-sex marriage, as it becomes a part of our lived reality, may facilitate familial and community acceptance for same-sex relationships through social witnessing, legal sanction and the symbolic weight that marital status, rightly or wrongly, accords relationships. Marriage holds automatic access to legal protections that might otherwise be financially costly or personally difficult to negotiate. But while the list of the virtues of marriage is substantial, have we adequately interrogated the role and function of marriage? And, is the entry into a conservative, patriarchal, heterosexist convention not the price we pay for full social and legal relationship status?

Although activists have always maintained that the struggle for same-sex marriage was about the right to have the *choice* to marry and not necessarily an endorsement of marriage as the only and preferential relationship form, have we not, through our struggles, ensured the primacy of heterosexual-style marriage as an institution worth attaining?[11] Some of the interviewees in this book argue that same-sex couples will 'do marriage differently', and that they hold the power to redefine the institution and its prescribed gender roles, hierarchy and inherent financial, sexual and social power dynamics. This would demand a conscious rejection of the heterosexual mould of marriage in favour of a form that is akin to the kinds of equitable relationships and family systems we may strive for.

High levels of prejudice and homophobia remain a barrier to marriage rights for many same-sex couples. Numerous stories of couples turned away by marriage officers invoking the "conscientious-objection clause" in the Act shows that the dignity of lesbian and gay people continues to be undermined, vitiating the impact of legal gains made. At the same time, there are many examples of positive experiences in accessing the Act, as covered in this book.

Former Cabinet Minster Kader Asmal recently noted that 'Human rights are never static; they are always dynamic. They are never completely won, just as they are never completely lost.'[12] There is little doubt that the progress of strategic litigation for the formal rights of lesbian and gay people has opened a space that marks a clear distinction from a prejudicial past, a space in which the legal recognition of diverse sexualities and relationship forms can take place. Time will tell whether same-sex marriage helps to transform the prejudices embedded in our society, and to facilitate the integration of LGBTI people into the social and legal fabric in a meaningful way. It may be that same-sex marriage contributes to the 'normalization' of homosexuality as such, while 'denormalizing' marriage itself.[13] At the same time, this normalizing effect may well serve to assimilate diverse sexualities into a heteronormative model, thereby undermining the real transformative potential of alternative sexualities to lead us closer to embracing difference rather than trying to dilute it.

But the price of difference in South Africa remains high. The outpourings of hate speech against lesbian and gay people embedded in the public debates on same-sex marriage, and often expressed in a vitriolic manner, bear testimony to this fact. As the escalation of the rape, torture and murder of black lesbian women and other LGBTI people demonstrate, we have a long way to go before the lived reality of LGBTI people is anywhere near the constitutional aspirations of human dignity, equality and freedom. Increased activism to address hate-motivated acts of violence that are underpinned by structural power imbalances will take our struggle beyond the honeymoon of formal equality and into the contested terrains of substantive equality and gender justice.

The debates around the making and meaning of marriage between people of the same sex must be deepened, as must the resistance against homophobia and prejudice, in a context of ongoing economic injustice (compounded by race and class), which continues to marginalize many LGBTI South Africans. Bridging the gap between the law and the social realms we inhabit on a daily basis is a vital task, as is the imperative to ensure that human rights and access to justice are made real for all South Africans.

As Justice Kate O'Regan recently put it, 'Social change is brought about not simply by changing the law or [by] landmark judicial decisions. It is brought about by the daily efforts of all citizens ... Social justice will only be achieved in South Africa by the ongoing efforts and struggle of all of us. We can rejoice that the law no longer represses and that the Constitution maps the way forward. But the Constitution is only the beginning. Achieving its vision is the task that lies ahead.'[14]

Notes

1 Speech at the opening night of the Out in Africa South African Gay and Lesbian Film Festival, Johannesburg, 1 March 2007
2 This formulation has become the accepted usage in referring to a diverse community united by self-identification with sexualities other than the traditional heterosexual norm. The 'LGBTI' acronym attempts to be as inclusive as possible, and hence we have adopted it as the standard usage in this book, though individual writers have used terms such as 'gay and lesbian people' where deemed appropriate. The 'I' for 'intersexed' is a relatively recent addition, hence the form 'LGBT' in some usages.

3 Over a number of years the Equality Project was to launch several court applications in their efforts to reform marriage laws so that same-sex couples could attain the right to marry. For more on the Equality Project's court cases, see pages 55-57 and 59.
4 See 'Judgment days', pages 58-69, for more detailed information on the *Fourie* case's journey through the courts.
5 The equality clause, Section 9 (3) in the Bill of Rights, prohibits discrimination by the state and persons on a number of grounds, including sexual orientation.
6 The Joint Working Group (JWG) is a national network of LGBTI organizations.
7 Speech at the opening night of the Out in Africa South African Gay and Lesbian Film Festival, Cape Town, 8 November 2007
8 Constitution of the Republic of South Africa, Act 108 of 1996 (Preamble)
9 Marc Epprecht, *Hungochani: The History of a Dissident Sexuality in Southern Africa* (McGill–Queen's University Press, 2004), 225
10 Of the total 1 070 civil unions registered thus far, 940 are designated as marriages, and 130 as civil partnerships. Of this total, 476 are gay male couples, 589 are lesbian couples, and 14 are heterosexual couples. These statistics are for the period 30 November 2006 to 29 February 2008, and were kindly supplied by the Department of Home Affairs, Chief Directorate: Population Register.
11 By the time of going to print, a draft Domestic Partnership Bill had been released by the Department of Home Affairs, for public comment. This is a progressive step toward potentially extending legal protection to a particularly vulnerable group – women who are unmarried, often not out of choice.
12 Kader Asmal, 'A New Chapter Opens in the Thick Tome of Struggle' (edited version of his retirement speech to the National Assembly, 26 February 2008), *Cape Times*, 28 February 2008
13 This notion is intriguingly raised in William N Eskridge and Darren R Spedale, *Gay Marriage: For Better or for Worse? What We've Learned From the Evidence* (OUP, 2006), 19. Eskridge and Spedale also discuss the long history of opposition to same-sex marriage in the US, where the arguments since the 1970s prefigure those deployed in South Africa: the 'definitional' argument (marriage is *by definition* heterosexual and dyadic); the 'stamp of approval' argument (the state should not give homosexuality the stamp of approval); the 'slippery slope' argument (same-sex marriage represents a line that, once crossed, will lead to all sorts of social degeneration, including acceptance of incest, polygamy and so on; interestingly, in South Africa, the 'slippery slope' argument is used by African traditionalists who often support polygamy). The evidence adduced by Eskridge and Spedale of social issues such as the 'decline of marriage' in Scandinavian countries since the legalization of same-sex marriage there tends to undermine these arguments.
14 Speech at the opening night of the Out in Africa South African Gay and Lesbian Film Festival, Johannesburg, 1 November 2007

1: AND WE WENT A-COURTING
The legal steps to same-sex marriage

Getting to the Constitutional Court on time: A litigation history of same-sex marriage

Jonathan Berger

The accidental hero

On 4 August 1997, Gordon Kampher made history when his conviction on a charge of sodomy – for which he had been 'sentenced to 12 months' imprisonment suspended for three years on condition that he … [was] not again convicted of sodomy' – was set aside on review by Justices Ian Farlam and Sandile Ngcobo of the Cape High Court.[1] It was not because Kampher had not engaged in the then unlawful sexual practice that his conviction and sentence were set aside – indeed he had pleaded guilty to the charge 'that on or about 10 January 1997 and at or near Knysna Correctional Services, in the district of Knysna, he had wrongfully and intentionally had sexual intercourse *per anum* with another male person, one Ignatius Jones' – but rather because the common-law crime of sodomy was declared inconsistent with the interim Constitution and therefore invalid.[2]

Kampher's account of having sex in a holding cell, part of which is set out in the High Court judgment, makes for interesting reading: Kampher proposed, Jones consented, Kampher penetrated and Jones 'only received'. When asked by the prosecutor where he had penetrated Jones, Kampher replied 'from behind'. Disturbingly, but not particularly uncommon in the prison context, he admitted that they had not used a condom. When asked if he knew that his conduct was 'wrong' and that he could be punished, he agreed. '*Ons het maar 'n kans gevat*,' he replied – 'We simply took a chance.'

Kampher's case represents the first time a court pronounced on the express constitutional protections for lesbian and gay people in South Africa. Ironically, it was not part of the organized and largely successful programme of the National Coalition for Gay and Lesbian Equality (NCGLE) to rid the statute books of discriminatory laws – a well-orchestrated and executed series of cases designed to address a 'shopping list' of necessary law reform – nor was it even something Kampher had necessarily thought about himself. Instead, legal history was made by accident.

An unmarried father of two who had completed Standard 4 and was working at Knysna Concrete for the meagre sum of R320 per week, Kampher had simply wanted to have sex with Jones when they were both behind bars at a prison in Knysna. But, upon conviction, when the case came before the High

Court on automatic review, Justice Farlam 'asked the magistrate for his reasons for conviction and specifically raised the question as to whether the crime of sodomy continue[d] to exist since the coming into operation of the Interim Constitution, Act no 200 of 1993'. The rest is indeed history, with Justices Farlam and Ngcobo striking down the common-law crime of sodomy – which drew no distinction between consensual and non-consensual anal intercourse – on the basis that it unreasonably and unjustifiably limited the right to be free from unfair discrimination on the basis of sexual orientation.

Let's go shopping
After *Kampher* – which deserves to receive significant credit for helping to open the doors of the High Courts to a barrage of sexual-orientation cases – the litigious road that culminated in the Constitutional Court decision in the same-sex marriage cases began. But despite the existence of a well-developed litigation strategy (the so-called 'shopping list' to which reference has already been made), the road to Constitution Hill was paved with a combination of unexpected obstacles and opportunities, which appeared at times to threaten and at other times to support the goal of ensuring the full legal recognition of marriages between persons of the same sex ('same-sex marriages'). These cases are discussed below.

This essay has a modest agenda – simply to chart the litigation course that enabled the Constitutional Court to pave the way for same-sex marriage. Importantly, it recognizes that while same-sex marriage would not have become a reality in the absence of such litigation, the existence of the Civil Union Act of 2006 owes a significant debt to other processes and developments. Simply put, the cases did not happen in a vacuum. Instead, a combination of civil-society advocacy and activism, legislative developments[3] and other processes all coalesced to provide the space and legal basis for the court to rule (largely) favourably in the same-sex marriage cases.

But before looking at the cases in more detail, it is important to consider the 'shopping list' referred to earlier. That list, based largely on a litigation strategy presented by then Professor (now Justice) Edwin Cameron[4] to a meeting of the newly formed NCGLE in 1994, started with the decriminalization of sodomy and ended with the legal recognition of same-sex marriage. From the very beginning, the right to choose whether or not to get married was seen as the ultimate goal.

In large part, the litigation agenda was based on Cameron's seminal article 'Sexual Orientation and the Constitution: A Test Case for Human Rights' (published in the *South African Law Journal* in 1993[5]), which argued that adequate constitutional protection for people facing discrimination on the basis of sexual orientation would include:
• The decriminalization of sex between consenting adults, by abolishing the

common-law crimes of sodomy and 'unnatural sexual offences' and provisions of the Sexual Offences Act of 1957 which also criminalized such acts;
- Equalizing the age of consent for heterosexual and homosexual sex acts;
- The legislative enforcement of non-discrimination, including in areas such as employment and the provision of public resources;
- Rights of free speech, association and conduct; and
- Formal recognition of permanent domestic partnerships, including the extension of partner benefits; rights to intestate inheritance; and fair and non-discriminatory assessment of abilities in relation to adoption and child care.
- In the main, the list has been achieved. In terms of the 'pink (law reform) agenda', legal equality – no unfair discrimination on the basis of sexual orientation – has largely been achieved. There are, however, a few key unresolved matters. These are addressed later.

Painting the courts pink

Formed in 1994 by a group of lesbian and gay activists and organizations under the slogan 'equality and justice for all', the NCGLE was 'a voluntary association of gay, lesbian, bisexual and transgendered people in South Africa and of 70 organizations and associations representing gay, lesbian, bisexual and transgendered people in South Africa'.[6] Among other things, it sought to achieve the retention of the interim Constitution's equality clause in the final Constitution,[7] to scrap unjust laws, to challenge discrimination through constitutional litigation, and to train a representative and effective lesbian and gay leadership.

Largely based on Cameron's shopping list, the NCGLE's litigation strategy envisaged a cautious, incremental approach. In short, it contemplated beginning with a challenge to the criminalization of sodomy, followed by various aspects of same-sex family relationships and culminating in same-sex marriage.[8] Each case would build on what came before, so that if and when same-sex marriage was finally litigated, it would merely put 'the final touch on the process of incremental legal development that the Constitution has already ordained'.[9] But despite the NCGLE's carefully hatched plans, unaffiliated litigants brought some of their own cases in a different order. Even the NCGLE departed from the programme, with two initial challenges to employment-related discrimination.[10]

Luckily, none of these cases was overly problematic, with most in fact complementing the 'official' cases significantly. As Beth Goldblatt points out, 'In general, the plan ran its course and proved to be highly successful, both in changing the law, and in shifting (sections of) public opinion towards the rights of lesbian and gay people.'[11] Importantly, running largely in parallel to the litigation was a 'legislative trend ... evincing Parliament's commitment to equality on the ground of sexual orientation'.[12] In a key 1999 decision, for example, the Constitutional Court cited no fewer than ten statutes in support of this commitment, including landmark legislation such as the Basic Conditions of Employment Act of 1997, the Employment Equity Act of 1998 and the Medical Schemes Act of 1998.[13]

Sex before marriage

Although same-sex marriage was always viewed as the holy grail, as if full legal recognition of their relationships is all that lesbian and gay people need to live their lives as equal citizens, the somewhat 'conservative'[14] approach to litigation chose to pick up the baton from where *Kampher* had left it – to decriminalize gay[15] sex – before dealing with the legal recognition of same-sex relationships. While groundbreaking, *Kampher* was nevertheless limited: it only applied to the geographic area falling under the jurisdiction of the Cape High Court and it only addressed sodomy. Untouched was the common-law crime of 'unnatural sexual offences', the infamous 'men at a party' clause of the Sexual Offences Act (Section 20A)[16] and a couple of technical provisions.

In the first of three seminal cases that the NCGLE – and its successor the Lesbian and Gay Equality Project – took all the way to the Constitutional Court, the two common-law crimes and Section 20A were targeted in *National Coalition for Gay and Lesbian Equality and the South African Human Rights Commission v Minister of Justice and Others* ('the decriminalization case'). In addition, the case challenged the inclusion of sodomy in Schedule 1 of the Criminal Procedure Act of 1997,[17] a particularly pernicious provision that effectively gave law-enforcement officers the power to use force – lethal if necessary – to stop a fleeing suspect. Simply put, as a gay man you could be shot dead if you ran away after being apprehended under suspicion of having had consensual sex.[18]

Ironically, it was the designation of sodomy as a scheduled offence that permitted the Constitutional Court to consider the constitutionality of sodomy's criminalization. After the Johannesburg High Court declared all the impugned provisions unconstitutional,[19] it only referred the orders striking down provisions of statute to the Constitutional Court for confirmation, as the Constitution requires. Given that the state did not appeal the High Court's judgment, the declarations of constitutional invalidity in respect of the common-law crimes were not before the court. However, the constitutionality of the designation of sodomy as a scheduled offence could only be adjudicated once the constitutionality of the common-law crime itself had been established.

In its judgment, the Constitutional Court found that the impugned provisions unreasonably and unjustifiably limited three separate but interlinked rights: equality, privacy, and dignity. Although important in its own right, the judgment – as the late Professor Ronald Louw[20] eloquently noted – 'created a jurisprudential foundation on which to build far-reaching gay and lesbian rights to equality'.[21] As Justice Albie Sachs remarked in his separate concurring judgment:

> At a practical and symbolical level ... [this case] is about the status, moral citizenship and sense of self-worth of a significant section of the community. At a more general and conceptual level, it concerns the nature of the open, democratic and pluralistic society contemplated by the Constitution.[22]

Simply put, the decriminalization case was to provide the substantive basis upon which further rights for lesbian and gay people were to be claimed through litigation. In this case, sex before marriage proved to be a wise choice indeed.

There's more to a relationship than sex

In a letter to the NCGLE dated 9 January 1998, the Director-General (DG) of Home Affairs unwittingly set off a chain of events that was eventually to culminate in the promulgation of the Civil Union Act a month short of nine years later. In that letter, the DG informed the NCGLE that the department had effectively decided to renege on an earlier agreement in terms of which foreign same-sex partners of South African citizens were granted statutory exemptions to remain in the country. At that time, the legislation governing immigration – the inappropriately named Aliens Control Act of 1991 – did not recognize same-sex relationships, effectively denying the family life of lesbian and gay South Africans who had chosen foreign partners.

The DG's explanation for the u-turn displayed a remarkable disdain for the Constitution:

> [T]he Minister may only grant exemptions where there are **special circumstances** which justify such a decision ... The mere fact that the Aliens Control Act, 1991, does not cater for same-sex relationships cannot be considered as 'special circumstances' for the purposes [of] exercising the powers of exemption under that Act. In view of the above consideration, it has been decided not to grant exemptions ... merely to accommodate alien partners in same-sex relationships.

Under Zackie Achmat's leadership, the NCGLE turned to the courts for relief. Its successful application to the Cape High Court – which was joined by six South Africans, their foreign partners and the Commission on Gender Equality – resulted in, among other things, Section 25 (5) of the Aliens Control Act being declared unconstitutional. That provision, which allowed for immigration permits to be granted to the spouses and dependent children of South African citizens and permanent residents, did not cover same-sex partners. As such, it unfairly discriminated on the basis of sexual orientation.

In confirmation and appeal proceedings before the Constitutional Court, the government's lawyers argued that South Africa,

> as a sovereign independent state, was lawfully entitled to exclude any foreign

nationals from the Republic; that it had an absolute discretion to do so which was beyond the reach of the Constitution and the courts; and that, to the extent that Parliament legislated to permit foreign nationals to reside in South Africa, it did so in the exercise of such discretion and that the provisions of such legislation were equally beyond the reach of the Constitution and the courts.[23]

In its judgment in *National Coalition for Gay and Lesbian Equality and Others v Minister of Home Affairs and Others* ('the immigration case'), however, the Constitutional Court focused instead on the rights of the South African partners:

Such an argument, even if correct, would not assist the respondents, because in the present case we are not dealing with such a category of foreign nationals, but with persons who are in intimate life partnerships with ... South Africans ... This is a significant and determinative difference. The failure of the Act to grant any recognition at all to same-sex life partnerships impacts in the same way on the South African partners as it does on the foreign national partners.[24]

Simply put, the case was to be decided on whether Section 25 (5) of the Aliens Control Act unreasonably and unjustifiably limited the rights of South Africans involved in 'permanent same-sex life partnerships' with foreign nationals, not on the basis of whether the rights of foreign nationals had been impermissibly limited. Importantly, the judgment makes it plain that lesbian and gay people in same-sex life partnerships 'have the same ability [as heterosexual couples] to establish a *consortium omnis vitae*', defined as 'a physical, moral and spiritual community of life'[25] made up of '[c]ompanionship, love, affection, comfort, mutual services ... [and] sexual intercourse'[26] – what our law has historically understood as the very essence of marriage.

The immigration case was not the first superior court decision to guarantee partnership benefits on the basis of the legal recognition of same-sex relationships. That honour goes to *Langemaat v Minister of Safety and Security*,[27] an earlier case brought on behalf of a lesbian police officer and her partner by a legal team that was given direction and funded by the NCGLE. In that case, the failure of the rules of the Police Medical Aid Scheme (Polmed) to accord beneficiary status to same-sex partners of police officers – as was accorded to heterosexual spouses – was successfully challenged.

The immigration case was, however, the foundational case upon which partnership benefits were demanded – and secured – in cases such as *Satchwell v President of the Republic of South Africa and Another*[28] and *Du Plessis v Road Accident Fund*.[29] In *Satchwell*, the partnership benefits under scrutiny were those accorded to the spouses of judges, whereas in *Du Plessis*, they were those that accrued to spouses of road-accident victims. In both cases, the rights claimants were successful – same-sex relationships were granted legal recognition and benefits were accordingly granted. Equally successful were rights claimants in cases brought before dispute resolution bodies such as the Pension Funds Adjudicator.[30]

Perhaps the most interesting – albeit disturbing – case of the batch is *Farr v Mutual & Federal Insurance Co Ltd*,[31] in which a same-sex couple sought to deny their relationship in a misguided attempt to benefit from an insurance policy. In terms of the policy, family members of the insured were excluded from claims against the insurance company in the event that they were injured in a car accident in which the insured was driving. In quite uncharacteristic style, a gay couple proudly proclaimed that they were 'not family'. The court was not convinced, denying the claim on the basis of its express recognition of the same-sex relationship. Good for the gays; not particularly fine for Farr!

What about the children?
So if same-sex couples constitute family, given that 'families come in many shapes and sizes',[32] what about the children? In an early-1990s custody case, a particularly homophobic judgment resulted in a mother's rights of access to her then dependent children being severely curtailed on the basis of her stable and committed lesbian relationship. Disingenuously, the so-called 'best interests of the child' were used as a smokescreen for decision-making on the basis of prejudice. That case – *Van Rooyen v Van Rooyen*[33] – was decided prior to the introduction of a justiciable Bill of Rights, is no longer good law, and has been strongly criticized in the post-1994 decision of *V v V*.[34]

Subsequently, the parental rights of lesbian and gay people were strongly affirmed by the Constitutional Court in two key decisions: *Du Toit and De Vos v Minister for Welfare and Population Development*,[35] and *J and Another v Director-General of Home Affairs*.[36] In both cases, the relevant legal principles were easy to establish. The facts in *Du Toit* were particularly straightforward, dealing primarily with the rights of same-sex couples to adopt children jointly. *J and Another*, however, provided a somewhat more challenging set of facts. In that case, a woman had given birth to a child conceived through *in vitro* fertilization. What complicated the matter was that both gametes – the sperm and the egg – had been 'donated', with the latter being provided by the birth-mother's lesbian partner. The law had simply not anticipated such a situation.

In both cases, the Constitutional Court once again rose to the challenge. In *Du Toit*, it amended the Child Care Act so that same-sex couples could adopt *qua* couples, further making provision for the permanent same-sex life partners of a child's biological mother or father to become a second parent by way of adoption. In *J and Another*, the law was amended to recognize the 'genetic mother' as a parent, with the 'biological mother' retaining her status as mother. In both cases, the rights of the child featured prominently. In *Du Toit*, for example, the Court found that failure of the law to permit same-sex couples to adopt jointly served simply to 'deprive children of the possibility of a loving and stable family life as required by Section 28 (1) (b) of the Constitution'.[37]

The wedding planner

Having amassed a series of court decisions and legislative amendments, lesbian and gay people were finally able to focus their attention on the grand prize – the right to choose whether or not to enter into a marriage with another person of the same sex. Marriage had the potential to do two things: first, to provide automatic legal recognition for all purposes where relationship status was at issue; and second, to accord equal status to same- and opposite-sex relationships. Given that the first goal could equally be achieved through domestic-partnership legislation, the primary goal in pursuing marriage was to achieve the desired equal status. As lesbian and gay activists argued, anything less than marriage was simply not equal.

Yet, by the time activists decided it was appropriate to challenge the marriage laws, at least two lesbian couples had already decided to take action themselves. Only one of these couples – Marié Adriaana Fourie and Cecelia Johanna Bonthuys – managed to get to court. The other – a South African and her French life partner – had wanted to launch and conclude a case in the late 1990s before emigrating to France, where the couple hoped to be able to rely on their South African marriage for full legal recognition under French law. Swift action by the organized lesbian and gay community managed to persuade the women not to proceed with what was very risky litigation at the time.

Fourie and Bonthuys, however, were determined to have their day in court. But a combination of badly drafted legal papers and judicial reluctance to ensure that rights were indeed vindicated resulted in a judgment that essentially refused to engage with the substantive issues. In his judgment of 18 October 2002, Justice Pierre Roux of the Pretoria High Court held that he could not order the Department of Home Affairs to recognize the applicants' 'marriage' because the law recognized marriage as a union between a man and a woman. He refused to acknowledge that the applicants' request for their 'marriage' to be recognized was in effect an application to declare the common-law definition of marriage unconstitutional. In short, he deliberately avoided the issue.[38]

Without any legal precedent and most likely in conflict with Section 34 of the Constitution (which guarantees the right of access to the courts), Justice Roux ordered the Equality Project – as *amicus curiae* – to pay costs. He argued that it had gone beyond the bounds of what was ordinarily permitted, having tried to convince him that the applicants' case was essentially a constitutional challenge to the exclusion of same-sex couples from the institution of marriage. This aspect of the judgment was to be argued on appeal, but at the eleventh hour the state abandoned its costs order against the Equality Project and the need for an appeal on this point disappeared.

Separately, the applicants applied to the High Court for leave to appeal against Justice Roux's decision. Their first choice – the Constitutional Court – was denied, but with leave to the Supreme Court of Appeals (SCA) being granted. The applicants, however, were determined to get to the Constitutional Court, approaching it for leave to appeal directly to it against the judgment and order of the High Court. The Constitutional Court was not convinced,[39] refusing the application on the basis 'that the interests of justice required that the appeal first be heard by the SCA'.[40]

But before it could be argued before the SCA, the Equality Project filed an application asking the High Court to declare the common-law definition of marriage and the prescribed marriage formula in Section 30 (1) of the Marriage Act of 1961 unconstitutional.[41] That case, which made reference to the rapidly emerging international jurisprudence on the topic, nevertheless took great care to place emphasis on the Constitution and South African case law. In so doing, it recognized that a foreign case may be helpful but cannot provide any definitive answers. Simply put, the applicants' confidence in their case derived largely from the knowledge that the domestic building blocks were firmly in place.

The *Equality Project* case was brought for two reasons. First, it was unclear whether the *Fourie* case would succeed before the SCA, particularly given certain discouraging statements made by the Constitutional Court in its judgment dismissing the application for direct access. Second, even if successful, the *Fourie* case would not be able to address the prescribed marriage formula, without which most civil marriages – all except those conducted by religious marriage officers using their own formulae approved by the Minister – cannot go forward. The High Court's inability to grant a timeous hearing date meant that events forced the Equality Project to rethink its strategy. It had no option but to approach the SCA to be admitted as *amicus curiae* in the *Fourie* case, with its application including its entire set of High Court papers.

Had the state simply accepted the SCA's decision in *Fourie and Another v Minister of Home Affairs and Another*, which declared the common-law definition of marriage unconstitutional and therefore invalid, the Civil Union Act may very well have not yet come into force. But by applying for leave to appeal against the SCA's judgment, the state opened the door for the Equality Project and its allies to bring their case directly to the Constitutional Court.[42] In that way, it allowed the Constitutional Court to determine the constitutionality of the prescribed marriage formula in addition to addressing the common substantive issues raised in both cases. Had this not happened, there would have been no direct pressure on Parliament to act.

Happily ever after

So where are we now? Are we ready to live happily ever after? In terms of formal legal equality, we are indeed almost there. With the coming into force on 16 December 2007 of certain sections of the Criminal Law (Sexual Offences and Related Matters) Amendment Act of 2007, we now have an equal age of consent (at 16) and a gender-neutral definition of rape. But we are still missing domestic-partnership legislation, and the Civil Union Act is an unfairly discriminatory statute.

The first of these unresolved issues is expected to be addressed by the Domestic Partnerships Bill, which is likely to be tabled in Parliament in April 2008 and may very well arise out of the excised portions of the Civil Union Bill originally tabled in the National Assembly. The other unresolved issue – a constitutionally suspect Civil Union Act – is addressed elsewhere in this book. In my view, however, the three key problematic provisions of the Civil Union Act are the need for religious organizations and denominations to apply to be designated before religious marriage officers are able to apply to conduct civil unions;[43] the unjustifiably broad scope of the conscientious-objection clause;[44] and Section 8 (6), which appears to limit the Act's application to same-sex couples.

But 'happily ever after' won't come simply by ensuring that the 'shopping list' is completed. Instead, we need to go further in at least two ways. First, rights claims need to be made real by ensuring broad access to legal services. Second, the legitimate needs of lesbian and gay people demand an equitable share of state resources. These broader social-justice concerns must be addressed if the gains achieved to date are not to remain the sole preserve of the relatively privileged.

Notes

1 *S v Kampher* 1997 (4) SA 460 (C). Justice Farlam now sits as a judge of appeal in the Supreme Court of Appeal (SCA) and was part of the five-judge panel that declared the common-law definition of marriage unconstitutional in *Fourie and Another v Minister of Home Affairs and Another* 2005 (3) SA 429 (SCA); 2005 (3) BCLR 241 (SCA), hereafter '*Fourie* (SCA)'. Justice Ngcobo now sits as a judge of the Constitutional Court and was part of the *en banc* panel that upheld the SCA's finding regarding the unconstitutionality of the common-law definition of marriage and declared the marriage formula in Section 30 (1) of the Marriage Act (Act 25 of 1961) to be unconstitutional in *Minister of Home Affairs and Another v Fourie and Another* 2005 (3) BCLR 355 (CC); 2006 (1) SA 524 (CC), hereafter referred to as '*Fourie*'; *Lesbian and Gay Equality Project and Others v Minister of Home Affairs and Others* 2006 (1) SA 524 (CC) ('the Lesbian and Gay Equality Project case').

2 The Constitution of the Republic of South Africa, 1993 ('the interim Constitution'), came into force on 27 April 1994 and remained in operation until the Constitution of the Republic of South Africa, 1996, came into force on 4 February 1997. The effect of *Kampher* was to strike down the common-law crime of sodomy in the geographic area under the jurisdiction of the Cape High Court.

3 The first legislative recognition of same-sex relationships came indirectly in the Independent Media Commission Act of 1993 and the Independent Broadcasting Authority Act of 1993, both of which predate the interim Constitution and were enacted by the apartheid Parliament. In both statutes, a spouse is defined to include 'a *de facto* spouse'. The first statute to define spouse expressly to include same-sex couples was the Special Pensions Act of 1996, which defined spouse to include 'continuous cohabitation in a homosexual or heterosexual partnership for a period of at least 5 years'.
4 Justice Cameron wrote the majority decision in the SCA's judgment in *Fourie*. He also sat on the *en banc* Constitutional Court panel in *National Coalition for Gay and Lesbian Equality and Others v Minister of Home Affairs and Others* 2000 (2) SA 1 (CC) ('the immigration case')
5 *South African Law Journal* 110 (1993), 450. See also page 125 of this book.
6 *National Coalition for Gay and Lesbian Equality and the South African Human Rights Commission v Minister of Justice and Others* 1999 (1) SA 6 (CC) ('the decriminalization case'), paragraph 4
7 Constitution of the Republic of South Africa, 1996
8 Beth Goldblatt, 'Case Note: Same Sex Marriage in South Africa – The Constitutional Court's Judgment', *Feminist Legal Studies* 3 14:2 (2006), 265
9 Justice Sachs in the *Fourie* and *Lesbian and Gay Equality Project* cases, op. cit., paragraph 14, summarizing the SCA's majority decision in the *Fourie* case. A glance at the list of authorities cited by the applicants in the *Lesbian and Gay Equality Project* case shows nine South African superior-court judgments dealing with sexual orientation, the majority of which had gone to the Constitutional Court.
10 The first case – against Eskom – was settled. The second case – dealing with medical scheme membership for a same-sex partner – was successfully litigated in *Langemaat v Minister of Safety and Security* 1998 (3) SA 312 (T), also known as 'Polmed'.
11 Goldblatt, op. cit., 265
12 Immigration case, op. cit., paragraph 37
13 Ibid., note 41
14 The term 'conservative' is deliberately placed in inverted commas because the NCGLE's project of large-scale law reform can hardly be termed as inherently conservative. Nevertheless, the cautious and strategic approach to litigation is somewhat conservative relative to other more ambitious – but often less successful – approaches followed in other jurisdictions.
15 South African law did not criminalize lesbian sex *per se*. It only treated lesbian sex unfairly in relation to the issue of the age of consent, which until recently, was 19 (as opposed to 16 for heterosexual sex). As mentioned above, this has been addressed by the Criminal Law (Sexual Offences and Related Matters) Act of 2007, relevant provisions of which came into force on 16 December 2007.
16 Section 20A (1) provided that '[a] male person who commits with another male person at a party any act which is calculated to stimulate sexual passion or to give sexual gratification, shall be guilty of an offence'. A party was defined in Subsection 2 as 'any occasion where more than two persons are present'.
17 In addition, the inclusion of sodomy as an item in the schedule to the Security Officers Act of 1987 was also challenged.
18 As noted in paragraph 7 of the Constitutional Court's judgment: 'Section 49 (2) of the … [Criminal Procedure Act] allows a person authorized to arrest an individual suspected of having committed sodomy to kill the suspect if, upon attempting to arrest the suspect, such person cannot arrest the suspect, or the suspect flees, and there is no other way to arrest the suspect or to prevent him from fleeing.'
19 The common-law crime of unnatural sexual offences was declared unconstitutional only 'to the

extent that it criminalizes acts committed by a man or between men which, if committed by a woman or between women or between a man and a woman, would not constitute an offence'. Given that the offence was ordinarily used to criminalize gay sexual acts other than anal sex, it is unclear what – if anything – remains.
20 Louw, who served as an executive committee member of the NCGLE for many years, died of an AIDS-related illness in 2005.
21 Ronald Louw, 'A Decade of Gay and Lesbian Equality Litigation', in Max du Plessis and Steve Pete (eds.), *Constitutional Democracy in South Africa 1994-2004* (LexisNexis Butterworths, 2004), 65-79
22 Decriminalization case, op. cit., paragraph 107
23 Immigration case, paragraph 27
24 Ibid., paragraph 28
25 *Peter v Minister of Law and Order* 1990 (4) SA 6 (E) at 9G
26 *Grobbelaar v Havenga* 1964 (3) SA 522 (N) at 525 E
27 *Langemaat*, op. cit.
28 2002 (6) SA 1 (CC)
29 2004 (1) SA 359 (SCA)
30 See, for example, *Martin v Beka Provident Fund* (case number PFA/GA/563/99, 8 June 1999), available online at http://www.pfa.org.za/sitesmart/uploads/files/D3F0F73D-531C-4ABF-9ACD-CA9223822BAB.pdf (last accessed 7 February 2008), and *Muir v Mutual & Federal Pension Fund* (case number PFA/WE/2932/01/SM, 13 May 2002), available online at ftp://ftp.fsb.co.za/public/pfa/MuirR.pdf (last accessed 7 February 2008).
31 2000 (3) SA 684 (C)
32 *Dawood, Shalabi and Thomas v Minister of Home Affairs* 2000 (3) SA 936 (CC), paragraph 31
33 1994 (2) SA 325 (W)
34 1998 (4) SA 169 (C)
35 2003 (2) SA 198 (CC)
36 2003 (5) SA 621 (CC)
37 Paragraph 22
38 *Fourie and Another v Minister of Home Affairs and Another* (the Lesbian and Gay Equality Project intervening as *amicus curiae*), unreported case number 17280/02
39 *Fourie and Another v Minister of Home Affairs and Another* 2003 (5) SA 301 (CC)
40 Ibid.
41 The Triangle Project, the Durban Lesbian and Gay Community and Health Centre, the Forum for the Empowerment of Women (FEW), OUT LGBT Well-being and six same-sex couples joined the case.
42 The Equality Project's legal representatives in its various marriage cases were as follows: in the Pretoria High Court *amicus* application, Daniel Berger and Refilwe Thulare (as counsel) and Nicholls, Cambanis and Associates (as instructing attorneys); and in the Johannesburg High Court application, the Supreme Court of Appeal *amicus* application, and the Constitutional Court direct access application, Daniel Berger SC and Fayeeza Kathree (as counsel) and Nicholls, Cambanis and Associates (as instructing attorneys). For more information on the Equality Project's case in the Constitutional Court, see pages 55-57, 59.
43 Section 5
44 Section 6

Difference and belonging:
The Constitutional Court
and the adoption of the Civil Union Act

Pierre de Vos

It is a curious fact that the Constitutional Court judgment which led to the adoption of the Civil Union Act by Parliament in December 2006 never explicitly ordered Parliament to extend the institution of *marriage* to same-sex couples. Instead, the Court argued that same-sex couples were constitutionally entitled to a legal institution that would grant them the same rights and the same status as that associated with traditional heterosexual marriage.[1] It nevertheless came as a great shock to constitutional lawyers and members of the LGBTI community when the original version of the Civil Union Bill[2] was tabled in Parliament at the end of August 2006. The Bill proposed the creation of a separate and exclusive institution for same-sex couples – called a 'civil partnership' – which purported to comply with the Constitutional Court judgment by bestowing exactly the same legal rights on same-sex civil partners as on heterosexual married couples.[3] There were, however, three pivotal ways in which the proposed civil partnership differed from traditional marriage: it would not be called a marriage (except at the ceremony if the partners so choose);[4] marriage officers – even those not related to a religious institution – would have a right to refuse to solemnize a civil partnership;[5] and it would only be open to same-sex couples, not to heterosexual couples.[6]

Constitutional lawyers and LGBTI activists rallied against this Bill, arguing that it represented an attempt to create a 'separate but equal' marriage regime that would protect 'real' marriage from so-called contamination and defilement by same-sex couples, while pretending to provide such couples with equal partnership rights. Given the general antagonism in South African society towards the recognition of same-sex marriage, such arguments against the first draft of the Bill would not have succeeded on their own. But lawyers and activists came to Parliament armed with a powerful weapon: the Constitutional Court judgment in the case of *Fourie*. Despite the fact that the judgment never orders Parliament to provide same-sex couples with access to an institution called *marriage*, I would argue that the judgment nevertheless gave politicians very little room to manoeuvre. It was therefore the (belated) realization by politicians that the draft Bill failed to comply with the clear instructions of the Constitutional Court which led to the last-minute revision of the

Bill and the ultimate adoption of the much-improved Civil Union Act. At the same time it is important to realize that the *Fourie* judgment did not appear on our legal landscape out of the blue, but was really the culmination of a long line of decisions in which the Constitutional Court developed a body of jurisprudence around discrimination based on sexual orientation.

The jurisprudence on sexual orientation predating *Fourie*

Reading the Constitutional Court's judgment in the *Fourie* case, it is striking to note that it contains six pages of discussion on the Court's precedent regarding discrimination on the grounds of sexual orientation.[7] It is as if Justice Albie Sachs, who wrote the majority opinion, was saying to the public and to his fellow judges that the outcome of the case had indeed become inevitable, given the nature of the jurisprudence developed by the Court in previous cases. By the time it had to decide on the same-sex marriage question, the Constitutional Court had given such a ringing endorsement of the rights of gay and lesbian people that it became very difficult to present a constitutionally persuasive argument against the full recognition of same-sex marriage. Constitutional Court judges who might have wished to provide same-sex couples with partnership rights that fell short of full marriage[8] were thus roped in by the long list of precedent and may therefore have been forced to go along with the decision by Sachs.

In the first case on sexual orientation to make it to the Constitutional Court the judges[9] produced a moving and powerful endorsement of the rights of individuals who experience an emotional and sexual attraction to members of their own sex. In *National Coalition for Gay and Lesbian Equality and the South African Human Rights Commission v Minister of Justice and Others*,[10] they declared invalid the common-law crime of sodomy as well as several legislative provisions dealing with male same-sex sexual activity.[11] In the process, the Constitutional Court daringly associated respect for the rights of gay men and lesbian women with the acceptance of the significance of difference in society. The court linked the equality guarantee in the Constitution to the anti-subordination principle, arguing that the 'desire for equality is not a hope for the elimination of all differences', but, indeed, a rejection of subordination. The court thus argued that any justification for differently treating individuals who are viewed as 'different' from the norm would produce or perpetuate the subordination of that group and it is exactly this subordination of groups which the right to equality is trying to root out. In our constitutional order, equality and uniformity are far from synonymous but instead mean 'equal concern and respect across difference'.[12] In one of the most astonishing passages to ever have appeared in a judicial decision, Justice Albie Sachs went even further, arguing that this meant that

> the concept of sexual deviance needs to be reviewed. A heterosexual norm was established, gays were labelled deviant from the norm and difference was located in them. What the constitution requires is that the law and public institutions acknowledge the variability of human beings and affirm the equal respect and concern that should be shown to all as they are. At the very least, what is statistically normal ceases to be the basis for establishing what is legally normative. More broadly speaking, the scope of what is constitutionally normal is expanded to include the widest range of perspectives and to acknowledge, accommodate and accept the largest spread of difference. What becomes normal in an open society, then, is not an imposed and standardised form of behaviour that refuses to acknowledge difference, but the acceptance of the principle of difference itself, which accepts the variability of human behaviour.[13]

One could therefore interpret the judgement as a rejection of the discourse of normality around sexuality. What is rejected (perhaps) is the very notion of heteronormativity that has been deeply entrenched in South Africa's legal culture and society. A heteronormative society is one in which it is assumed that heterosexual culture is the elemental form of human association, the very model of relations between the genders, the indivisible basis of all community and the means of reproduction without which society would not exist.[14] It is a society in which heterosexuality is unreflexively viewed as the main and dominant category of sexual orientation,[15] while homosexuality has come to be understood as an hierarchically inferior deviation from this category. At first glance, this profoundly progressive moment in Sachs's judgment thus embodies a rejection of conformity and an embrace of diversity. It suggests that we are all different from each other, heterosexuals as much as homosexuals. In this view, then, homosexuals cease to be 'failed heterosexuals' and become fully human beings with the same right to self-realization as all other groups in society.

The fact that the state may not impose orthodoxies of belief systems on the whole of society has two consequences. The first is that gay men, lesbian women and bisexual people cannot be forced to conform to heterosexual norms. They can now break out of their invisibility and live as full and free citizens of South Africa. The second is that those persons who, for reasons of religious or other beliefs disagree with or condemn homosexual conduct, are free to hold and articulate such beliefs. Yet, while the Constitution protects the right of people to continue to hold such beliefs, it does not allow the state to endorse such beliefs in any way.[16]

The second significant judgment, discussed at length in the *Fourie* case, dealt with the immigration rights of same-sex couples. In *National Coalition for Gay and Lesbian Equality v Minister of Home Affairs*[17] – the second National Coalition case – the Constitutional Court endorsed the view that in the absence of same-sex marriage, the state has a duty to protect same-sex couples who live in same-sex life partnerships.[18] In the process it created a new legal entity, namely the same-sex life partnership, which is 'a conjugal relationship between two people of the same sex'.[19] The decision made it clear that not all relationships of same-sex couples would be considered constitutionally worthy of protection. However, same-sex couples who could demonstrate that they had entered a life partnership, in which they had undertaken a mutual duty of support to one another, would qualify for constitutional protection.[20] The importance of this decision was that the Court made significant findings about the nature of same-sex relationships, finding that 'gays and lesbians in same-sex life partnerships are as capable as heterosexual spouses of expressing and sharing love in its manifold forms, including affection, friendship, eros and charity ... [that] they are likewise as capable of forming intimate, permanent, committed, monogamous, loyal and enduring relationships; of furnishing emotional and spiritual support; and of providing physical care, financial support and assistance in running the common household ... [that] they are individually able to adopt children and in the case of lesbians to bear them ... [and that] finally, ... they are capable of constituting a family, whether nuclear or extended, and of establishing, enjoying and benefiting from family life which is not distinguishable in any significant respect from that of heterosexual spouses.'[21]

In several other decisions handed down between 2000 and 2006 the Constitutional Court extended the legal protection for same-sex couples in permanent life partnerships.[22] The most important of these decision was that handed down in *Du Toit and De Vos v Minister of Welfare and Population Development and Others*[23] in which the Constitutional Court declared invalid the provision in child-care legislation that confined the right to adopt children jointly to married couples, and would thus have prohibited same-sex couples from jointly adopting children. The Court held that the prohibition on joint adoption by same-sex life partners conflicted both with the best interests of the child and the right to dignity of same-sex couples, and pointed to recent legislative and jurisprudential developments in South Africa indicating the growing recognition afforded to same-sex relationships.[24] Many of those who opposed the adoption of the Civil Union Act (as well as Members of Parliament on the Home Affairs Portfolio Committee) lost sight of this slew of Constitutional Court judgments affirming that the relationships of same-sex couples were just as worthy of legal protection as those of different-sex couples. These opponents of the recognition of same-sex marriage thus tried to argue that same-sex relationships were inherently different or inferior from heterosexual relationships – high divorce rates notwithstanding. It thus came as a big surprise to them that their arguments about the unsuitability of same-sex couples to adopt and raise children had become legally and constitutionally irrelevant by the time the Constitutional Court came to hear the *Fourie* case.

The Constitutional Court judgment in *Fourie*

Back in 2002 Marié Adriaana Fourie and Cecelia Johanna Bonthuys decided they had waited long enough to tie the knot and lodged an application in the Pretoria High Court asking the Court for an order declaring that the law recognize their right to get married and instructing the relevant authorities to marry them.[25] Until that point no same-sex couple had been able to get married in South Africa – despite the constitutional prohibition against discrimination on the grounds of sexual orientation. The legal impediments to concluding such a marriage were twofold. First, the common-law definition of marriage developed over the centuries by the ordinary courts *defined* marriage as the union of one man and one woman to the exclusion of all others for as long as it lasts. Second, such a marriage had to be officially concluded in terms of the Marriage Act,[26] which prescribed a specific marriage formula that contemplated marriage only between a man and a woman.[27] Unfortunately Bonthuys and Fourie did not challenge the constitutionality of either the common-law definition of marriage or the gender-specific marriage formula in the Marriage Act, and their application was therefore turned down by the High Court. A subsequent application to challenge the High Court decision in the Constitutional Court was also turned down on technical grounds.[28] The couple therefore had to re-launch their application in the correct legal format in the High Court, and it took almost four years for the case to wend its way up to the Constitutional Court for a final decision. It was therefore only towards the end of 2005 that the Constitutional Court handed down judgment in the case. First, it invoked the rich jurisprudence on sexual-orientation discrimination described above, declaring that the common-law definition of marriage was invalid to the extent that it did not permit same-sex couples to enjoy the status and the benefits coupled with responsibilities it accorded to heterosexual couples. Second, it declared that the Marriage Act – in terms of which marriages are concluded in South Africa – was invalid because it refers only to marriage between a 'husband' and 'wife', and not between 'spouses'.[29]

In doing so the Court again endorsed the notion that, at the heart of the prohibition on discrimination based on sexual orientation, is an acceptance of the right to be different.[30] It also confirmed its previously expressed view that individuals in same-sex relationships should not be defined exclusively in terms of sexuality but should be viewed as more complex beings whose sexuality does not tell the whole truth about who they are as human beings,[31] and that same-sex couples are equally as capable of forming intimate lasting relationships and raising children as heterosexual couples.[32]

The Court situated its analysis of the case within the broader perspective of South Africa's oppressive and discriminatory past, noting that gay and lesbian people have suffered considerably in the past because of their sexual orientation. This was not a new development: South Africa's Constitutional Court has often emphasized that one can only grasp the far-reaching, progressive effect of the constitutional protections if one remains aware of the dark apartheid past and understands that the Constitution was drafted in great part to prevent a recurrence of the dehumanizing oppression and marginalization that so characterised the apartheid state.[33] The apartheid legislation that contributed to this oppression included the Immorality Act,[34] which criminalized sexual intercourse between white and black people, and the Prohibition of Mixed Marriages Act,[35] which prohibited marriage between white and black people in South Africa. There has therefore been a long history in South Africa of interference with the all-important life-enhancing choices people make about their intimate actions and relationships, interference that was based on a disregard for the human dignity of black citizens.

The Constitutional Court further noted that during the apartheid era gay men and lesbian women had suffered a particularly harsh fate, having been branded as criminals and rejected by society as outcasts and perverts. It also pointed out that this exclusion and marginalization, and the concomitant hatred and violence that it produced, was experienced more intensely by those South Africans already suffering under the yoke of apartheid because of their race and/or sex and/or economic status. It is within this historical context that the reasoning of the Constitutional Court in the *Fourie* case should be understood. The Court's reasoning – building on its earlier jurisprudence – follows a logical route which suggests that at least some of the fears expressed about the creation of a second-class recognition for same-sex couples, through the recognition of same-sex life partnerships, were unfounded. The Court emphasized that marriage is an important and unique institution and constitutes 'much more than a piece of paper'.[36]

On the one hand, it pointed out that marriage until recently was the only source of socio-economic benefits such as the right to inheritance, medical-insurance coverage, adoption, access to wrongful-death claims and the like. On the other hand, the Court noted that marriage also bestows a myriad *intangible* benefits on those who choose to enter into it. As such, marriage entitles a couple to celebrate their commitment to each other at the kind of public event so celebrated in our culture. They are showered with presents and throughout their lives they will be able to commemorate this event at anniversaries while pictures of the day can be displayed in their house and in the houses of their families. Given the centrality attributed to marriage and its consequences in our culture, to deny same-sex couples a choice in this regard 'would be to negate their right to self-definition in a most profound way'.[37] This is an important point because it endorses the view that marriage is about far more than legal rights. It is about symbolic acceptance and belonging in a society, about accessing an institution that has a specific status in our society. To deny same-sex couples access to *marriage* would therefore deny them the right to *belong*.

Thus, the Court argued, that where the law fails to recognize the relationship of same-sex couples 'the message is that gays and lesbians lack the inherent humanity to have their families and family lives in such same-sex relationships respected or protected'. It serves in addition to perpetuate and reinforce existing prejudice and stereotypes. 'The impact constitutes a crass, blunt, cruel and serious invasion of their dignity'.[38] The Constitutional Court then concluded that the exclusion of same-sex couples from the benefits and responsibilities of marriage was not

> a small and tangential inconvenience resulting from a few surviving relics of societal prejudice destined to evaporate like the morning dew. It represents a harsh if oblique statement by the law that same-sex couples are outsiders, and that their need for affirmation and protection of their intimate relations as human beings is somehow less than that of heterosexual couples. It reinforces the wounding notion that they are to be treated as biological oddities, as failed or lapsed human beings who do not fit into normal society, and, as such, do not qualify for the full moral concern and respect that our Constitution seeks to secure for everyone. It signifies that their capacity for love, commitment and accepting responsibility is by definition less worthy of regard than that of heterosexual couples.[39]

The important conclusion is therefore that the exclusion of same-sex couples from marriage has both a *practical* and *symbolic* impact, which means that the problem cannot be rectified through the recognition of same-sex unions outside the law of marriage. According to the Court, in responding to the unconstitutionality of the existing marriage regime, *both* the practical and the symbolic aspects have to be responded to: 'Thus, it would not be sufficient merely to deal with all the practical consequences of exclusion from marriage. It would also have to accord to same-sex couples a *public and private status* equal to that which heterosexual couples achieve from being married.'[40]

In the light of the fact that the judgment never explicitly states that Parliament has to extend *marriage* rights to same-sex couples, the point that marriage has a symbolic power is of pivotal importance. Because of this symbolic power of the institution of marriage, a 'separate but equal' regime for same-sex couples would therefore not be sufficient.[41] The judgment refers per illustration to the apartheid-era case of *S v Pitje*, in which the appellant (a candidate attorney with the law firm of Nelson Mandela) occupied a place at a table in court that was reserved for 'European practitioners'. The Appeal Court at the time upheld the appellant's conviction for contempt of court as it was 'clear that a practitioner would in every way be as well seated at the one table as at the other, and that he could not possibly be hampered in the slightest in the conduct of his case by having to use a particular table'. This approach, Justice Sachs remarked, would be 'unthinkable in our constitutional democracy' today.[42]

The Court then proceeded to consider (and then to reject) some of the arguments put forward by religious groups against the recognition of same-sex marriage.[43] Because these arguments were put forward to try and convince the Court of the need to recognize same-sex relationships in a way not associated with marriage, it is important to highlight some of the reasoning here. First, the Constitutional Court confirmed its rejection of the age-old argument that the constitutive and definitional characteristic of marriage is its procreative potential and can therefore never include same-sex couples.[44] This argument, it said, was deeply demeaning to heterosexual married couples who, for whatever reason, either choose not to procreate or are incapable of procreating when they enter a relationship or become so at any time thereafter.[45] It was also demeaning to couples who start a relationship at a stage when they no longer have the capacity to conceive, or for adoptive parents. Although this view might have some traction in the context of a particular religious worldview, from a legal and constitutional point of view, the Court found, it could not hold.[46]

Second, it rejected the other familiar argument that marriage is by its very nature a religious institution and that to change its definition would violate religious freedom in a most fundamental way. Although the Court recognized that religious bodies play a large and important part in public life and are part of the fabric of our society,[47] it endorsed the view that in the open and democratic society contemplated by the Constitution there must be mutual respect and co-existence between the secular and the sacred. It rejected the notion that the extension of marriage rights to same-sex couples would in any way be inconsistent with the rights of religious organizations to continue to refuse to celebrate same-sex marriages. 'The constitutional claims of same-sex couples can accordingly not be negated by invoking the rights of believers to have their religious freedom respected. The two sets of interests involved do not collide, they co-exist in a *constitutional realm* based on accommodation of diversity.'[48] This means that 'the religious beliefs of some cannot be used to determine the constitutional rights of others'. In other words, put more bluntly, prejudice inspired by religion – no matter how sincerely held – cannot justify unfair discrimination. The Court argued that in an open and democratic society there should be a capacity to accommodate and manage difference and not to enforce the view of the (religious) majority on marginalized minorities.[49] Any contrary view smacks unpleasantly of the authoritarian and totalitarian tactics so characteristic of the National Party government during the apartheid era.

The judgment provided Parliament with the opportunity to fix the problem within one year. What was required was for Parliament to adopt new legislation that would accord same-sex couples the same rights and status as heterosexual married couples. If Parliament failed to do so within a year, the existing Marriage Act would automatically be amended to include same-sex couples and would extend all the rights associated with marriage to such couples. Many activists and ordinary gay men and lesbian women were deeply upset by this remedy offered by the majority, arguing that the majority of the Court[50] failed to provide an effective remedy and condemned same-sex couples to another year in legal limbo.[51] Because the judgment never used the word 'marriage', there was also some anxiety that Parliament would try to avoid its responsibilities by providing a 'separate but equal' regime of legal protection that would not comply with the letter and spirit of the majority judgment.

The Civil Union Act

As pointed out above, the first draft of the Civil Union Bill did not comply with the judgment of the Constitutional Court in *Fourie*. Because the Court endorsed the notion that the concept of marriage has a profound symbolic, emotional and political power in our culture, it was clear that by refusing same-sex couples the right to enter into an institution called 'marriage', the Bill would deprive same-sex couples of the right to access to the status associated with the term 'marriage'. Thus, after political intervention, the ANC members of the Home Affairs Portfolio Committee decided, at the last possible moment, that it would be necessary to amend the draft Bill, and early in November 2006 the National Assembly adopted a substantially amended Bill which provided for same-sex couples to enter into a 'marriage' or a 'civil partnership'[52] that would accord them all the rights associated with traditional heterosexual marriage.[53] The Civil Union Act thus amends all existing legislation in which references are made to 'marriage', 'husband', 'wife' or 'spouse', so that it applies equally to those couples who register a marriage or a civil partnership in accordance with the Civil Union Act. The Act now provides for the recognition of same-sex relationships in a way that extends to same-sex couples the same rights and duties and the same status as that traditionally enjoyed by different-sex couples. The new Act provides for both same-sex and different-sex couples to enter into a marriage or a civil partnership[54] and prescribes the formal requirements for entering into such a civil-union marriage. This means that the Act allows both same-sex and different-sex couples to register their relationship in terms of this legislation. It also means that such couples have a choice either to register a 'marriage' or a 'civil partnership'. Whichever is chosen, the legal consequences are exactly the same.

At first blush, it seems somewhat perplexing that this choice was provided at all. Given the special status that marriage has in our society, most couples would probably not choose to register 'civil partnerships' if they have the choice of registering a 'marriage'. Yet, given the contested nature of heterosexual marriage and feminist critiques regarding the alleged patriarchal nature of the institution,[55] the inclusion of this option seems like a net gain for progressives. It allows those couples who do not wish to be associated with an institution specifically called 'marriage' to enter into a union that will provide them with the full range of legal rights and duties associated with that institution. Some more conservative same-sex couples, who view marriage as an institution exclusively associated with heterosexual relationships, may well also choose to enter into a civil partnership instead of a marriage.

With the adoption of the Civil Union Act, same-sex couples will, in effect, now have additional legal rights, over and above those of different-sex couples. Over the past ten years the Constitutional Court has extended many of the rights enjoyed by married heterosexual couples to (obviously unmarried) same-sex couples in life partnerships.[56] These rights include the right of same-sex couples to adopt children, to enjoy immigration rights, pension benefits and the right to inherit from a same-sex life partner. Limiting these rights to heterosexual married couples was found to be discriminatory precisely because same-sex couples could not get married and were thus automatically excluded from enjoying these rights. Given the fact that the extension of these rights to same-sex couples was based on the absence of same-sex marriage, the question was raised whether same-sex couples who did not marry on 1 December 2006 would automatically lose these rights where the court had read the words into existing legislation to include same-sex life partners. In a recent judgment the Constitutional Court, in the case of *Gory v Kolver and Others*, confirmed that these hard-won rights would not *automatically* be amended merely because same-sex couples are now allowed to get married. Even if same-sex couples do not get married they have, for example, the right to inherit from their life partner – even where no will is left. They also retain the right to jointly adopt children – even when they are not married. But, as the Court pointed out, Parliament will have the right to amend this kind of legislation in the future to take away the rights of unmarried same-sex couples so that they are treated the same as unmarried heterosexual couples.[57]

In at least one important aspect, however, the Civil Union Act remains problematic. As with the original Marriage Act, the Civil Union Act allows for the designation of ministers of religion as marriage officers, if that religious denomination as a whole makes application for them to do so (though individual ministers may opt out). Unlike the Marriage Act, the Civil Union Act allows non-religious marriage officers appointed by the state to refuse 'on the grounds of conscience, religion and belief to solemnise a civil union between two persons of the same-sex'.[58] Marriage officers are designated by the state in terms of

Section 2 of the Marriage Act and, as such, are state officials. This provision thus clearly endorses discrimination on the basis of sexual orientation by state officials, and would probably be struck down by the Constitutional Court if challenged. It may make it more difficult, especially for less wealthy and less educated same-sex couples who live in small towns in South Africa, to get married. Such a couple would typically go to the local magistrate's court where that magistrate would act as the state's designated marriage officer. If such a magistrate refused to marry a couple, they might not pursue the matter – out of ignorance or a lack of resources. This clause has therefore been strongly criticized by activists in the LGBTI community.

Notes
1 *Minister of Home Affairs and Another v Fourie and Another* 2005 (3) BCLR 355 (CC), paragraphs 71-72 (hereinafter referred to as '*Fourie*')
2 First draft of the Civil Union Bill, published in the *Government Gazette* 29169, 31 August 2006
3 Ibid., Section 13
4 Ibid., Section 11
5 Ibid., Section 6
6 Ibid., definition Section 1
7 *Fourie*, op. cit., paragraphs 49-58
8 There is no way of knowing whether some of the Constitutional Court judges who took part in the *Fourie* case harboured doubts about the full extension of marriage rights to same-sex couples. It is my contention, however, that if there were such judges they would have been boxed in by previous precedent.
9 Now-retired Justice Laurie Ackermann wrote the opinion and Justice Albie Sachs wrote a concurring opinion in this case.
10 1998 (12) BCLR 1517 (CC)
11 This included Section 20A of the Sexual Offences Act of 1957; the inclusion of sodomy in Schedule 1 of the Criminal Procedure Act of 1977; and the inclusion of sodomy in the schedule to the Security Officers Act of 1987.
12 *National Coalition for Gay and Lesbian Equality and the South African Human Rights Commission v Minister of Justice and Others* 1999 (1) SA 6 (CC) ('the decriminalization case'), paragraph 130. According to Sachs the success of the whole constitutional endeavour in South Africa will depend in large measure on how successfully 'sameness' and 'difference' are reconciled.
13 Ibid., paragraph 134
14 Michael Warner, introduction, in Warner (ed.), *Fear of a Queer Planet: Queer Politics and Social Theory* (University of Minnesota Press, 1993), xxi
15 Monique Wittig, *The Straight Mind* (Beacon, 1992), 40, 43
16 Decriminalization case, op. cit., paragraph 137
17 2000 (1) BCLR 39 (CC)
18 Ibid., paragraph 57
19 Ibid., paragraph 36
20 Ibid. See *Peter v Minister of Law and Order* 1990 (4) SA 6 (E) at 9G
21 Ibid., paragraph 53

22 See *Satchwell v President of the Republic of South Africa and Another* 2002 (9) BCLR 986 (CC) (judges in same-sex life partnerships have the same right to pension benefits as married heterosexual judges); and *J and Another v Director General, Department of Home Affairs and Others* 2003 (5) BCLR 463 (CC) (permanent same-sex life partners have a right to access to artificial insemination equivalent to married heterosexual couples).
23 2002 (10) BCLR 1006 (CC)
24 Ibid., paragraph 32
25 *Fourie and Another v Minister of Home Affairs and Another*, case number 17280/02, handed down on 18 October 2002, unreported
26 Act 25 of 1961
27 Ibid., Section 30 (1)
28 *Fourie and Another v Minister of Home Affairs and Another* 2003 (10) BCLR 1092 (CC)
29 *Fourie*, op. cit., order of the court, section 2
30 Ibid., paragraphs 59-62
31 Ibid., paragraph 52
32 Ibid., paragraph 53
33 *Prinsloo v Van der Linde* 1997 6 BCLR 759 (CC), paragraph 19
34 Act 21 of 1950
35 Act 55 of 1949
36 *Fourie*, op. cit., paragraph 70
37 Ibid., paragraph 72
38 Ibid., paragraph 54
39 Ibid., paragraph 71
40 Ibid., paragraph 81
41 It is intriguing to note that the judgment never uses the term 'marriage' itself when speaking of the need for the legal recognition of same-sex relationships. However, the fact that the court emphasizes that marriage provides not only tangible legal rights, but also intangible benefits and status, implies that extending anything less than marriage rights to same-sex couples would constitute disregard for the human dignity of same-sex couples and would thus be discriminatory.
42 *Fourie*, op. cit., paragraph 151
43 Many groups intervened as *amici curiae* (friends of the court) to oppose the application by Fourie and Bonthuys. These were Doctors for Life International and its legal representative, John Smyth; and the Marriage Alliance of South Africa, supported on affidavit by Catholic Cardinal Wilfred Napier.
44 *Fourie*, op. cit., paragraph 51
45 Ibid., paragraph 86
46 Ibid., paragraph 90
47 Ibid., paragraphs 90-93
48 Ibid., paragraph 98
49 Ibid., paragraph 94
50 O'Regan J dissenting. See pages 68-69 of this book.
51 Many of us who had criticized the majority in this regard changed our minds. Although the public participation process that accompanied discussions about the adoption of the Civil Union Act was deeply flawed, it did open up a conversation about sexual orientation and provided an unprecedented platform in the media for those arguing in favour of respect for gay and lesbian people.
52 Civil Union Act (Act 17 of 2006), Section 1, which defines a civil union as 'the voluntary union of two persons who are both 18 years of age or older, which is solemnised and registered by way of either a marriage or a civil partnership, in accordance with the procedures prescribed in this Act, to the exclusion, while it lasts, of all others'.

53 Ibid., Section 13, which states:
    (1) The legal consequences of a marriage contemplated in the Marriage Act apply, with such changes as may be required by the context to a civil union.
    (2) With the exception of the Marriage Act and the Customary Marriages Act any reference to –
       (a) marriage in any other law, including the common law, includes with such changes as may be required by the context, a civil union: and
       (b) husband, wife or spouse in any other law, including the common law, includes a civil union partner.
54 It has been suggested that Section 8 (6) of the Act muddies the waters in this regard and may be interpreted to restrict marriage under the new Act to same-sex couples. Section 8 (6) states:
    A civil union may only be registered by prospective civil union partners who would, apart from the fact that they are of the same sex, not be prohibited by law from concluding a marriage under the Marriage Act or the Customary Marriages Act.
    I contend that it is clear from the context that this section does not prohibit different-sex couples from entering a marriage in terms of the Civil Union Act. It merely states that such different-sex couples would only be able to enter into a civil union marriage if they had also been allowed to enter into a marriage in terms of one of the two other laws regulating marriage in South Africa.
55 See Paula Ettelbrick, 'Since When Is Marriage a Path to Liberation?', in Robert M Baird and Stuart E Rosenbaum (eds.), *Same-Sex Marriage: The Moral and Legal Debate* (Prometheus, 1997), 164–168
56 *National Coalition for Gay and Lesbian Equality and the South African Human Rights Commission v Minister of Justice and Others* 1999 (1) SA 6 (CC); 1998 (12) BCLR 1517 (CC); *National Coalition for Gay and Lesbian Equality and Others v Minister of Home Affairs and Others* 2000 (2) SA 1 (CC); 2000 (1) BCLR 39 (CC); *Satchwell v President of the Republic of South Africa and Another* 2002 (6) SA 1 (CC); 2002 (9) BCLR 986 (CC); *Du Toit and De Vos v Minister of Welfare and Population Development and Others* (Lesbian and Gay Equality Project as *amicus curiae*) 2003 (2) SA 198 (CC); 2002 (10) BCLR 1006 (CC); *J and Another v Director General, Department of Home Affairs, and Others* 2003 (5) SA 621 (CC); 2003 (5) BCLR 463 (CC); *Gory v Kolver NO and Others* 2007 (3) BCLR 249 (CC)
57 *Gory v Kolver*, op. cit., paragraph 28
58 Civil Union Act, Section 6

'A logical next step'
Interview with Beverly Palesa Ditsie

Bev Ditsie was a close friend of Simon Nkoli, and, with him, was a founder member of the Gay and Lesbian Organization of the Witwatersrand (GLOW), which became the public face of gay and lesbian rights activism, particularly that involving people of colour, in the late 1980s and early 1990s. GLOW organized the first gay and lesbian Pride marches in South Africa (beginning 1990) and helped lobby for gay and lesbian rights at a time when the country's new post-apartheid Constitution was under discussion and negotiation. Now a filmmaker, Ditsie reflects here on the early stirrings of a campaign for same-sex marriage.

In the gay and lesbian rights movement in the late 1980s and early 1990s, was the recognition of gay and lesbian relationships part of the agenda?
We knew that same-sex relationships should be recognized in the Constitution. The non-discrimination clause [Section 9 (3) of the Bill of Rights in the Constitution, also known as the equality clause], as it is, is very clear. There shall be no discrimination against anyone – any South African citizen – based on gender, race, age, all those things, including sexual orientation, and that flat-out means everything that we wanted it to mean. It means that you can't be discriminated against at work. It means that you can't be discriminated against at the church. It means all of those things, including that you can't be discriminated against if you want to get married. So for me marriage is a logical next step.

But, obviously, we knew at the time there had to be the campaigns for each one of the little things we wanted to undo. First of all, we had to decriminalize homosexuality, based on that clause, because there can't be a clause that says you can't be discriminated against and yet legally speaking it is illegal to be gay. So we knew then that there had to be individual campaigns for each one of the things that needed to be decriminalized, and the ones that had to be legalized as well. Same-sex marriage had always been one of them. And so we started to talk about same-sex relationships and same-sex unions, and all of that that had to be legalized. It came from knowing that there were far too many of us who would get into long-term relationships but those people pass on, or if anything happens that hurts them, then we find ourselves outside of the system. As a loving partner to somebody, you couldn't go to the hospital – that became clear to many of us, that it is one of those things that you do not want see happen, to be in love with someone and they get hurt and they are in a coma and you can't visit them. You can't sit there with them when you know that they are dying. So all those things made perfect sense. It was with the full knowledge that, as time went on, there would be a need for either the same group of people or a different group of people to take the campaign further, because I think everybody ultimately had their roles to play.

Do you think it was important to go for same-sex marriage?
I think that we have, right from the beginning, been fighting for the ability to live the way we want to live. That is what this fight has always been about. Therefore same sex-marriage has been the natural part of the next level. If you can't marry legally, what is the point of what we were doing then? We were not just having fun. We were fighting for something.

'A space to challenge the norms'
Interview with Wendy Isaack

Wendy Isaack is currently Manager of the Legal Department at People Opposing Women Abuse (POWA). She was born in Ladysmith in KwaZulu- Natal and came out as lesbian at age 14 (she reports that her father, son of an Indian father and a black African woman, said, 'Ja, maybe you are a lesbian. It's fine'). She studied law but found it hard to get articles ('I've been shaving my hair and wearing trousers since I was 14. So I would wear a suit and a tie, and I would go to the interviews dressed like that ...'). She moved to Johannesburg, where she joined the Lesbian and Gay Equality Project and worked on the campaign for same-sex marriage.

How did you get involved with the Equality Project?
I was walking through the streets of Yeoville, and I saw a sign for the Equality Project. I walked in and I met the staff. They were very welcoming, and I started to go there often. Eventually I was asked if I wanted to volunteer, because the person who was doing legal advice had a political science degree, not a law degree. Soon I was offered a position as a paralegal in the organization.

Tell us about the work you did on same-sex marriage at the Equality Project.
The litigation for same-sex marriages was always on the agenda of the Equality Project, and on the 'shopping list' of its predecessor, the National Coalition for Gay and Lesbian Equality [NCGLE]. Marriage was a logical step after having won the right to medical aid, pensions, immigration and adoption, and having tested the waters. There were activists at the time of the writing of the Constitution who were very clear about what they wanted. The first step – get sexual orientation in the Constitution. When you have that, decriminalize homosexual conduct, and, after that, challenge the state on issues that will not cost the state much money – medical aid, pensions and immigration. These are also issues that are not necessarily that controversial. Over a period of ten years it built up the jurisprudence that we relied on when we litigated for same-sex marriage. And if, at the end, we did not get marriage, we would still have something else. There were people who were saying from 1996, 'You have sexual orientation in the Constitution, you should go for marriage now.' We said, 'No, we're still criminal in this country – we need to change the Sexual Offences Act first.'

We would have lost if we'd gone for marriage earlier, because as much as we would like to think that the law is an independent institution, it is informed by social discourse. There would have been social pressure not to give lesbian and gay people same-sex marriage. People needed to get accustomed to the human rights culture after 1994 – to move from institutionalized discrimination into a space of respecting each other's diversity. This was entrenched in the Constitution, but it wasn't necessarily a reality in people's lives. We needed to do the groundwork and build the foundation for making a final argument for same-sex marriage.

The actual same-sex marriage litigation and advocacy work had started about two years before we filed our papers in the High Court. We did a lot of public education work in the provinces of KwaZulu-Natal, Mpumalanga, Western Cape, Eastern Cape and Gauteng. The only three provinces we didn't go to were Limpopo, Northern Cape and Northern Province. We always knew that we had a mandate as an organization, but that mandate was reinforced with the public education work that we did. We engaged with communities and asked, 'How do you feel about the topic?' Of course people had very strong feelings that they wanted marriage. Beyond having the legal protection, it gave our relationships a certain social recognition and we wanted that. We were engaging broadly with both lesbian and gay people and with other sectors. Everywhere we went we would say, 'This is a right that lesbian and gay people are entitled to.'

An aspect of the more formal advocacy work was getting involved in the South African Law Reform Commission's review of domestic partnerships and marriage. We made submissions on the discussion paper, and we attended the public workshops and the hearings, and made inputs. We were clear that the bottom-line was marriage and anything else was unequal and gave us second-class citizenship.

We were doing this work very carefully and very slowly. For four years, I had a big file of couples who'd come in for partnership contracts. For the marriage case, we were looking for couples who would represent the diversity of this country – white, black, Indian, coloured, poor, rich. There were about 18 of these couples in our files. I spoke to them and they met with the attorneys. While we were doing that, Fourie and Bonthuys filed their application with the Pretoria High Court, and we had to get our act together really fast. There were a number of strictly legal decisions and strategies. The most interesting aspect of it was actually living the practical exclusion. We took a trip to the Home Affairs office with two couples who were part of the litigation and said, 'These couples want to get married.' The person at Home Affairs sat there trying to type in the ID numbers. The system wouldn't accept the ID numbers, because the system is designed to accept the numbers according to gender. The guy really tried, and he said, 'Sorry, I can't marry you because your ID numbers are both female, so it's not working.' That was a necessary step in the arguments we were going to make in court – that there was no other possible avenue of redress of this issue.

What was your experience working on domestic-violence issues at the Equality Project?

We always think the root-problems of domestic violence are patriarchy and masculinity, and we want to perceive ourselves as being quite different, that we do not carry that heterosexist baggage, and so our relationships are based on equality and respect. But my experience in that office was quite different. There is a lot of domestic violence in same-sex relationships – sufficient to warrant the application for protection in legislation. The brilliant thing about the Domestic Violence Act is that the Act makes it possible to include a range of relationships. If people come in and say, 'Listen, my partner and I are fine, but we're being abused by her family,' then even the partner can apply for a protection order on the basis of that relationship. The Domestic Violence Act is sufficiently progressive and it makes provision for people who are involved in same-sex relationships.

What impact will the legalization of same-sex marriage have on domestic violence?

I'm bound to think it will increase it. The reasons for the high levels of domestic violence in same-sex relationships are not fundamentally different from the reasons for domestic violence in heterosexual relationships. Domestic violence is about power and control, and about exercising some legal control over another person. These dynamics are relevant in any relationship. I'm afraid that the Civil Union Act institutionalizes the relationship and with the institutionalization of the relationship you carry that baggage.

Will same-sex marriages be more equal because the partners are of the same sex?

The basis of inequality, or the way in which people exercise power in personal relationships, is not only through the difference in sex or gender. Lesbian and gay people are not growing up in a vacuum isolated from social processes and systems. We're living in a society which is patriarchal, which is sexist. Now is the time to think about the consequences of having same-sex marriage, and educating ourselves so we do not carry the baggage pertaining to heterosexual marriage into our relationships.

What does same-sex marriage mean for you as a black African woman?

Following the adoption of the Constitution, we had legal recognition of customary marriages. Legislation was drafted that acknowledged relationships that were negotiated around customary rules and traditional values. Unfortunately the process has been limited to protecting heterosexual relationships. I think the Constitution gives potential to open up the debate on customary marriages to include lesbian and gay people. The lesbian and gay sector has been centred on sexual identity in the face of claims that 'homosexuality is unAfrican, it's against tradition, it's against culture'. It's time to be more challenging, and to say that we have multiple identities. I am a lesbian. I can access the Civil Union Act. But I am also a black Zulu woman, and there is a law in this country which makes provision for Zulus in terms of recognizing marriage. Why should I not have that? The Constitution has offered us a space to challenge the norms of how we do relationships and how we do politics and how we engage with the Constitution itself.

Would you get married yourself?
Right now, I'm in a committed relationship, and my partner and I are having that conversation about marriage. I believe that it's not only a legal institution – it's also about social recognition and communicating certain social values. So I would like to do it properly. I might take the Zulu aspect of my tradition: the lobola needs to be paid, and there needs to be negotiation around how that is done. I know of lesbian couples who talk about paying lobola for each other – they pay the same portion to each other's families. One can work around these things. But what we have so far is not enough. I want to have all the options. I want to have the option of using the Customary Marriages Act. I want to have the option of just living in a domestic relationship, and having that relationship protected.

'Reforming and renewing'
Interview with Dominee André Muller

André Muller studied theology at the University of Pretoria and became a minister in the Dutch Reformed Church at Witbank-Panorama. When his gay orientation became known he was ostracized and expelled from his church community. (The church synod even demanded immediate repayment of his study bursary!) In 1992 Muller started a gay and lesbian church in Pretoria, the Reforming Church. Muller conducted ceremonies of commitment for congregants as well as non-church-members. He was approached by Marié Fourie and Cecelia Bonthuys to solemnize their union, which led in due course to their legal challenge to the common-law definition of marriage in the courts. Muller is a designated religious marriage officer under the Civil Union Act, and since the Act's promulgation he has performed 182 civil unions, of which eight are registered as civil partnerships and 174 as marriages.

What is the ethos of the Reforming Church?
We could be described as a conservative gay Afrikaans church. We are just like any other traditional Afrikaans congregation, except that we say it's OK to be gay. We condemn promiscuity, we're against so-called open relationships, and try to promote togetherness, relationships, and being celibate while you're single. So it's quite traditional.

How did the church come by its name?
In 1991 Hendrik Pretorius started the first gay church in this country, called the Reforming Congregations of Equals in Christ. It sadly lasted only eight months and ended when Hendrik accused his congregation of spinelessness in an article in the Afrikaans Sunday newspaper *Rapport* [19 July 1992].

When I started the Reforming Church on 3 August 1992, I thought that, as a gesture to acknowledge his work, we would retain the word 'reforming', because it is a positive and lively word. It denotes constant change – not something stagnant, but reforming and renewing. The word is in the present-continuous tense, not in the past tense like in 'reformed church'. We are a church that wants to grow and renew all the time.

How big is your congregation now?
We have about 400 people. Other Dutch Reformed Church congregations

average between 3 000 and 7 000 members. In our congregation, the youngest member is 19 and the oldest is in his eighties. I'd say the majority are in their thirties.

You said that the church emphasizes stable relationships. Did the subject of marriage came up in discussions early on?
From the earliest times we had marriages in our church. We didn't refer to them as marriages but as life-commitment ceremonies. People always had the wish to have some kind of ceremony to formalize their relationship. From the beginning I had requests from my church members and from people outside the church.

What did those life-commitment ceremonies mean for you?
It was wonderful. In the gay community, so many people just have one-night stands. I wanted to break that cycle and establish new norms, and I thought the best way to do it was to promote permanent relationships through life-commitment ceremonies. At the Pride march in 1998, the theme was 'Recognize Our Relationships'. That was when it really became a driving force for myself to make the church instrumental in getting this dream realized – that gay marriages could actually take place. I wrote letters to the South African Law Reform Commission, requesting the legalization of gay marriages on behalf of my church, and saying that we as a Christian church support gay marriages.

When you wrote to the Law Reform Commission, was that part of a bigger initiative by gay and lesbian organizations?
No, not really. I discussed it with my church council, and I said that as a church we can play a role by sending an official letter on the church's letterhead and requesting the whole process be discussed. So we drew up a letter and we sent it to the Law Reform Commission. It was favourably accepted, and after that we were invited to take part in talks and workshops. It was an information-sharing experience. My impression was they were testing the waters at first. The next thing was a huge workshop where there were about 200 people – Home Affairs delegates and representatives from various churches made themselves heard. There was a black pastor from a Lutheran church, and he had a very strong voice. He said gay marriages were totally against the will of God. He made the announcement, and got up and left. The whole atmosphere was that he spoke on behalf of all Christians and that he had said everything that could be said.

Did the National Coalition for Gay and Lesbian Equality and its successor, the Equality Project, interact with your church?
No, they never really tried. I think the gay community was against religion,

because they viewed religion, the Christian church in particular, as opposing them and who they were. It was the church – *we* had the longing to be part of the process.

How many life-commitment ceremonies you were doing at that time?
In the busiest year there were about 20. In total I had conducted 131 ceremonies from 1993 to 2005. We still have the registers in our church office.

What would a typical commitment ceremony be like?
Like a typical wedding ceremony, nothing different, except on two occasions where the two grooms appeared in dresses. But apart from that the ceremony is like any other marriage ceremony. There's an entrance, there's music, there's a message, a prayer, vows are exchanged, rings are exchanged, and then the pronouncement. At that stage I pronounced them as life partners. That's the term I used.

When did you become aware of the campaign to make same-sex marriage legal?
The 1998 Pride march, where the theme was 'Recognize Our Relationships'. When Marié [Fourie] and Cecelia [Bonthuys] approached me and asked me to marry them, that was really my first introduction to the whole legal side of things. I accompanied them to the Constitutional Court in 2005 and witnessed what was going on. That awoke strong feelings of the need, because it wasn't just about Marié and Cecelia, they were only symbols, they were representing the rest of the community. I was there just to observe and be educated.

How did you feel about this attempt to legalize gay and lesbian marriage?
I thought it was the absolutely right thing to do. Having life-commitment ceremonies was only halfway. It was a religious thing, but it had no legal consequences. Most of those couples eventually broke up. I thought that if we as a community wanted to be taken seriously, we ourselves had to consider our relationships in a more serious light. When you enter into marriage it should be the full marriage, with all the legal consequences. If you want to separate, it must be done in a legal way. You will have to go through divorce. You can't just pack your things and go.

Had Marié and Cecelia been part of your congregation beforehand?
No, they joined because they wanted to get married. They thought that if I married them we could take the life-commitment register to Home Affairs and inform them that their ceremony took place, here's the proof of it, and could Home Affairs convert that into a marriage certificate? We followed that route, but it was not accepted. The official there thought it was a joke. She just laughed and said it cannot be done.

What were your next steps? Or did Marié and Cecelia do things independently?
They did that independently. They had a law professor who acted as their guide through the whole process and his recommendation was that they should take it to the next court. I wasn't part of that decision. I didn't suggest to them that they take it further.

Did you attend the Constitutional Court on the day the Fourie judgment was handed down?
I accompanied Marié and Cecelia. I actually drove them to the Court. There was electricity in the air – very exciting. I think we all knew what the outcome was going to be. There was a large group of supporters of same-sex marriage who made their feelings known. At one point the court had to silence them. A very solemn atmosphere, but also this electricity and this expectation that we were going to get a favourable answer. Marié and Cecelia looked quite tense. From where I sat I only saw their hands, and both of them were clenching their fists all the time. Their hands were sweaty – they often dried their hands on their clothes. And Marié had a frown on her face all the time, looking very concerned.

How did you feel about the verdict?
We were jumping up and down with joy.

How did you feel about the court giving Parliament a year to pass legislation?
I was a little bit disappointed. We had adhered to all the legal requirements for a marriage, so I thought we shouldn't have to wait for another year. Following Justice Edwin Cameron's judgment in the Supreme Court of Appeal, we had complied with all the provisions under the existing Marriage Act and regulations, namely that I was a registered marriage officer, there were no legal objections to the marriage – of Marié and Cecelia – and two witnesses had signed the register. While Home Affairs couldn't provide us with an official same-sex marriage register at that stage, I really hoped that they would have accepted the ecclesiastical marriage register as a source document and proof that such a marriage had taken place.

'It was a privilege to be involved in the case'
Interview with Sharon Cox and Diane Holdsworth

Sharon Cox and Diane Holdsworth have been in a relationship for seventeen years. Sharon is a volunteer at the Triangle Project in Cape Town and a pastoral worker for the Good Hope Metropolitan Community Church; Diane is a financial broker. They were among the couples in the Equality Project's case for the legalization of same-sex marriage. They have answered the questions put to them with one voice.

Why did you decide to join the Equality Project's court application for the right to marry?
We came to be involved in the case through the Triangle Project. We chose to be involved in the case for two reasons. Firstly, we felt it important that all people of this country, regardless of sexual orientation, should have the right to have their relationships legally recognized if they wished and, secondly, it was important as a couple who are practicing Christians to be part of the case. Having done media interviews over the years, it has always been clear that the religious right is very vocal on any issue that involves LGBTI people and we knew that this case would be no different. In this democratic country with a progressive Constitution, we all have the right to pursue the faith of our choice and the state has a responsibility to ensure that no one person's belief, religious or otherwise, should interfere with another's basic civil rights. We felt that legislation should reflect a tolerance for diversity and move past discrimination based on sexual orientation, and so it was important to us that by being involved in the case we would have the opportunity to make it known that the prevailing prejudiced Christian voice was not the only Christian voice. It was important for us to ensure that people knew that these people do not speak for all Christians.

How would you describe the experience of challenging the law? What impact did it have on your lives, both as individuals and as a couple?
It was a very exciting process. We were a little removed from the physical presence at the Constitutional Court in Johannesburg because we live in Cape Town, but we were kept up to date every step of the way by Crystal Cambanis and others from Nicholls, Cambanis and Associates – the lawyers handling the case. It was frustrating and maddening at times to hear the comments being made – especially those made at the public hearings at the Woodstock town hall, but

it was a great to be able to speak up and speak out against the loud voices of discrimination. It was a privilege to be involved in the case and, after the passing of the Civil Union Act, it was awesome to think that our names were linked to the case and a great feeling to be in possession of all the documentation that was part of the case.

Are there particular memories that stand out? At the courts? Media coverage?
There are several memories that stood out in the lead-up to the outcome of the case. One of these was an invitation to speak at a conference at Stellenbosch University, arranged by the Beyers Naudé Centre for Public Theology, in co-operation with Inclusive and Affirming Ministries. The conference was entitled 'Same Sex Marriages: Responding with Integrity'. In attendance were theologians and theological students who will have the opportunity in the future to make an impact on people's lives. The church universal over decades has caused great damage in the lives of many LGBTI people. It dawned on me that it is important for them especially to hear our stories and perhaps the next generation of outspoken theologians may think differently and, in turn, their congregations may also begin to think and act differently. Sharon received a wonderful e-mail after the conference from a student who said that, after listening to all the speakers and after hearing personal stories, he pledged never to stand in a pulpit and preach messages of hate, intolerance and discrimination. We decided after that wonderful day that it may takes decades to change attitudes and perceptions, but we could do it one person at a time.

One memory that really stands out is at the public hearings held at the Woodstock town hall. Speaker after speaker seemed to be from one or another denomination or faith group who were vocal and mostly hateful in their attitudes about granting us the right to marry. As the speakers lined up, we were guessing as to where they may be from. A woman then got up and approached the mic. We decided that she was probably someone in the mission field and was going to add to the prejudice that was so prevalent. She approached the mic and said that she was engaged to be married. She said how she had looked forward to this day and to the rights and responsibilities of marriage but she could not find it in her conscience to go ahead with her wedding until all people were granted the same right. The next at the mic was a young man. He was her fiancé and added to what she had said. It's hard to forget how it felt to have some relief from the prejudice and to hear two people, whose lives would not be affected one way or another by the outcome of the case, say what they did.

We will also always remember several members of clergy, both heterosexual and homosexual, who spoke up on our behalf. They were far more eloquent and what they said far more powerful than anything else said on that day.

How did you feel when the Civil Union Act was finally passed and same-sex marriage was legalized?
We always felt confident, even in the face of all that was being said, that we would be granted the right to marry, but it took nothing away from the excitement that we felt when it passed.

What do you think of the Civil Union Act itself?
We think it is a far better version than the initial Bill was. We opposed the first version on the grounds that it was a separate piece of legislation and 'separate but equal' is not equal at all. We are proud that, unlike some other countries, we did not just accept the first draft with an attitude of being grateful for what we could get. It is disappointing that there was not just one Act for all people and that the Marriage Act wasn't just adapted to make the language gender-neutral. It was confusing as to why there should be a whole new piece of legislation created. Another aspect of the Act that is troubling is that civil marriage officers are allowed to refuse to marry a couple if they so choose.

Have you married, or do you plan to marry?
Just after the Act was passed, the media attention was overwhelming. We had several offers from the media asking if they could cover the occasion and we realized that for us it was not about the occasion but about what marriage means to us, so we chose not to do it straight away.

Sharon's brother was marrying in the weeks following the Act's passing and he suggested that we have a combined wedding. We did not want to detract from his wedding, and by the time their wedding was over we had had enough of weddings for one year, so decided to leave it till a later date. We still haven't got married but plan to do so in 2008.

Legal milestones for gay and lesbian rights in South Africa

Bill of Rights of the South African Constitution

Section 9 (1) states that 'Everyone is equal before the law and has the right to equal protection and benefit of the law.'

Section 9 (3), also known as the equality clause, states: 'The state may not unfairly discriminate directly or indirectly against anyone on one or more grounds, including race, gender, sex, pregnancy, marital status, ethnic or social origin, colour, sexual orientation, age, disability, religion, conscience, belief, culture, language and birth.'

In keeping with the equality clause, Parliament has passed legislation to prevent discrimination in a range of areas. The Promotion of Equality and Prevention of Unfair Discrimination Act of 2000 requires the government to 'promote equality' on all the grounds in the equality clause. Other statutes that give recognition to the rights of gays and lesbians include the Domestic Violence Act of 1999, the Rental Housing Act of 1999, the Employment Equity Act of 1998, the Medical Schemes Act of 1998 and the Labour Relations Act of 1995.

Key court cases

Below is a list of significant High and Constitutional Court judgments which served to repeal or reform a range of laws that had previously discriminated against gay and lesbian people. These judgments were a result of legal challenges brought by the National Coalition for Gay and Lesbian Equality (which later became the Lesbian and Gay Equality Project) as well as by independent lesbian and gay couples and/or individuals.

1997
State v Kampher

The Cape High Court set aside a conviction and sentence for the crime of sodomy on the basis that it was unconstitutional. The order applied only to the limited geographical area that falls under the jurisdiction of the Cape High Court.

1998
Langemaat v Minister of Safety and Security and Others (also known as 'Polmed')

The High Court ordered that a state medical scheme recognize the same-sex relationship of its member and extend beneficiary status to her lesbian partner.

1998
National Coalition for Gay and Lesbian Equality and Another v Minister of Justice and Others
The High Court declared unconstitutional the common law offence of sodomy, certain discriminatory aspects of the common law offence of unnatural sexual offences, and the inclusion of sodomy as a crime in schedules to certain criminal law statutes. The finding on unnatural sexual offences did not form part of the subsequent confirmation and appeal proceedings in the Constitutional Court, and is therefore applicable only in the geographic area that falls under the jurisdiction of the Witwatersrand Local Division.

1998
National Coalition for Gay and Lesbian Equality and the South African Human Rights Commission v Minister of Justice and Others ('the decriminalization case' or 'the sodomy case')
The Constitutional Court decriminalized sodomy and removed it from some schedules to certain criminal law statutes.

1999
Martin v Beka Provident Fund
The Pension Funds Adjudicator ordered that a pension fund change its rules so that permanent same-sex life partnerships are recognized and surviving same-sex life partners receive the same benefits as surviving heterosexual married partners. It also ordered the fund to process Martin's claim in accordance with the revised rules.

1999
National Coalition for Gay and Lesbian Equality and Others v Minister of Home Affairs and Others
The High Court ruled that the exclusion of permanent same-sex life partners of South African citizens and permanent residents from certain immigration rights is unconstitutional. It also declared the conduct of Home Affairs officials in refusing to grant same-sex couples exemptions from the discriminatory laws unlawful.

1999
National Coalition for Gay and Lesbian Equality and Others v Minister of Home Affairs and Others ('the immigration case')
The Constitutional Court ruled that the permanent same-sex life partner of a South African citizen or permanent resident should be granted the same rights as a spouse when it comes to immigration rights.

2002
Satchwell v President of Republic South Africa and Another
The Constitutional Court ruled that the permanent same-sex life partner of a judge is entitled to the same pension payout as a spouse.

2002
Fourie and Another v Minister of Home Affairs and Another (the Lesbian and Gay Equality Project as *amicus curiae*)
The High Court dismissed the case because it did not expressly challenge the constitutionality of the relevant marriage laws.

THE LEGAL STEPS TO SAME-SEX MARRIAGE

2002
The Lesbian and Gay Equality Project and Others v the Minister of Finance
The case established the right to equal benefits from pension funds for the same sex partners of state employees. (The matter was settled out of court.)

2002
Du Toit and De Vos v the Minister of Welfare and Population Development and Others
The Constitutional Court ordered the insertion of words into the Child Care Act and the Guardianship Act so that same-sex couples can be joint legal parents of a minor adopted child.

2003
J and Another v Director General, Department of Home Affairs and Others
The Constitutional Court ruled that both parties in a same-sex couple should be allowed to be registered as the parents of a child born to one of the parties by way of *in vitro* fertilization.

2004
Du Plessis v Road Accident Fund
The Supreme Court of Appeal determined that a permanent same-sex life partner of a deceased person has the right to claim damages for loss of support.

2004
Fourie and Another v Minister of Home Affairs and Others (the Lesbian and Gay Equality Project as *amicus curiae*)
The Supreme Court of Appeal declared the common-law definition of marriage unconstitutional.

2005
Minister of Home Affairs and Another v Fourie and Another
The Constitutional Court largely upheld the Supreme Court of Appeal decision and declared the unconstitutionality and invalidity of both the common-law definition of marriage and the current marriage formula. This declaration was suspended for 12 months from the date of judgment to allow Parliament to correct the defects in the law.

2006
Gory v Kolver NO
The High Court granted equal benefits to the surviving partner of a same-sex relationship in the case of his or her partner dying without a will (intestate). This judgment was confirmed by the Constitutional Court.

Judgment days:
The journey through the courts

The *Fourie* case: Challenging the common-law definition of marriage

In 2002 Marié Adriaana Fourie and Cecelia Johanna Bonthuys, a lesbian couple, approached the High Court in Pretoria with the desire to marry and thereby acquire the status, benefits and responsibilities that flow from marriage between heterosexual couples. They asked the court to recognize their relationship as a marriage. The Court dismissed the application on the basis that the common law, at the time, defined a marriage as a union between a man and a woman. Because the couple had not expressly sought to challenge the constitutionality of the marriage laws, the Court could not grant the relief they sought. Yet implicit in their papers, as the *amicus curiae* argued and the Supreme Court of Appeal (SCA) was later to find, was a direct constitutional challenge to these laws.

Later, the couple was granted leave to appeal to the SCA. Their application for leave to appeal to the Constitutional Court was however denied. Nevertheless, Fourie and Bonthuys approached the Constitutional Court directly in 2003. However this court refused their application on the ground that the case should first be heard by the SCA.

On 23 August 2004 the couple stated their case before the SCA. The Lesbian and Gay Equality Project intervened as *amicus curiae*. On 30 November 2004 the SCA handed down its judgment. The court concluded that the exclusion of same-sex couples from existing marriage laws amounted to unfair discrimination against gay and lesbian people. See extracts from this judgment below, on pages 60–63.

Both parties to the case approached the Constitutional Court for leave to appeal the SCA decision. The State's primary reason was its view that Parliament, rather than the judiciary, should be tasked with reforming marriage laws. Fourie and Bonthuys were still unable to get married due to the unchanged Marriage Act (the marriage formula in the Marriage Act only referred to 'husband' and 'wife'), and so also sought leave to appeal the SCA decision.

The next step was for the Constitutional Court to hear the *Fourie* case.

The Lesbian and Gay Equality Project (Equality Project) cases:
Challenging the common-law definition of marriage and Section 30 (1) of the Marriage Act

At the same time as the *Fourie* case, the Equality Project acted on the need for both the common law and the Marriage Act itself to be challenged and so launched an application in the Johannesburg High Court (in mid-2004). This application was made on behalf of the Equality Project and sixteen others (including Triangle Project, OUT LGBT Well-being, Forum for the Empowerment of Women, The Durban Gay and Lesbian Community and Health Centre and six same-sex couples).

The applicants asked the court to order the following, among other things:
- To declare the common-law definition of marriage and the prescribed marriage formula in Section 30 (1) of the Marriage Act (Act 25 of 1961) unconstitutional in that they violate the rights of lesbian and gay people to:
    - Equality in terms of Section 9 of the Constitution of the Republic of South Africa
    - Dignity in terms of section 10 of the Constitution
    - Privacy in terms of section 14 of the Constitution
- To amend the common-law definition of marriage to be read as follows:
  'Marriage is the lawful and voluntary union of two persons to the exclusion of all others while it lasts.'
- To declare that the words 'or spouse' be read into the prescribed marriage formula in Section 30 (1) of the Marriage Act immediately after the words 'or husband'

This case was originally due to be heard in the High Court in October 2005, and was subsequently set down for January 2006. However, as a result of the developments in the *Fourie* case at the time, and as outlined above, the Equality Project applied for direct access to the Constitutional Court. This would allow for their challenge to the Marriage Act to be heard together with the appeal and cross-appeal of the SCA judgment in the *Fourie* case.

As such the Equality Project and 18 others (including Triangle Project, OUT LGBT Well-being, Forum for the Empowerment of Women, The Durban Gay and Lesbian Community and Health Centre and seven same-sex couples) made an application to the Constitutional Court.

The Equality Project had also intervened as *amicus curiae* in the *Fourie* case, at both the Pretoria High Court and the SCA.

On the 14 May 2005 the Constitutional Court, the highest court in South Africa, heard the *Fourie* case and the Equality Project direct application. On 1 December 2005 the decision of this court was handed down. See extracts from this judgment below, on pages 63–69.

The Supreme Court of Appeal judgment

Case name: *Fourie and Another v Minister of Home Affairs and Others (the Lesbian and Gay Equality Project as* amicus curiae*).*
Appeal: *Monday 23 August 2004*
Judgment: *Tuesday 30 November 2004*

Below are a series of edited extracts from the majority judgment of the Supreme Court of Appeal, written by Justice Edwin Cameron. All footnotes have been excluded for the sake of brevity. Where the text has been shortened, elisions are indicated by an ellipsis (...). The original numbering of clauses has been retained for reference purposes. The full judgment is available at: wwwserver.law.wits. ac.za/sca/files/2322003/2322003.pdf (last accessed 27 February 2008).

The majority judgment, written by Justice Edwin Cameron

[*Justice Cameron reflects on the strides that equality jurisprudence has taken in respect of gay and lesbian people over the last decade and prior to same-sex marriage. These legal developments included the decriminalization of sodomy; the extension of immigration rights, and pension and medical aid benefits to same-sex couples; as well as the right to co-parent and to adopt children. He quotes from these cases; see pages 55-57.*]

[13] The importance of these cases lies not merely in what they decided, but in the far-reaching doctrines of dignity, equality and inclusive moral citizenship they articulate. They establish the following:

(a) Gays and lesbians are a permanent minority in society who in the past have suffered from patterns of disadvantage. Because they are a minority unable on their own to use political power to secure legislative advantages, they are exclusively reliant on the Bill of Rights for their protection.

(b) The impact of discrimination on them has been severe, affecting their dignity, personhood and identity at many levels.

(c) 'The sting of past and continuing discrimination against both gays and lesbians' lies in the message it conveys, namely that, viewed as individuals or in their same-sex relationships, they 'do not have the inherent dignity and are not worthy of the human respect possessed by and accorded to heterosexuals and their relationships'. This 'denies to gays and lesbians that which is foundational to our Constitution and the concepts of equality and dignity', namely that 'all persons have the same inherent worth and dignity', whatever their other differences may be.

(d) Continuing discrimination against gays and lesbians must be assessed on the basis that marriage and the family are vital social institutions. The legal obligations arising from them perform important social functions. They provide for security, support and companionship between members of our society and play a pivotal role in the rearing of children.

(e) Family life as contemplated by the Constitution can be constituted in different ways and legal conceptions of the family and what constitutes family life should change as social practices and traditions change.

(f) Permanent same-sex life partners are entitled to found their relationships in a manner that accords with their sexual orientation: such relationships should not be subject to unfair discrimination.

(g) Gays and lesbians in same-sex life partnerships are 'as capable as heterosexual spouses of expressing and sharing love in its manifold forms' ... They have in short 'the same ability to establish a *consortium omnis vitae*'. Finally, they are 'capable of constituting a family, whether nuclear or extended, and of establishing, enjoying and benefiting from family life' in a way that is 'not distinguishable in any significant respect from that of heterosexual spouses'.

(h) The decisions of the courts regarding gays and lesbians should be seen as part of the growing acceptance of difference in an increasingly open and pluralistic South Africa that is vital to the society the Constitution contemplates.

(i) Same-sex marriage is not unknown to certain African traditional societies.

[Justice Cameron outlines the impact of an exclusionary legal definition of marriage on gay and lesbian people.]

[15] The current common law definition of marriage deprives committed same-sex couples of this choice. In this our common law denies gays and lesbians who wish to solemnise their union a host of benefits, protections and duties. Legislation has ameliorated, but not eliminated, the disadvantage same-sex couples suffer. More deeply, the exclusionary definition of marriage injures gays and lesbians because it implies a judgment on them. It suggests not only that their relationships and commitments and loving bonds are inferior, but that they themselves can never be fully part of the community of moral equals that the Constitution promises to create for all.

[16] The vivid message of the decisions of the last ten years is that this exclusion cannot accord with the meaning of the Constitution, and that it 'undermines the values which underlie an open and democratic society based on freedom and equality'. In the absence of justification, it cannot but constitute unfair discrimination that violates the equality and other guarantees in the Bill of Rights.

[Justice Cameron contemplates how the unconstitutionality of the common-law definition of marriage should be dealt with by the court. Here reference is made to the minority judgment, written by Justice Farlam, which held that the development of the common law to bring it into line with the Constitution

should be suspended to enable Parliament to enact appropriate legislation. He pointed out that the South African Law Reform Commission had indicated three possible legislative responses to the unconstitutionality of the marriage laws, and that it should be Parliament and not the judiciary that should choose the appropriate remedy.[1]]

[38] Having concluded that the common law should be developed, Farlam JA proposes to suspend the order for two years. I cannot agree. The suggested suspension is in my respectful view neither appropriate nor in keeping with principle, the justice of this case, or the role the Constitution assigns to courts in developing the common law ...

[39] First the Constitution. As suggested earlier, development of the common law entails a simultaneously creative and declaratory function in which the court perfects a process of incremental legal development that the Constitution has already ordained. Once the court concludes that the Bill of Rights requires that the common law be developed, it is not engaging in a legislative process. Nor in fulfilling that function does the court intrude on the legislative domain.

[40] It is precisely this role that the Bill of Rights envisages must be fulfilled, and which it entrusts to the judiciary ... in order to give effect to a right in the Bill of Rights a court must – subject to limitation – 'apply, or if necessary develop, the common law to the extent that legislation does not give effect to that right' ... the Constitution deliberately assigns an imperative role to the court ... And this role is particularly suited to the judiciary, since the common law and the need for its incremental development are matters with which lawyers and judges are concerned daily.

[41] ... the incremental development that the Bill of Rights envisages is entrusted to the courts. It will be rarely, if ever, that an order pursuant to such incremental development can or should be subjected to suspension.

[*The order of court is then outlined.*]

[48] In all these circumstances I conclude that the appellants are entitled to immediate declaratory relief regarding the development of the common law, and to a declaration that their intended marriage is capable of recognition as lawfully valid subject to compliance with statutory formalities.

[49] The following order is made:

1. The appeal succeeds with costs.

2. The order of the court below [Pretoria High Court] is set aside. In its place is substituted:

'(1) It is declared that:

(a) In terms of sections 8 (3), 39 (2) and 173 of the Constitution, the common law concept of marriage is developed to embrace same-sex partners as follows:

'Marriage is the union of two persons to the exclusion of all others for life.'

(b) The intended marriage between the appellants is capable of lawful recognition as a legally valid marriage, provided the formalities in the Marriage Act 25 of 1961 are complied with.

(2) The respondents are ordered to pay the applicants' costs.'

[*In summary, the SCA ruled that the common-law definition of marriage discriminated unfairly against same-sex couples. Justice Cameron, for the majority, believed that the common-law definition should be developed immediately, so as to include same-sex couples.*]

The Constitutional Court judgment

Case names: *Minister of Home Affairs and Another v Fourie and Another; Lesbian and Gay Equality Project and 18 Others v Minister of Home Affairs and Others*
Heard on: *17 May 2005*
Decided on: *1 December 2005*

Below are a series of edited extracts from the majority and majority judgments of the Constitutional Court. All footnotes have been excluded for the sake of brevity. Where the text has been shortened, elisions are indicated by an ellipsis (...). The original numbering of clauses has been retained for reference purposes. The full judgment is available at: www.constitutionalcourt.org.za/Archimages/5257.PDF (last accessed 27 February 2008).

The majority judgment, written by Justice Albie Sachs
[*Justice Sachs reflects on unfair discrimination on the basis of sexual orientation and the response of the courts preceding the same-sex marriage cases.*]

[59] This Court has thus in five consecutive decisions highlighted at least four unambiguous features of the context in which the prohibition against unfair discrimination on grounds of sexual orientation must be analysed. The first is that South Africa has a multitude of family formations that are evolving rapidly as our society develops, so that it is inappropriate to entrench any particular form as the only socially and legally acceptable one. The second is the existence of an imperative constitutional need to acknowledge the long history in our country and abroad of marginalisation and persecution of gays and lesbians ... The third is ... there is no comprehensive legal regulation of the family law rights of gays and lesbians. Finally, our Constitution represents a radical rupture with a past based

on intolerance and exclusion, and the movement forward to the acceptance of the need to develop a society based on equality and respect by all for all.

[*Justice Sachs points to the notion of* difference *in relation to the constitutional principle of equality.*]

[60] A democratic, universalistic, caring and aspirationally egalitarian society embraces everyone and accepts people for who they are ... Equality means equal concern and respect across difference. It does not presuppose the elimination or suppression of difference ... Equality therefore does not imply a levelling or homogenisation of behaviour or extolling one form as supreme, and another as inferior, but an acknowledgement and acceptance of difference. At the very least, it affirms that difference should not be the basis for exclusion, marginalisation and stigma. At best, it celebrates the vitality that difference brings to any society. The issue goes well beyond assumptions of heterosexual exclusivity, a source of contention in the present case. The acknowledgement and acceptance of difference is particularly important in our country where for centuries group membership based on supposed biological characteristics such as skin colour has been the express basis of advantage and disadvantage ... The Constitution thus acknowledges the variability of human beings (genetic and socio-cultural), affirms the right to be different, and celebrates the diversity of the nation. Accordingly, what is at stake is not simply a question of removing an injustice experienced by a particular section of the community. At issue is a need to affirm the very character of our society as one based on tolerance and mutual respect. The test of tolerance is not how one finds space for people with whom, and practices with which, one feels comfortable, but how one accommodates the expression of what is discomfiting.

[*Justice Sachs reflects on the impact of the exclusion of same-sex couples from being able to marry if they chose.*]

[71] The exclusion of same-sex couples from the benefits and responsibilities of marriage, accordingly, is not a small and tangential inconvenience resulting from a few surviving relics of societal prejudice destined to evaporate like the morning dew. It represents a harsh if oblique statement by the law that same-sex couples are outsiders, and that their need for affirmation and protection of their intimate relations as human beings is somehow less than that of heterosexual couples ... It signifies that their capacity for love, commitment and accepting responsibility is by definition less worthy of regard than that of heterosexual couples.

[72] ... the intangible damage to same-sex couples is as severe as the material deprivation ... they are not entitled to celebrate their commitment to each other in a joyous public event recognised by the law. They are obliged to live in a state of legal blankness in which their unions remain unmarked by the showering of presents and the commemoration of anniversaries so celebrated in our culture ...

Yet what is at issue is not the decision to be taken, but the choice that is available. If heterosexual couples have the option of deciding whether to marry or not, so should same-sex couples have the choice as whether to seek to achieve a status and a set of entitlements and responsibilities on a par with those enjoyed by heterosexual couples. It follows that, given the centrality attributed to marriage and its consequences in our culture, to deny same-sex couples a choice in this respect is to negate their right to self-definition in a most profound way.

[*Justice Sachs addresses religious freedom in relation to same-sex marriage.*]
 [92] ... It is one thing for the Court to acknowledge the important role that religion plays in our public life. It is quite another to use religious doctrine as a source for interpreting the Constitution. It would be out of order to employ the religious sentiments of some as a guide to the constitutional rights of others. Between and within religions there are vastly different and at times highly disputed views on how to respond to the fact that members of their congregations and clergy are themselves homosexual. Judges would be placed in an intolerable situation if they were called upon to construe religious texts and take sides on issues which have caused deep schisms within religious bodies.
 [94] In the open and democratic society contemplated by the Constitution there must be mutually respectful co-existence between the secular and the sacred. The function of the Court is to recognise the sphere which each inhabits, not to force the one into the sphere of the other. Provided there is no prejudice to the fundamental rights of any person or group, the law will legitimately acknowledge a diversity of strongly-held opinions on matters of great public controversy. I stress the qualification that there must be no prejudice to basic rights. Majoritarian opinion can often be harsh to minorities that exist outside the mainstream ... The test, whether majoritarian or minoritarian positions are involved, must always be whether the measure under scrutiny promotes or retards the achievement of human dignity, equality and freedom.
 [95] The hallmark of an open and democratic society is its capacity to accommodate and manage difference of intensely-held world views and lifestyles in a reasonable and fair manner. ...
 [97] State accommodation of religious belief goes further ... no minister of religion could be compelled to solemnise a same-sex marriage if such a marriage would not conform to the doctrines of the religion concerned. There is nothing in the matters before us that either directly or indirectly trenches in any way on this strong protection of the right of religious communities not to be obliged to celebrate marriages not conforming to their tenets.
 [98] ... acknowledgement by the state of the right of same-sex couples to enjoy the same status, entitlements and responsibilities as marriage law accords to heterosexual couples is in no way inconsistent with the rights of religious

organisations to continue to refuse to celebrate same-sex marriages. The constitutional claims of same-sex couples can accordingly not be negated by invoking the rights of believers to have their religious freedom respected. The two sets of interests involved do not collide, they co-exist in a constitutional realm based on accommodation of diversity.

[Justice Sachs contemplates how the unconstitutionality of existing marriage laws could be rectified.]

[138] This is a matter that touches on deep public and private sensibilities. I believe that Parliament is well-suited to finding the best ways of ensuring that same-sex couples are brought in from the legal cold. The law may not automatically and of itself eliminate stereotyping and prejudice. Yet it serves as a great teacher, establishes public norms that become assimilated into daily life and protects vulnerable people from unjust marginalisation and abuse. It needs to be remembered that not only the courts are responsible for vindicating the rights enshrined in the Bill of Rights. The legislature is in the frontline in this respect ...

[139] ... it is my view that it would best serve those equality claims by respecting the separation of powers and giving Parliament an opportunity to deal appropriately with the matter. In this respect it is necessary to bear in mind that there are different ways in which the legislature could legitimately deal with the gap that exists in the law. On the papers, at least two different legislative pathways have been proposed. Although the constitutional terminus would be the same, the legislative formats adopted for reaching the end-point would be vastly different ... What might appear to be options of a purely technical character could have quite different resonances for life in public and in private ... Provided that the basic principles of equality as enshrined in the Constitution are not trimmed in the process, the greater the degree of public acceptance for same-sex unions, the more will the achievement of equality be promoted.

[Justice Sachs outlines key principles that should guide the legislative process in correcting the legal defect in existing marriage laws.]

[149] ... in exercising its legislative discretion Parliament will have to bear in mind that the objective of the new measure must be to promote human dignity, the achievement of equality and the advancement of human rights and freedoms. This means in the first place taking account of the fact that in overcoming the under-inclusiveness of the common law and the Marriage Act, it would be inappropriate to employ a remedy that created equal disadvantage for all ... the achievement of equality would not be accomplished by ensuring that if same-sex couples cannot enjoy the status and entitlements coupled with the responsibilities of marriage, the same should apply to heterosexual couple ... The law concerned with family

formation and marriage requires equal celebration, not equal marginalisation; it calls for equality of the vineyard and not equality of the graveyard.

[150] ... Parliament be sensitive to the need to avoid a remedy that on the face of it would provide equal protection, but would do so in a manner that in its context and application would be calculated to reproduce new forms of marginalisation. Historically the concept of 'separate but equal' served as a threadbare cloak for covering distaste for or repudiation by those in power of the group subjected to segregation. The very notion that integration would lead to miscegenation, mongrelisation or contamination, was offensive in concept and wounding in practice. Yet, just as is frequently the case when proposals are made for recognising same-sex unions in desiccated and marginalised forms, proponents of segregation would vehemently deny any intention to cause insult. On the contrary, they would justify the apartness as being a reflection of a natural or divinely ordained state of affairs. Alternatively they would assert that the separation was neutral if the facilities provided by the law were substantially the same for both groups ...

[152] It is precisely sensitivity to context and impact that suggest that equal treatment does not invariably require identical treatment. Thus corrective measures to overcome past and continuing discrimination may justify and may even require differential treatment ... The crucial determinant will always be whether human dignity is enhanced or diminished and the achievement of equality is promoted or undermined by the measure concerned. Differential treatment in itself does not necessarily violate the dignity of those affected. It is when separation implies repudiation, connotes distaste or inferiority and perpetuates a caste-like status that it becomes constitutionally invidious.

[*The order made by the Constitutional Court:*]

1. In the matter between the Minister of Home Affairs and the Director-General of Home Affairs and Marié Adriaana Fourie and Cecelia Johanna Bonthuys, CCT 60/04, the following order is made:

The order of the Supreme Court of Appeal is set aside and replaced by the following order:

- The common law definition of marriage is declared to be inconsistent with the Constitution and invalid to the extent that it does not permit same-sex couples to enjoy the status and the benefits coupled with responsibilities it accords to heterosexual couples.
- The declaration of invalidity is suspended for twelve months from the date of this judgment to allow Parliament to correct the defect.
- The Minister of Home Affairs and the Director-General of Home Affairs are ordered to pay the costs of the respondents.

2. In the matter between the Lesbian and Gay Equality Project and eighteen

Others and the Minister of Home Affairs, the Director General of Home Affairs and the Minister of Justice and Constitutional Development, CCT 10/05, the following order is made:

a) The common law definition of marriage is declared to be inconsistent with the Constitution and invalid to the extent that it does not permit same-sex couples to enjoy the status and the benefits coupled with responsibilities it accords to heterosexual couples.

b) The omission from section 30(1) of the Marriage Act 25 of 1961 after the words 'or husband' of the words 'or spouse' is declared to be inconsistent with the Constitution, and the Marriage Act is declared to be invalid to the extent of this inconsistency.

c) The declarations of invalidity in paragraphs (b) and (c) are suspended for 12 months from the date of this judgment to allow Parliament to correct the defects.

d) Should Parliament not correct the defects within this period, Section 30 (1) of the Marriage Act 25 of 1961 will forthwith be read as including the words 'or spouse' after the words 'or husband' as they appear in the marriage formula.

e) The Minister and Director-General of Home Affairs and the Minister of Justice and Constitutional Development are ordered to pay the applicants' costs.

The minority judgment of Justice Kate O'Regan

[Justice O'Regan dissents from the Sachs judgment on the issue of legal remedy.]

[165] The difference between his [Justice Sachs] judgment and this, therefore, lies solely in one significant area, namely, that of remedy. How best should these clear constitutional infringements be remedied by this Court? ... [in the past] this Court held that it is an important principle of the law of constitutional remedies that successful litigants should ordinarily obtain the relief they seek. ... A court must consider in each case whether there are other considerations of justice or equity which would warrant an exception to this key precept ... Sachs J concludes that this case does involve considerations which warrant such an exception, and he accordingly proposes an order suspending the declaration of invalidity for twelve months. The effect of this order is that gay and lesbian couples will not be permitted to marry during this period. ...

[169] ... this Court should develop the common-law rule as suggested by the majority in the Supreme Court of Appeal, and at the same time read in words to section 30 of the Act that would with immediate effect permit gays and lesbians to be married by civil marriage officers (and such religious marriage officers as consider such marriages not to fall outside the tenets of their religion). Such an order would mean simply that there would be gay and lesbian married couples at common law which marriages would have to be regulated by any new marital

regime the legislature chooses to adopt ... The fact that Parliament faces choices does not, in this case, seem to me to be sufficient for this Court to refuse to develop the common law and, in an ancillary order, to remedy a statutory provision, reliant on the common law definition, which is also unconstitutional.

[171] ... The power and duty to protect constitutional rights is conferred upon the courts and courts should not shrink from that duty. The legitimacy of an order made by the Court does not flow from the status of the institution itself, but from the fact that it gives effect to the provisions of our Constitution. Time and again, there will be those in our broader community who do not wish to see constitutional rights protected, but that can never be a reason for a court not to protect those rights.

[172] ... It does not seem to me that an order developing the common law, as ordered by the majority in the Supreme Court of Appeal, coupled with an order reading in the words 'or spouse' to the relevant provisions of the Marriage Act would undermine the institution of marriage at all. ... Permitting those who have been excluded from marrying to marry can only foster a society based on respect for human dignity and human difference. Nor will it undermine the special role of marriage as recognised by different religions. Such marriages draw their strength and character from religious beliefs and practices. The fact that gay and lesbian couples are permitted to enter civil marriages should not undermine the strength or meaning of those beliefs.

[173] ... I dissent from the judgment of Sachs J in one respect. I would not suspend the order of invalidity as proposed by Sachs J. In my view, the Court should make an order today which has immediate prospective effect. Such an order would not preclude Parliament from addressing the law of marriage in the future, and would simultaneously and immediately protect the constitutional rights of gay and lesbian couples pending parliamentary action.

Note

1 Discussion Paper 104, Project 118, published by the South African Law Reform Commission, contains proposals aimed at bringing family law in line with the Bill of Rights and the constitutional principles of equality and dignity. With specific reference to the lack of legal recognition of same-sex relationships, the Commission proposed three alternative ways of effecting law reform in this area: 1. opening up the common-law definition of marriage to same-sex couples by inserting a definition to that effect in the Marriage Act; 2. separating the civil and religious elements of marriage, by amending the Marriage Act so that it only regulates the civil aspect of marriage, for both same- and opposite-sex couples); 3. providing a 'marriage-like alternative' to accord same-sex couples (and possibly also opposite-sex couples) the right to conclude civil unions with the same legal consequences as marriage.

2: TAKING IT TO THE PEOPLE
The national debate

'This thing' and 'that idea': Traditionalist responses to homosexuality and same-sex marriage

Graeme Reid

This essay draws on two 'archives'. One is my own doctoral research, which took place in small towns, urban peripheries and rural areas in the Mpumalanga province, beginning in December 2003, and continuing, with varying degrees of intensity, until 2005. In this essay, I focus on an engagement ceremony that took place at the beginning of my fieldwork, marking a threshold of my research experience in the region. Through a description of the engagement ceremony, I highlight the importance of gender dichotomies for the organization of male same-sex relationships in the ambit of my fieldwork. The second archive is a series of hearings that were organized by the National House of Traditional Leaders (NHTL) in the early part of 2005. These hearings took place in the aftermath of the Supreme Court of Appeal judgment in the *Fourie* case and prior to the deliberations of the Constitutional Court that led ultimately to the Civil Union Act. The prospect of same-sex marriages provided an ideal opportunity to mobilize a constituency and to raise the public profile of the NHTL. This was a road show with a tight schedule: over the course of a fortnight, representatives from the NHTL (specifically from the Traditions and Customs Committee, headed by Chief Mathebe from Mpumalanga) held hearings in six provinces – Limpopo; Mpumalanga; KwaZulu-Natal (KZN); Eastern Cape; North West and the Free State. I attended the hearing in Mpumalanga, on Valentine's Day, 14 February 2005. This and all other hearings were visually recorded and the digital tapes were made available to me by an official at the NHTL. These I have had copied, translated and transcribed. I draw on this material to analyze some of the public rhetoric around same-sex marriage. I also compare these perspectives with other public perceptions of gays[1] gleaned though my research experience. In so doing I explore the ambiguous position that gay people occupy in the social imaginary, one that can be the source of condemnation, but also veneration; exclusion but also integration. Through a close reading of these archives I suggest that gays embody many of the fears and anxieties – as well as some of the hopes and aspirations – associated with rapid social and political change, especially as these effect gender roles and norms.

An engagement: An ethnographic account

On 12 December 2003, in the early evening, a group of *ladies* find themselves outside the local supermarket in Ermelo, Mpumalanga, surrounded by shopping bags, looking tired, a trifle stressed, primarily exuberant. These *ladies* are, in fact, young men. I arrive and my car is soon loaded with as many *ladies* and groceries as can fit in. I drive to Wesselton township situated on the outskirts of Ermelo and park the car outside Bhuti's place. Bhuti stays in a room next to a busy, noisy shebeen. Arrangements are in full swing for the engagement that is to take place in Ermelo tomorrow afternoon. Once the groceries are offloaded I again drive back towards town. A symphony of cell phone ring tones and snippets of conversation – 'Hello sweetheart! Thank you darling! Ntombazane!' – accompanies the 'jolly-talk' in the car.

Meanwhile the groom, Thabo, is hungry. He calls Andrew several times on his mobile, demanding to know when supper will be ready. In the car there is talk of divorce before marriage. Andrew pacifies Thabo over the phone until we get back to Bhuti's place. At Bhuti's place the groom and his friends are sitting separately from the ladies, smoking, drinking Hunter's Gold and waiting for supper. These are the *gents*, and the room is a very masculine space. It is in this room that the groom tells his friends that he is only doing it for the money. In the next room, the kitchen is a hive of activity as groceries are unpacked and supper prepared by the *ladies* amid laughter and chatter. Bhuti leaves his guests to get on with preparations while he steals some time to have his hair plaited by a neighbour in readiness for the big day. 'Is the groom still angry?' he asks, grimacing as his hair is tugged and deftly woven by a young woman who keeps an eye on *The Bold and the Beautiful*, a popular television soap opera, while working with his hair.

Wandile, who has travelled from Standerton, is relieved to have made it to Ermelo at all. His boyfriend did not want him to come and had argued with him before he left. Wandile told him that the bride-to-be was 'not just anybody, he is my friend'. The boyfriend eventually relented on condition that Wandile ironed his clothes and made him supper before he left. The boyfriend reminded Wandile that 'when we are married, then you will have to obey me'. But Wandile is not so keen on marriage; he does not completely trust his boyfriend. He explains that his boyfriend is 'straight' and he suspects that he also has a girlfriend, because he sometimes comes home very late at night or even early in the morning without a plausible explanation.

That night I am accommodated in a nearby house, sharing a small room and large bed with Henry, who in Ermelo is seen as a *lady*, and who has recently moved from Soweto to Standerton. Henry is struck by differences and similarities between gay life in his Soweto home and in Mpumalanga, and is keen to share these insights with me so we talk late into the night. 'Most Zulus are gay,' Henry observes, having lived in Standerton, a predominantly Zulu-speaking area, for little over a month and having received many propositions from men. Yet he explains that 'Here it is unlike in Johannesburg or Cape Town where you find a gay partner who does not have a girlfriend. Here maybe he is gay but he has a girlfriend. You start to ask "Is this person gay, or what?"'

The next day, several hours later than planned, the engagement ceremony takes place on the outskirts of Ermelo. Thulani starts the formal proceedings by welcoming the guests and asserting that the engagement gives expression to 'something that is within us. We are not faking it.' He introduces Pastor Nokuthula Dhladhla from a gay Pentecostal-style church community in Johannesburg, who officiates at the ceremony. She has strong family connections in the town of Volksrust, not far from here, so the ceremony has special resonance for her, even though she has conducted several similar services in her Johannesburg congregation. She expresses regret that the bride and groom's family members are not present. 'Part of me feels so disappointed when I don't see the family. It kills me somehow.' She bewails the fact that marriage is not yet legal but says that she hopes and prays that one day God will make it possible. She gives advice to the assembled guests on the nature of true love – and the obstacles and pitfalls in its path. Engagement rings are exchanged and to end the day's formal proceedings a bouquet of flowers is thrown to the single *ladies* present and much pleasure and enjoyment is derived from the fact that Emmanuel, who caught the bouquet, is ignorant of its meaning and significance. Unwittingly he (or she) has placed herself next in line for engagement and, possibly, marriage.

Ladies and gents; town and country

The engagement ceremony was a particularly dramatic enactment of the dichotomies that were pervasive in the small towns where I undertook my research, towns such as Ermelo, Bethal, Standerton and Piet Retief. These are the gender dichotomies, and some of the ways in which they are dramatized in this vignette: bride and groom; *ladies* and *gents*; a male space occupied by *gents*; a feminine space occupied by the *ladies*; *ladies* waiting on *gents*; *gents* drinking and smoking; *ladies* cooking and gossiping. *Ladies* and *gents* were shorthand for the imaginative ideals that set the parameters for appropriate behaviour among gays, between gays and their boyfriends and between gays and the wider community. *Ladies* and *gents* were central to gay self-identification and to the ways in which 'being gay' was enacted in the wider community. These categories, *ladies* and *gents*, thus set the stage for the ways in which gays imagined themselves and interacted with their world.

These gender ideals were strongly informed by another locally evoked dichotomy – that between 'city' and 'country'. In 'jolly-talk' (the local gay lingo) this separation between the imagined worlds of city and small town were evoked through the terms 'country style' and 'city style'. This is what newcomer Henry was alluding to when he said, 'Here it is unlike in Johannesburg or Cape Town …' This is not to suggest that there was not a great deal of interaction between the hinterland and the metropole. Gays in Ermelo and surrounding towns were mobile. For one thing, there was a lot of interaction between gays in various small towns, who gathered for parties, pageants, workshops, funerals and other events. There was also a lot of exchange with Johannesburg and Durban – the movement of boyfriends, shopping, visiting friends or relatives, attending church or simply partying. City and countryside interacted in an ongoing exchange of people, ideas and goods. Gays were also linked up through the media – television, magazines and, to a lesser extent, the internet. Yet 'country style' was shorthand for appropriate behaviour in a local setting. And the hallmark of this was that same-sex relations were organized around *ladies* and *gents*.

This arrangement superficially echoed hegemonic notions of masculinity and femininity and, as such, replicated heterosexual norms, just as the engagement ceremony drew on archetypal images of 'bride' and 'groom'. But there were significant differences. One was economic. It was the bride who covered the costs of the engagement. It was not uncommon that *ladies* were the main breadwinners who supported their *gents*. The other difference was that among *ladies* there was a great deal of overt gender performance, whether in the demure role of the churchgoer or the extravagant self-presentation of the hairstylist. Whether implicit or overt, there was a playfulness with gender roles and norms that was subtly subversive. What it meant to be a *lady* or a *gent* was contested terrain and this played itself out in everyday interactions, through camp playfulness and gossip as well as in more formal events such as activist workshops and beauty pageants which sought to grapple with what it meant to be gay in contemporary South Africa. But while there may have been a lot of humour, especially in the form of 'jolly-talk', which acknowledged that nothing was set in stone, this did not mean that gender was only a realm of lighthearted play. On the contrary, gender roles and norms were taken very seriously. For one thing, gender difference and hierarchy were seen as central to erotic charge and sexual excitement. The idea of two gays having an affair was met with disdain or thigh-slapping hilarity. When a *lady* was bemoaning the fact that his *gent* was getting married to a woman, my research assistant asked him why he did not have a relationship with someone more suitable, mentioning his gay friend, Henry. 'Oh, I love him very much,' he replied, 'but I am not a lesbian!'

And take Clive's predicament, for example. Clive was confused about whether he was a *lady* or a *gent*. It was an experience that caused great personal frustration and distress in a context in which he understood that unambiguous choices needed to be made:

> Mostly in the black community there is a man and a woman. A man is a man completely and a wife is a wife completely. Myself, I do perform both sides completely. But I think that there must be a final decision. If I am a man, I must be a man ... I am confused about that, whether to be a man or a wife.

The instability of gender categories was played out in disagreements among gays about appropriate forms of self-styling. On the one hand, more activist-minded people urged gays to dress down and to come out, using a human-rights discourse to encourage *ladies* to be more discreet in their style of dress and more assertive in relation to *gents*. On the other hand were those who regarded cross-dressing as synonymous with being gay: the more flamboyant queens, hyper-feminine hairstylists, for example, who combined extravagant dress, mannerisms and style with a political project, as the legendary coming-out story of three hairstyling friends testified. In the immediate aftermath of the first democratic elections in 1994, the three friends 'came out' by wearing make-up and adaptations of the girls' uniform to school. All three would go on to become well-known hairstylists.

Inequality in the social sphere meant that *ladies* occupied a vulnerable place, in many respects analogous to the role of women in that environment. Bhuti evicted young men from his home because one of them was suspected of theft and attempted rape. Gays were often perceived to be better-off and to carry the most up-to-date and desirable accoutrements, such as cell phones. During the course of my fieldwork several gays were mugged, had their bags snatched and their cellphones stolen. In the domestic sphere male authority tended to dictate the terms of the relationship, as in the case of Wandile, who was expected to iron and cook, before being reluctantly permitted to attend the engagement party. During the course of my fieldwork there were several incidents of domestic violence and one lady was the victim of sexual assault. On the other hand, several hairstylists, through a hyper-feminine form of self-styling, enjoyed widespread popularity and had achieved something of a celebrity status in the region. And gays were also integrated into conservative church communities, as fully-fledged 'female' members of the congregation. So femininity could be a source of integration as well as a site of vulnerability.

A marriage

On Valentine's Day, 14 February 2005, a charismatic Christian pastor and a disgruntled local chief enacted a brief same-sex marriage on the stage of the Nhlazatshe community hall in a rural settlement not far from the village of Badplaas, Mpumalanga. The largely middle-aged and elderly group of men and women who had gathered in the hall exclaimed in dismay as Pastor Manana and Chief Nkosi walked hand-in-hand along the stage. The chief seemed uncomfortable with this theatrical display and the performance was drawn to a brisk close.

Through this dramatic vignette, the pastor was trying to spell out the implications of the then recent Supreme Court of Appeal ruling on the definition of marriage to a small crowd that appeared to be both perplexed and outraged at the prospect of legally sanctioned same-sex unions taking place in South Africa. Chief Mabandla outlined the purpose of the visit:

> There is a law, which does not exist amongst us black people that says same-sex couples have a right to marry each other ... As Swazi people do you have such a thing in your culture and tradition?

In the circumstances, it was a largely rhetorical question that was nevertheless answered by a resounding 'no' from the audience. The MC made it clear that the National House of Traditional Leaders, organizers of the event, were there to gather the views of ordinary people and not to impose their own ideas: 'The nation must be free to talk,' he said.

What followed was an outpouring of strongly held views on a wide range of topics including Christianity, morality, parental authority, the nature of democracy, culture, human rights, the role of women, teenage pregnancy, abortion, divorce, AIDS, prostitution and witchcraft. Homosexuality was never mentioned by name but always referred to as 'this thing', while same-sex marriage was referred to as 'that idea'.

Government policies were lambasted and cast in a morally dubious, even evil, light; they were bound to bring calamity to the country. A man suggested that the government's laws on gender equality had produced stubborn women who talk of 'rights and do not respect their men'. One speaker delivered a tirade against child-support grants, claiming that this had led to a wave of teenage pregnancies. Another thanked democracy for 'bringing witches to light so that you could know that this one is a witch' and illustrated her point with reference to the termination-of-pregnancy legislation: 'Our children would do abortion and you would not know.' Gender and generational reversals were at the heart of the articulation of a collapsing moral order and apocalyptic visions of divine destruction inspired, in this instance, by Sodom and Gomorrah. The government and its laws had set children against parents, learners against teachers, women against men, good against evil, Christian and traditional values against secular laws. And now the measure that was indeed 'trying our patience' was the proposal that men would be allowed to marry men, and women marry women.

'These people are like a stone or a dry piece of wood'

The main objection to homosexuality and same-sex marriage expressed at the six provincial hearings, including the one in Mpumalanga, was the non-procreative nature of same-sex coupling. As one of the organizers of the events put it

THE NATIONAL DEBATE

in an interview with me, 'My understanding is that our belief all along is that a woman and a man they are kind of made for each other. They need each other so that they can procreate.' This objection was closely linked to the erosion of gender roles and norms. As the chief of the Zembeni district in KZN put it, 'If you want to destroy the male and female categories, just marry each other ... Just say it if you no longer want to reproduce.'

The Bible was frequently used to stress the importance of procreation. 'Multiply in the world'; 'reproduce and fill the earth'; 'have children and multiply' – these were phrases that echoed through the hearings, but there were also more practical considerations. 'How are you going to get her pregnant?' a woman asked a lesbian from the Equality Project who addressed the audience at the KZN hearing. 'How would two men make children? Can they get pregnant to multiply that family?' asked a participant in Limpopo. A man in North West who had 12 children by his three wives exclaimed: 'I have children with these women. So where will children come from if I marry another man?'

This discussion is important because many *gents* are fathers. Having girlfriends or wives, and children, is part of their heterosexual identity – which fits in with their sense of self and is also an important aspect of their allure for *ladies*. *Ladies* are attracted to *gents* precisely because they are regarded as straight men. In a context in which 'gay' is synonymous with being effeminate, the *gents* confirm (through their masculine and heterosexual self-presentation) *ladies*' sense of themselves as both effeminate and gay. Thabo, the groom at the engagement ceremony, had a child with his girlfriend, and Andrew, the bride-to-be, contributed financially through the money that he gave to Thabo on a monthly basis. Another *gent*, Brian, was deeply moved by the birth of his first child, an experience that was tied to his sense of masculinity: 'In February 2000 when my child was born, I realized that maybe God was telling me something about that. Maybe he showed me that I am a real man.' At the time his girlfriend was pregnant with their second child. It seems that *gents* evade social opprobrium because they continue to fulfill their social roles as husbands and fathers.

The parallel with a childless heterosexual couple was drawn at the KZN workshop where one participant reflected that after seven childless years the family would start to get concerned, asking why their daughter-in-law had not become pregnant. While a man in Limpopo put it in these terms:

> If a woman marries another woman are they going to make children the way we do or what? These people are like a stone or a dry piece of wood. Have you ever heard of a pregnant stone or dry wood that bore children?

Reproductive sexuality was given a particular urgency in the face of the AIDS pandemic. The MC in Mpumalanga made the link explicit when he said:

79

AIDS is finishing people. So if people do not reproduce what would become of us – who are the chiefs going to rule over?

'A gay person does not have relatives'

A closely related factor was that children were the embodiment and confirmation of family alliances, set in motion through the marriage between two individuals, and family and kinship were fundamental to an understanding of marriage. Same-sex partnerships were seen as contrary to kinship ties: 'A gay person does not have relatives, because he cannot give birth,' said a male participant at the KZN workshop. Or as the MC at the Limpopo workshop put it: 'A marriage amongst us is intended to bring two families together.' It is this idea that is contained in the later Congress of Traditional Leaders of South Africa (Contralesa) submission to Parliament during the hearings on the Civil Union Bill:

> Marriage is between two families, two clans, two tribes and even two nations. It is about the establishment of blood ties between the two entities through, among others, the birth of children. A same-sex marriage cannot bring about the birth of children.[2]

In this framework, same-sex marriage is seen to break family and kinship ties and to threaten social cohesion. As one of the organizers observed:

> If you come to think about it they are afraid more than anything. If you compare the rural with the urban you will find that urban people are more accommodating and rural people are more conservative.

In the hearings the idea of procreation and family alliances was contrasted with European-style weddings, and became a focal point for framing the debate as one between African culture/tradition and foreign/Eurocentric values, often articulated in racial terms. The MC in Limpopo, for example, explained to the group who had gathered:

> Marriage amongst us black people is not the same as amongst the white people ... In our system of marriage we are actually bringing two families together. That is what marriage means to us ... So with whites it is just the two concerned people getting married ... So that is not how we do things amongst us blacks.

A speaker in KZN expressed the view that 'gays were not in existence amongst the Zulus. Gays were prevalent amongst whites and coloureds. They are the ones who are gay. They walk around in tight pants.' When a lesbian speaker from the Equality Project addressed the hearing in KZN she was shouted down for drawing a parallel between years of apartheid oppression and the social position of gays and lesbians.[3]

It was apparent from the hearings that the discussions about same-sex marriage were an opportunity to express deeper concerns about changing gender roles, the erosion of masculine authority and the increased autonomy of women and of youth. Discussions about 'this thing' meandered seamlessly into other terrains such as reflections on teenage pregnancy, legal abortion, the ordination of women priests, the Beijing conference on the rights of women,[4] infidelity and 'troublesome girls'. The erosion of patriarchy and gerontocracy was summed up in a pithy statement made by a male speaker at the KZN hearing:

> And you girls as you say you have rights, fine, go ahead and destroy us because you want to do what you want. Children make their own laws. Women make their own laws.

A speaker at the Mpumalanga hearing laid the blame squarely at the door of government:

> Today parents no longer feel like they are parents because of people in Parliament, police today no longer feel like they are policemen because of people in Parliament, teachers no longer feel like they are teachers because of people in Parliament.

The NHTL leaders present at the hearings were sensitive to the criticism about gender equality and urged women to participate in the hearings, although in practice it was mostly the men who spoke. The women who did speak reiterated the views of the men, especially when it came to the question of 'unruly' young people.

'I have never seen a cock chasing another cock'

There were several clear messages emanating from the workshops: non-procreative marriages were unacceptable; gays were excluded from networks of family and kinship and the authority of men and elders was seen to be in decline. How then did this fit into perceptions of homosexuality and same-sex marriage?

The discussions about gays followed familiar lines of enquiry: to paraphrase, the history of homosexuality, its etiology, the nature/nurture debate, the cultural variation of same-sex sexualities, indigenous terms for same-sex practices, and the difference between God-made, inborn sexual inverts – called *stabane* and *ungqingili* – and 'democracy's gays', who were seen to represent a youth trend, a fashion. There was a discussion, for example, on the role of prisons and single-sex schools and hostels on the mines. 'This thing' was associated with cities and 'locations', not rural areas. A speaker from Limpopo acknowledged that 'There are boys who behave like girls. Boy-girls, we see them around here.' A chief from the Free State drew a distinction between those who had two sexual organs and those who did not, thus suggesting that same-sex unions should be granted to those whose 'nature is different', but not to 'democracy's gays':

> Their nature is different from us who only have a single sex organ. But that opportunity should not be given to those people who were doing this thing in prison and now want to do it in the community even if they can see that it is wrong. I'd like to say to this committee that it should only be afforded to those people who have been created differently with two organs, because they were created by God.

A common conception about gays is that they are hermaphrodites: the Zulu terms *stabane* and *ungqingili* both refer to intersexed people. The idea that there are genuine gays and others for whom being gay is 'a fashion', or the result of circumstance, is pervasive. It also suggests that same-sex desire can and will proliferate, especially among the youth, who, according to several speakers, are easily led astray. The MC at the Mpumalanga hearing claimed that youth, left to do as they please, 'will eventually engage in such things'. A male speaker in Limpopo suggested that 'We should have included the youth because we are grown-ups here and we are not familiar with this thing.' A woman at the Mpumalanga hearing said, 'Young people like this thing.' And in North West, a speaker claimed that 'This thing has been spread amongst the young people.'

The difference between the present and the past was summed up by a woman speaker in Mpumalanga, who said: 'Even under the previous government the same-sex relationships were in existence. It does not happen now just because we have democracy. Democracy made it possible for people to choose.' This was a perceptive remark. But what many may laud as desirable – in this case the freedom to choose – others see as regrettable. What the woman was bewailing was the triumph of individual desire over social responsibility. And the quintessential marker of this, repeated *ad nauseam* at the hearings, is the non-procreative nature of 'this thing'. The emergence of gay people is seen to coincide with the dawn of democracy and to be inextricably tied with human rights that have undermined a set of hierarchical relations. And, especially in relation to traditional male authority, this is seen to fly in the face of 'tradition and custom'. Chief Diragadibonwe reflected on the Free State hearings:

> One speaker said that for the past 2 000 years there has never been such a strange thing. Even amongst the animals, I have never seen a cock chasing after another cock.

And yet, anachronistic though these debates may seem, they also touch on issues fundamental to the nature of the democratic order in South Africa. The participants in the workshops were correct in the assertion that 'this thing' was unpopular and did not represent the wishes of the majority of the population

– the very reason for Constitutional protection of a vulnerable minority. In this respect the equality clause goes to the heart of the role of a Constitution set up to protect 'the weakest amongst us'.[5] The protection afforded to gays and lesbians as marginal and vulnerable members of society ('the weakest') becomes a measure of the success of a social order based on principles of human rights and equality before the law. In the opinion of the workshop participants, however, a small group of elected officials was imposing legislation counter to majority opinion. In this scenario it was traditional, unelected chiefs who presented themselves as listening to the views of the people and were hence portrayed as the true voice of participatory democracy. This was made explicit in an exchange at the conclusion of the Mpumalanga hearing:

> MC: When I started I asked you not to ask me to ask the chief to speak. But with your permission I would let him speak – that as a chief who is anointed, not a voted chief, he must tell us what he thinks. A voted chief would say same-sex marriages are OK.
>
> CHIEF DLAMINI: Thanks to the MC. The nation has spoken. As a creation of God and your leader I am not going to go against the word of God and come up with my own things.
>
> APPLAUSE
>
> CHIEF DLAMINI: I agree with the nation because there would never be a leader without a nation that supports him. So I am not going to go against what the people of God had to say. What we are hearing shocks me as well.

The participants are thus left with the impression that the traditional leaders will convey their wishes to parliamentarians who are unlikely to listen or take their views into account.

The hearings held by the NHTL provided a glimpse, on a micro-level, of widespread discomfort with the ideals enshrined in the South African Constitution, particularly those relating to gender and sexuality. Speaker after speaker articulated, in various ways, two central tropes on homosexuality in the region: that homosexuality is intrinsically 'unAfrican' and is also 'unChristian'. In the hearings, same-sex marriage was seen as the inevitable outcome of tampering with 'natural, God-given' laws governing gender and sexuality. Give women equal rights, the argument seemed to go, and before you know it men will want to marry men and women, women.

The annual conference of the National House of Traditional Leaders, held at the Sanbonani hotel in Hazyview in December 2005, aimed to reflect on the 'Influence of African Traditional Values in Realising a Peaceful Development in Modern Africa'. The bland theme invoked contrasting images of 'tradition' and 'modernity' – these framed the deliberations on same-sex marriage. Drawing on the NHTL hearings held earlier that year, it was no surprise that the first resolution of the conference dealt with this issue. In summing up, African beliefs and customs were contrasted with decadent Western practices:

> The practice of same-sex marriages is against most of [sic] African beliefs, cultures, customs and traditions, and this in turn goes against the mandate of traditional leaders which is to promote and protect the customs of communities observing a system of customary law.
>
> Traditional leaders have vowed to make it their mission for the coming five years to campaign against this wicked, decadent and immoral Western practice.[6]

Conclusion

To reiterate, in the hearings the three most striking issues that were raised were: first, the problem of procreation, linked to ideas about family alliances and social cohesiveness; second, there were concerns about the erosion of hierarchical gender roles, and the undermining of parental and, in particular, male authority; and, third, gays were seen to be not only associated with, but a product of, an individualistic rights-based political order. Gays were also associated with foreigners – American television programmes, for example, or a Eurocentric Constitution. It is whites and coloureds who wear tight pants. Gays disrupt the categories of male and female: they were described as 'girl-boys', 'men who want to be women', *ungqingili* and *stabane*. In a context in which 'tradition' is pitted against 'modernity' (and the NHTL hearings were emblematic of this dichotomy, as it was imagined and articulated by the participants) then gays are a particularly potent symbol of 'modernity'. And in a context in which a patriarchal gender order is hegemonic and there is deep anxiety about the crisis of gender roles and norms, gays also become a focal point for these more pervasive concerns. The prospect of same-sex unions generated such ferment because it is seen as the embodiment and logical conclusion of a disrupted gender order. This is exacerbated by the public perception of gays as products of foreign influence, associated with new trends, current fashions, and with a modern, liberal Constitution. Gays embody the fears and anxieties of rapid social change and exemplify the faultlines of a Constitution in which individual rights are paramount and where custom and tradition have been accommodated only uncomfortably. Nowhere are these tensions more apparent than in contestations around gender and sexuality.

Gays occupy an ambiguous space in relation to gender and in relation to culture – they are *ladies*, but not women; they are *izitabane*, symbolically imagined as embodying both sexes. They are perceived to be 'unAfrican' and yet may access ritual power, as in the case of sangomas – the second most popular profession among gays in the ambit of my fieldwork, trumped only by hairstyling. And in the profession of hairstyling – informal and highly competitive

– gays enjoy a special niche precisely because of their close association with trend-setting fashions and a hyperfemininity that tap into small-town aspirations to urban sophistication. Although seen as 'unAfrican', gays are entrusted with producing quintessential African styles. Ambiguity is a potentially productive space and gays have found ways to negotiate the rules of gender associated with country style and to work these to social, economic and erotic advantage.

The question remains as to how civil unions will translate in a context such as small-town Mpumalanga. As the engagement ceremony shows, such ceremonies and rituals preceded the Civil Union Bill. The progress of the Bill was followed closely in small towns, and the gays of Ermelo celebrated the passing of the Act with a braai. Outside the *gents* tended to the meat, while indoors *ladies* made salad and gossiped. In a context where relationships are based on a *ladies/gents* model, and in which it is generally accepted that *gents* will eventually marry a woman, how will same sex-marriage translate? No doubt the gays of small-town Mpumalanga will find their own ways of occupying the space created by civil unions, on their own terms – and in a way that is loyal to their own 'customs and traditions', country style.

Notes
A version of the essay in this book was presented at the conference 'Paradoxes of the Postcolonial Public Sphere: South African Democracy at the Crossroads', University of the Witwatersrand, 28-31 January 2008. Research was funded by the Netherlands Foundation for the Advancement of Tropical Research (WOTRO) of the Netherlands Organisation for Scientific Research (NWO). Thanks to research assistant Phineas Riba for transcriptions and translations.

1 I use the term 'gays' because it is one that is in common usage in the ambit of my fieldwork. Another colloquial term for gays is *ladies*. 'Gay men' would be inappropriate in a context where gays regard themselves and are perceived by others as feminine.
2 Congress of Traditional Leaders of South Africa (Contralesa) submission to the public hearings of Parliamentary Portfolio Committee on Home Affairs, Cape Town, South Africa, 24 October 2006, 10. (See also pages 131-132 in this book.)
3 The KZN hearing was the only one where a gay or lesbian voice was heard.
4 The Beijing conference was seen as emblematic of a global discourse on gender rights which had a negative impact on traditional gender norms and practices, as one man speaking at the Mpumalanga hearing put it: 'A man does not have a right to do certain things because of the rights that women have. They then go to Beijing and say they want rights. In my culture it does not work like that.'
5 This concept was articulated by the then Chief Justice of the Constitutional Court, Arthur Chaskalson, who wrote the main judgment in the first case to come before the newly established Constitutional Court in 1995 (*State v Makwanyane*, to be found at http://www.concourt.gov.za/text/court/Langa.html; last accessed 13 December 2007). Ruling against the death penalty, he wrote:
    The very reason for establishing the new legal order, and for vesting the power of judicial

review of all legislation in the courts, was to protect the rights of minorities and others who cannot protect their rights adequately through the democratic process. Those who are entitled to claim this protection include the social outcasts and marginalized people of our society. It is only if there is a willingness to protect the worst and the weakest amongst us that all of us can be secure that our own rights will be protected [paragraph 88].

See also Edwin Cameron, 'Sexual Orientation and the Constitution: A Test Case for Human Rights', *South African Law Journal* 110 (1993), 450

6 'Statement on the Resolutions of the National Annual Conference of Traditional Leaders 2005', issued by National House of Traditional Leaders, 9 December 2005; http://www.info.gov.za/speeches/2005/05120914151004.htm (last accessed 7 February 2008)

In this essay I draw upon concepts of gender performativity as developed by Judith Butler, *Gender Trouble: Feminism and the Subversion of Identity* (Routledge, 1990). For comparative perspectives on gender roles and norms in male same-sex relationships see, for example, anthropologist Don Kulick, 'A Man in the House: The Boyfriends of Brazilian Travesti Prostitutes', *Social Text* 52/53 (1997), 133-160; and historian Dunbar Moodie, *Going for Gold: Men, Mines and Migration* (Witwatersrand University Press, 1994).

Lobbying for same-sex marriage:
An activist's reflections

Fikile Vilakazi

This essay is a personal reflection on my experience of lobbying, between 2004 and 2006, for the right of same-sex couples to marry in South Africa. I worked for the Lesbian and Gay Equality Project (the Equality Project) and OUT LGBT Well-being (OUT). This essay will outline my direct experience of a range of processes that formed part of the same-sex marriage campaign.

I will start with some background on the experiences that led to my involvement with lesbian and gay activism in 2004. I was born in 1977 in Soweto, a Johannesburg township. I grew up in an environment of apartheid repression where black people were discriminated against and oppressed on the basis of their skin colour. As a black person, I observed with concern as my parents and others around me suffered under apartheid. I learnt in my teens that racial segregation was legalized and institutionalized. It was lawful to treat black people as lesser citizens than their white counterparts. This was a painful and disturbing discovery. I got involved in neighbourhood and student politics, whether boycotting Afrikaans at school or fighting for better services in my local area.

Later I started to experience discrimination on the basis of sexuality – I was in loving relationships with women. I was a lesbian, a word I was unaware of at that time. My experiences of discrimination began in church, then became apparent at home and at work. This led to a growing desire within me to do something about the rights of sexual minorities in South Africa. I had eagerly followed the legal developments to secure rights for lesbian, gay, bisexual, transgender and intersexed (LGBTI) people in South Africa, led at the time by the National Coalition for Gay and Lesbian Equality and then by its successor the Equality Project. In 2003, while working in the youth-development sector, I decided that I was going to join the movement fighting for the rights of LGBTI people. For the first time in my life, I consciously identified myself as a lesbian as I came to understand the political and sexual meaning of this term.

After hearing in 2002 that a lesbian couple who had been living together for 11 years, Marié Fourie and Cecelia Bonthuys, had gone to court to have their union recognized as a marriage, I knew immediately that I wanted to be involved in ensuring that same-sex marriage was legalized in South Africa. The importance of marriage for same-sex couples was underlined for me when my partner fell seriously ill and my then employers refused me leave to take care of her. I saw my partner as my family, but my work did not recognize her as such. I felt the situation would have been different for a married heterosexual couple. I became involved in the same-sex marriage campaign when the Equality Project appointed me as their public education and advocacy officer.

What was the same-sex marriage campaign about?

The Marriage Act of 1961 and the common-law definition of marriage excluded same-sex couples from marrying. This left lesbian and gay couples on the margins of family law and perpetuated discrimination at different levels in society, including family, community, law, and politics. The same-sex marriage campaign was therefore about securing equality, dignity and freedom for LGBTI people who wished to marry and had been legally denied the right to do so. Marriage is an institution that is rooted in a patriarchal paradigm and has operated as a sphere of repression and discrimination for women. The campaign was therefore not about fighting for marriage as an institution, but rather about gaining access to it for sexual minorities who wished to enter the institution of marriage regardless of their sexual orientation and/or gender identity.

The Equality Project was a national organization that worked to promote legal and social justice and human rights for LGBTI people in South Africa. An important area of the Equality Project's work involved advocacy, and it had made same-sex marriage a key advocacy area. As part of its advocacy work, the Equality Project had engaged in strategic litigation to secure the right for LGBTI people to choose to marry. The Equality Project filed an application with the Johannesburg High Court challenging as unconstitutional both the common-law definition of marriage and the marriage formula in Section 30 (1) of the Marriage Act. Other LGBTI organizations and six LGBTI couples joined the application. The application subsequently journeyed through the courts, alongside the Fourie and Bonthuys case, and reached the Constitutional Court, where a final decision was taken on the matter in 2005.

The Equality Project also aimed to promote public education and advocacy on the merits of the strategic-litigation process. The aim of this area of work was to ensure that lesbian and gay people and other human-rights stakeholders throughout the country were aware of what the call for same-sex marriage was about. My role as public education and advocacy officer was to ensure that the Equality Project was in constant liaison with the LGBTI constituency and other stakeholders.[1] In 2005, operational reasons led to the suspension of the Equality Project, leaving a vacuum in advocacy leadership for same-sex marriage in the organized LGBTI sector. During this period, OUT, in collaboration with the Joint Working Group (JWG), provided leadership in the same-sex marriage campaign.

The JWG is a national network of lesbian, gay, bisexual and transgender organizations in South Africa.[2] OUT is an LGBTI organization that provides sexual and mental health services, conducts research, and implements mainstreaming and advocacy programmes. OUT, working with the JWG, took over the leadership of the campaign soon after the Constitutional Court judgment on the issue in December 2005. The JWG identified the marriage campaign as a shared national priority. Being no more than a network, the JWG did not have the capacity or infrastructure to coordinate the campaign on its own, so this responsibility was passed to member organizations. OUT took responsibility for leading the campaign in collaboration with the JWG. In January 2006, I was employed as an advocacy officer at OUT to be directly involved with the same-sex marriage campaign.

The Constitutional Court decision gave Parliament a year to develop legislation in response to the judgment. This meant that the process would be open for debate and consultation with the South African public (including political parties, faith-based and traditional institutions, influential individuals, and the general community). Given the high level of bigotry and antagonism that had risen against same-sex marriage, it was not clear whether the parliamentary process would eventually grant a full legal remedy.

Added to this challenge was the fact that lesbian and gay people were a political minority that would not, on its own, be able to influence the parliamentary process politically in such a way that would result in successful law reform. Hence the organized lesbian and gay sector, as represented by the JWG, needed to mobilize itself and develop a political strategy enabling the sector to build a legitimate and strong political voice for the parliamentary same-sex marriage campaign at that time.

The campaign's focus at that stage was to lobby Parliament and other key stakeholders directly. Thus a broad strategy was adopted by the JWG. OUT worked with the other JWG members to build a common position and a plan of action for implementation. This resulted in an OUT/JWG same-sex marriage campaign strategy that undertook the following activities:
- Direct lobbying of Parliament and key political individuals and structures
- Mobilizing lesbian and gay constituencies to support the campaign
- Building strategic partnerships with other human-rights organizations in support of the campaign
- Working with media to reflect the positions of the LGBTI sector on marriage

Working with the community
In 2004 and 2005, the Equality Project had conducted workshops with LGBTI people and organizations in several provinces in South Africa. The purpose of these workshops was to brief the LGBTI sector about the legal developments of the same-sex marriage court cases and to ensure that lesbian and gay people were constantly visible during court hearings and could engage with the merits of the

application and the legal process. The challenge at that time was that few LGBTI people in communities (who were not part of organized LGBTI groups) understood the legal language and technicalities of the Court's interpretation of the situation. Also, there were many LGBTI people who had no interest in engaging with the political discourse on the issue and just wanted to get married.

There was little political engagement and debate on the part of ordinary LGBTI people on what the same-sex marriage campaign was about and what the real political issues were at that time. The result was that the technicalities of the debate were for the most part dealt with by a small number of people, often academics and lawyers, who understood the language better than ordinary LGBTI people in communities. My feeling is that a political opportunity was lost here, in terms of locating and understanding the campaign as a fight for equality, dignity and freedom of lesbian and gay people within family law.

In 2006, the debate moved out of the courts to Parliament. OUT mobilized lesbian and gay voices to ensure visibility and engagement during the public debates in Parliament. We identified couples to make submissions to Parliament, and individuals to write opinion pieces and articles for possible publication in both the mainstream and the LGBTI press. We also prepared lesbian and gay people to respond to homophobic media articles and to participate in radio and television debates during the campaign. [3]

OUT also supported public demonstrations planned by members of the JWG and other lesbian and gay organizations during the campaign. These included the march to the Union Buildings organized by Jewish Outlook in September 2006 and a picket in front of Parliament organized by the Triangle Project during the stakeholder hearings in Parliament. These demonstrations were one of the ways in which lesbian and gay people could maintain visibility and a strong voice during the campaign.

The budget for the same-sex marriage campaign was extremely limited, and this was a challenge when it came to working with lesbian and gay people within communities. The majority of such people were left out of the process because of the lack of affordable transport to spaces where LGBTI voices were needed during the campaign. Consequently, visibility and presence were low at the provincial hearings conducted by the Parliamentary Portfolio Committee on Home Affairs, and such action on behalf of LGBTI people was left to a small number of people who were, at that time, either employed by LGBTI organizations or could afford to travel to the spaces where advocacy took place.

Working with human-rights organizations

The principle underpinning the marriage strategy was to work within a human-rights framework. There was a need to link the same-sex marriage campaign to broader issues of social and legal justice in South Africa. As such, a key element of the strategy was to target other human-rights organizations and lobby for their involvement in the campaign.

In view of the political task ahead, OUT and the JWG located this campaign within a broader human-rights framework. It was imperative that the same-sex marriage campaign be seen not just as a call for lesbian and gay people to enter the institution of marriage, but that it be seen as a call to advance equality, dignity and freedom for all people. This meant that we had a responsibility to ensure that the public, Parliament and the judiciary viewed the campaign in the same light. This meant lobbying strong human-rights voices and institutions responsible for holding Parliament accountable on the implementation of constitutional rights.

In view of this, we engaged with the South African Human Rights Commission (SAHRC); the Commission on Gender Equality; the Centre for Applied Legal Studies (CALS); the Women's Legal Centre; the South African Council of Churches (SACC); and many others. We encouraged these organizations to take a formal position on same-sex marriage, to make a submission to Parliament, and to actively support the campaign.

Working with the media

One of the biggest challenges during the same-sex marriage campaign was working with the media. The campaign received extensive media coverage both nationally and internationally, but it seemed to us that homophobic voices and hate-based attacks were given proportionally higher visibility in the media than voices in favour of equal marriage for all. The dominant view was that homosexuality is not African, and the notions that homosexuality was sinful, unnatural, intrinsically abnormal and merely a phase (ironically the faith-based organizations and traditionalists spoke largely in unison in this regard) were also expressed. These views dominated the media coverage of same-sex marriage, and the public was flooded with homophobia, hysteria, and hatred towards lesbian and gay people.[4]

Most members of the public who engaged with the discussion in the media were still stuck on the issue of whether homosexuality was African or not, whether it was right or wrong, whether lesbian and gay people should adopt children or not, and similar issues. The public did not engage with the issue of same-sex marriages as such, nor whether the law discriminates against lesbian and gay people or not. The result was that it was almost impossible to move the media debate towards a discussion of rights upheld and rights violated. The debate in the media degenerated to the point where lesbian and gay people had constantly to defend the fact that they were human and that their sexuality was as natural as heterosexuality. The opportunity for a robust discussion on human rights was lost. There is a need to look at the role of media in promoting democracy and human rights in Africa.

In view of this situation, it was strategic for us to ensure that the same-sex marriage campaign had an African face. This meant that dealing with the media would have to be done by a person who represented the public's limited understanding of what is African – that is, a black face. I was at the centre of dealing with media responses and representation of an LGBTI voice during the campaign.

Preparing a submission to Parliament

The process of writing and compiling a submission to Parliament required the establishment of a task team with legal capacity. A volunteer legal team worked closely with OUT staff in the drafting process.[5] The JWG submission to Parliament needed to respond creatively and robustly to the various amendments to the Civil Union Bill, as it moved through the legislative process. (See pages 124-127.)

It was imperative for all of us engaged in the campaign to understand how the law-making process worked in order to strategize accordingly.

The key objective for us was to understand and identify points and areas of impact in which we could lobby Parliament in favour of legalizing same-sex marriages in South Africa. This meant that, at all the stages in the legislative process, the influence of lesbian and gay people had to be exerted, directly and indirectly. This involved direct lobbying of officials in the Department of Home Affairs, ministerial legal advisors, members of the Portfolio Committee on Home Affairs, members of the National Assembly and the National Council of Provinces (NCOP), political parties, human-rights organizations, Chapter 9 institutions[6] and others.

Lobbying Parliament and politicians

It was identified as critical that we lobby lawmakers to ensure that they buy in to the position of the JWG. The aim was to identify possible allies and to build and develop these relationships to influence the outcome of the legislature's deliberations on legal remedy. Activities included one-on-one engagement with Members of Parliament (MPs); sending letters; development and dissemination of fact sheets and other information to inform policy-making; active participation at provincial public hearings; and maintaining the constant visibility and presence of LGBTI voices throughout the parliamentary process.

It became apparent that part of the success of the same-sex marriage campaign was dependant on the creative and political capability of the lesbian and gay sector to engage the African National Congress (ANC) as the ruling party in government and in Parliament. This required that those who led the campaign understood the decision-making processes, political landscape and positioning of the ANC in relation to the campaign. This was a daunting task given the conservatism of some in the ANC when it came to the understanding and interpretation of liberal democracy, the Bill of Rights and the Constitution itself. During the campaign, there were major divisions within the party over the potential legalization of same-sex marriage. Some in the ANC were seemingly convinced that there was a need to afford lesbian and gay couples the right to marry. Others imagined political and ethical catastrophe if same-sex marriages were legalized.

In view of the above, the campaign targeted strategic individuals within the ANC who were in influential leadership positions to establish support for same-sex marriages. Some of them were very supportive, pointing out the areas in which lobbying would be most effective – for instance, the National Executive Committee of the ANC; the Minister of Home Affairs (as a key figure in the implementation of any form of same-sex marriage legislation that Parliament would draft); parliamentary portfolio committees[7] (particularly the Home Affairs and Justice portfolio committees); and the two houses of Parliament, the National Assembly and the National Council of Provinces (NCOP). The idea was that targeting these individuals and structures would indirectly influence the ANC's decisions on the campaign, and that the views of the lesbian and gay sector would be heard and filter through the party and parliamentary structures.

It was very challenging to engage the NEC of the ANC during the period of the campaign. The only strategy that seemed to work was to target individual members of the NEC. The turning point of this work was the meeting that the Minister of Home Affairs (also a member of the NEC and the Chairperson of the ANC Women's League at that time) called with specific stakeholders, including the organized LGBTI sector. In this closed-door meeting, the lesbian and gay representatives (OUT, Jewish Outlook and the Equality Project) engaged with the Minister on the real issues at stake regarding the marriage campaign. It was clearly indicated to the Minister that the issue at stake was not simply that lesbian and gay people be given the right to marry. It was more than that: the fact that lesbian and gay people were treated as second-class citizens, and that their dignity and full enjoyment of all forms of equality were compromised by the existing marriage laws.

Parliamentary hearings on the Civil Union Bill
The Portfolio Committee on Home Affairs was responsible for engaging with the public, giving all South Africans the opportunity to share their opinions on the legalization of same-sex marriages. In September and October 2006 this committee held public hearings in all provinces on the Civil Union Bill. These hearings revealed the high level of ignorance, prejudice and homophobia among the citizens who participated. The platform for hearings became a pulpit for people who quoted verses in the Bible to condemn homosexuality as sin. Others used tradition and culture as an argument to oppose same-sex marriages claiming

that homosexuality is 'unAfrican'. Proponents of the latter view attempted to present homosexuality as an imperialist agenda from the West, claiming that there is no existence of same-sex relationships in Africa. The marriage campaign resulted in a civil pact between the religious and cultural fundamentalists who constantly supported each other's positions on legalizing same-sex marriages. This resulted in a rhetoric of ignorance, citing arguments such as: children's psychological well-being would be at stake if raised by two parents of the same-sex; that population growth is under threat with the rise of same-sex families because lesbian and gay people cannot bear children. This happened despite the fact that the law had long pronounced itself on the matter of adoption and children born of lesbian and gay couples.

The main opposition voices within Parliament included the African Christian Democratic Party[8] and the Pan African Congress[9]; at the parliamentary hearings, opposition came from groups such as the Marriage Alliance, the Kara African Institute, the National House of Traditional Leaders (NHTL), the Congress of Traditional Leaders of South Africa (Contralesa), and the Muslim Judicial Council, among others. Ironically, these organizations have major ideological differences among themselves, but same-sex marriage became a platform of convergence in their interpretation of ethics, morals, law and family.

We ensured the presence of LGBTI activists and individuals at every public hearing in the nine provinces and in Parliament. As part of planning for public hearings, JWG organizations mobilized lesbian and gay people within those communities to come in numbers to share their plight and voice out their support for same-sex marriages. Most provinces were a success, with the exception of Mpumalanga, Limpopo and Northern Cape. The presence at public hearings gave us an opportunity to lobby and engage members of the Portfolio Committee on Home Affairs, which was were conducting these public hearings.

The challenge with all the public hearings was that they degenerated into spaces and platforms for hate and homophobia. The platforms were not used constructively to engage on the Civil Union Bill, but rather to question the morality of homosexuality. In addition, the majority of people were not even aware of the fact that sexual orientation is included in the equality clause of the South African Constitution. The level of ignorance on the legal progress and transformation that has taken place regarding the rights and freedoms of lesbian and gay people in the past 12 to 13 years was not known, or was ignored. It also seemed that the majority of South Africans still did not understand how democracy works in terms of dealing with issues of majority versus minority rights.

It was disturbing that so few people were aware of the Bill of Rights in the Constitution and its protection against discrimination on the grounds of sexual orientation or marital status. The majority of those opposed to the Bill spoke from their religious and cultural convictions rather than from a constitutional perspective, even though the call for same-sex marriage was a constitutional matter concerning the right to dignity and equality for an excluded sexual minority. It was disturbing to discover that after 12 years of democracy there is still a lack of understanding of the culture of rights and freedoms in a democratic society, especially with regards to minority versus majority rights, and a lack of understanding of the role of public opinion in a constitutional democracy. The public hearings demonstrated a high level of verbal abuse and hate speech directed at sexual minorities in South Africa and on the African continent; they showed that there was still a violation of human rights on the basis of tradition, culture and religion. In this respect we need to condemn the negative use of tradition, culture and religion.

Conclusion

The same-sex marriage campaign was an extremely challenging political and ideological battle. It was confronted with antagonism, slander and hate.

The most important question we need to ask following the passage of the Civil Union Act is: Have we achieved equality for lesbian and gay people or not? The answer lies in the incongruity of South Africa's democracy, where an artificial notion of equality in law has been constructed, while intolerance and injustice in social interaction and association are entrenched. The real-life experiences of South Africans show that in many areas we are far from the realization of equality, dignity, privacy and freedom.

The Act was passed in November 2006, but many same-sex couples cannot be married by civil marriage officers as a result of Section 6 of the Act, which allows civil marriage officers to refuse to solemnize same-sex marriages on the basis of conscience. The greatest challenge remains the role of the Department of Home Affairs and its subsidiaries in ensuring that the Act becomes real for those who have been excluded for so long from the full range of rights provided by South African family law.

What emerged strongly during the debates about same-sex marriage was the complexity of the relationship between law and society. It became apparent that South African law reform and the national democratic revolution have moved ahead of the people of Umzantsi Afrika. The provincial hearings revealed this phenomenon clearly. There is a huge gap between the progress of law and public attitudes and understanding of social dynamics. There is a need for deepened public education on gender and sexual diversity if we are to make real our Constitution's promise of equality, dignity and freedom for LGBTI people and indeed all people in South Africa. *Aluta continua.*

Notes

1. I worked on this programme in collaboration with the legal advice officer (Wendy Isaack) and programme manager (Melanie Judge).
2. The JWG represents the organized LGBTI sector, and speaks and acts in the interest of its respective and diverse constituencies. The JWG aims to strengthen the LGBTI sector so as to maximize collective responses to LGBTI needs and rights. This is done through research; advocacy; constructive dialogue and collaboration; public education; social mobilization; and positive expressions of our diversity. JWG organizations collaborated closely during the public hearings and parliamentary lobbying process in the year that followed the Constitutional Court judgment in *Fourie*, culminating in the passing of the Civil Union Act.
3. Such articles, in support of same-sex marriage, appeared in the gay and lesbian media (Mambaonline, *Wrapped, Exit*) as well as the mainstream press (*Business Day, Pretoria News, Sunday Times, Cape Times, The Citizen, Sowetan*).
4. There were a number of homophobic opinion pieces in the mainstream press, for example, 'Same-sex Marriages a Foreign Aberration' by Motsoko Pheko (Leader of the Pan African Congress), *Pretoria News*, 1 December 2006; 'Reluctant Lawmakers' by Pathekile Holomisa (head of the Congress of Traditional Leaders of South Africa), *The Witness*, 7 September 2006.
5. The Joint Working Group submission was drafted by a team that included David Bilchitz, Kate Hofmeyr, Fikile Vilakazi, Melanie Judge, Michael Yarborough and Jonathan Swanepoel. Additional input was provided by Beth Goldblatt (Centre for Applied Legal Studies) and Sibongile Ndashe (Women's Legal Centre).
6. These are the institutions that were established in terms of Chapter 9 of the Constitution of the Republic of South Africa. The purpose of the institutions was to monitor government's role in the promotion and protecting of human rights and equality for all South African citizens. The institutions are the South African Human Rights Commission (SAHRC), the Commission on Gender Equality (CGE), the Commission for the Promotion and Protection of the Rights of Cultural, Religious and Linguistic Communities, the Public Protector, and the Public Service Commission (PSC).
7. Portfolio Committees were established by Parliament to assist with drafting and public debating of legislation before it is presented to the two houses of Parliament for debate and endorsement. They have the responsibility of engaging with the South African public and collect views, opinions and positions of the public regarding any piece of legislation that Parliament wants to develop.
8. See page 138 of this book for the statement to the National Assembly by the leader of the African Christian Democratic Party, the Reverend KRJ (Kenneth) Meshoe, on same-sex marriage.
9. See pages 140-141 of this book for the statement to the National Assembly by the leader of the Pan African Conference, Dr EM (Motsoko) Pheko, on same-sex marriage.

(Not) in my culture: Thoughts on same-sex marriage and African practices

Nonhlanhla Mkhize

The equal right to marry has been a major issue for lesbian and gay people across the world. In South Africa, this right has been achieved through the Civil Union Act. During the parliamentary hearings leading up to the passing of the legislation, objections were expressed by communities and religious and traditional African leaders. This leads us to ask the question: What is the contemporary cultural context for same-sex marriage in South Africa? In trying to respond to this question, I would like to address some of the things that same-sex marriage says about African history, the understanding of culture; and what same-sex marriage does to the definition of marriage.

It is important to acknowledge that the concept 'African culture' does not perfectly fit into one single definition or range of practices. On the African continent there are a variety of customs and traditions enforced either by one's family or ethnic group. For me, culture is the glue that holds both customs and traditions together – and protects and promotes these within families and ethnicities. While culture varies from region to region there are commonalities on certain practices. I will look at particular aspects of what is regarded as 'African culture' insofar as they relate to marriage, such as lobola (bride price[1]), within a broader context of attitudes towards marriage.

What is culture?

To understand the *contemporary cultural context* for same-sex marriage in South Africa we need to understand 'culture'. Between cultural and biological anthropologists there is an agreement that while culture is a term used to refer to 'learned patterns of thought and behaviour shared by a social group' the word 'culture' derives from a Latin term meaning 'to cultivate'.[2] This could mean that culture is a 'cultivation process': through culture people are assisted to grow in a certain way; to make sense of things in life from a particular point of view; to believe in and be guided by specific principles, which are then referred to as the morals and values of their families, societies and even of their particular grouping (to which they are affiliated through race, religion, or class).

In anthropology, 'culture' is used to refer to the universal human capacity to classify, codify and communicate his or her experiences through symbols. It is about the 'way people live and engage with other living things based on what they understand and believe'.[3] For Jane Goodall, a common way of understanding culture is to see it as consisting of specific elements that are 'passed on from generation to generation through learning alone: *values*; *norms*; *institutions*'.[4] *Values* are ideas; *norms* are behavioural standards expected and *institutions* are structures of a society within which values and norms are transmitted and enforced. Culture, thus, regulates relationships within society. How then, does this assist us in understanding the contemporary cultural context of same-sex marriage in South Africa, and what it says about African history and culture?

To understand the *contemporary context for same-sex marriage* in South Africa a walk down memory lane, highlighting a number of things about African history with regard to the concept of marriage and how this has changed over time, is necessary. To access this information, in July 2007 some young and old members of Zulu communities in KwaZulu-Natal (KZN) were interviewed about their perceptions and beliefs about marriage; what is known to be tradition and what is being practised today; and how they understand tradition and practice it in relation to marriage. These individuals were asked to reflect on what they know and understand to be 'African culture', in terms of marriage, related to both South African reality and other Africa country realities.

I interviewed Mrs Makhosazane Mkhize (67), wife, mother of three and grandmother of six, a traditionalist and preacher's wife; Mr Aron Mncwabe (96), widower, father, grandfather and great-grandfather and culturalist (both from Mpumalanga township, KZN); Mr Xolani Dlamini (54), married father of six and grandfather of four, from eNdwedwe; Tholakele Hadebe (42), single mother of three and grandmother of two, from KwaNongoma; and two individuals who identified themselves as single lesbian and gay, respectively: Thabisile Khumalo (31) from Umlazi and Senzo Ngobese (25) from KwaMashu. There were also two local chiefs who, like three other individuals, requested not to be referenced but their input utilized.

What is marriage (umshado)?

Most societies throughout Southern Africa are traditionally *patrilineal* and practice *patrilocal* residence at marriage. This means the wife is brought to her husband's father's home and through the payment of lobola the marriage is made legal and socially recognized. Lobola was, and still is, essentially a transfer of wealth from one group of men to another. Compared to all other regions in Africa, the eastern and southern African societies contract marriage with a substantially large bride price. In some west African matrilineal societies, the bride price value is relatively low. Important to remember is that patrilineal/patrilocal social system supported male dominance. In this system or social arrangement a woman's role was very clear. That was, 'loyalty, humility, silence and respect'[5] for her man. With the introduction of civil unions or same-sex marriages, it is a bit difficult to comprehend how these social arrangements would work, and this presents a 'cultural' challenge.

From conversations with Mkhize and Mncwabe, I also learned that marriage (*umshado*) '*ila imindeni emibili iganiselana; ukuveza emndenini umuntu ozimisele ukuphilisana naye; ukuxhumana kwemindeni eshadiselanayo. Abomfana bafike bayocela isihlobo esihle kubontombazana, kulotsholwe, kuphiwane izipho, kugcagcwe*'. ('Marriage is when two families wed their children; it is revealing to family who one intends to live with, it is the linking of two families who are marrying the two children. The boy's family would request "good relations" from the girl's family, bride price would be paid, gifts would be exchanged and then a public declaration of the union would be done.')

For Dlamini, marriage is a tradition through which a man declares a woman his own to love and cherish until they are separated by death. It is a vehicle for starting a family, thus, for him, children born outside wedlock have no legitimate claim to their father's estate after he dies. He was quick to explain that by this he did not mean the wife becomes property of her husband, but that she becomes one of his achievements, like his children and the homestead.

When asked about the implications of this definition when the husband is deceased, he replied that 'because she has left her home to be married into the man's family, when he dies, she cannot go back home or remarry to another family'. For him it makes sense for culture to have provisions for a widow '*ukuthi ingenwe*', 'to be taken in' by the late husband's brother, half-brother or any close male kin. A female relative, he chuckled, is not and has never been considered a candidate.

As for lobola, according to Mkhize and Mncwabe, unless you were marrying a princess, marriage was not as costly at it has become. Traditionally lobola comprised 11 cows, ten for the father and one *umqhoyiso*[6] for the mother. If you were marrying a chief's daughter you would expect to pay about 13 cows for lobola. If you were marrying a rich king's daughter, you would expect to pay about 16 or 17 cows, but if he were a poor king you could expect to pay more. Mkhize and Mncwabe indicated that in this day and age of poverty and diseases, lobola has increased significantly. Ironically, the level of education of the girl to be married pushes up lobola. Today, in calculating an appropriate amount for lobola, the girl's parents would calculate how much they have 'invested' in her education and upbringing. If she is already employed, and is paying monies into her parental household, as she would traditionally be required to do, they would calculate the loss of income to the family that would come with her getting married and starting a new family, and factor that into lobola. One of Mnwabe's grandchildren recently paid ten cows and two wedding rings worth R40 000. This excluded gifts for the girl's family and close kin.

Historically, marriage was about forging ties between two families. Mkhize and Mncwabe endorse this view. Typically, once a boy and girl agree on getting married, they would agree on the day when the boy's negotiators would arrive; she would tell her mother and together secretly prepare for it. The boy's negotiators would arrive, announce their presence, and if the girl admits to knowing them (that is, who sent them) and her father is willing, a date for negotiations would be set. When that day arrives, the girl's family and relatives would be present and would have prepared eats. The men would meet, and if they agree things proceed to wedding plans. If not, another date would be set. Once an agreement has been reached, the girl's father and his team would go and view the goods on offer. If they are happy, they would seal the deal. The process of exchanging gifts would follow, leading up to a public declaration of the union.

With modernization and a change in people's way of life, there has been a move away from doing things the traditional (or old-fashioned) way. For instance, lobola negotiations do not take as long as they used to. Young and old people do not hide their lovers or sexual partners from their families. Men now propose marriage with an engagement ring handy. If the families are not happy with it, the couple is likely to elope. Nowadays there are situations where bride price is not paid but there is, instead, a greater emphasis on the exchange of gifts. In many cases, bride price has become a means of showing off by the would-be husband and his family; in other societies it has simply been stripped down to a mere financial transaction.

Local chiefs I consulted agreed that traditions relating to lobola are, however, already under threat. They are made more complex in marriages across cultures. You find for example that if a black man marries a woman from another race, he is still expected to pay lobola for her. I also gather from Mkhize and Mncwabe that, even if the woman's family does not want lobola, the families need to at least exchange gifts and properly welcome the women into the man's family so that his ancestors can accept her. If this is not done she will always be known as *umfazi ongangeniswanga emadlozini asekhaya* (a wife who was never introduced to the family ancestors). It is also believed that this would have a negative effect on children born of the union.

Traditionally a woman marries into the husband's family; the children born from that marriage belong to his family, and hence take his family name. The woman takes on the husband's way of life, which she is expected to support. This persists in Western culture as it does in African culture. What seems to be a bit difficult to understand, and probably is further challenged by same-sex marriage, is what happens to children when their mother or father remarries into a different family, or if they had not been married before but now get married? It has been argued that if a woman has a child while not married, she is expected, upon getting married (unless if it was with the father of the child) to leave that child behind with her family and start a new life with the person she is marrying. Of course she will still be expected to maintain her child. Would this be the same in the case of a same-sex marriage?

In some African cultures, the traditional view on children born out of wedlock is that they are left with the maternal family when their mother marries another man. If it is the father who remarries, because they would have his surname, they would remain with him. South African law, at this point, looks at what is in the best interests of the child to determine who the child lives with. When it comes to one's being in a relationship with or marrying someone of the same sex, the law applies the same principle. Going back to tradition, it is not so clear what is culturally accepted. At the same time it is felt that if a child is male he would stay with his father, but what if he is not seen as such a great role model after entering into a relationship with another man? This is yet another challenge that same-sex marriage poses.

By contrast with the traditional outlook symbolized by lobola, Hadebe said that she 'always imagined marriage to be a celebration of love between two people and their commitment to spending their lives together'. She made it clear, though, that as far as she can see 'traditionally marriage is part of a patriarchal system invented by men as "heads of households" and as "leaders of society" to oppress women'. She referred to South Africa's high divorce rate and questioned the major reasons for it. 'It is not irreconcilable differences,' she argued. 'It is this being a virtuous wife while your husband pimps around as "The Man"!' Such marriages are about limiting the rights of women and reinforcing patriarchy and sexism. Similar questions surround the traditional institution of polygamy. A recent television show, *Muvhango* (SABC2), had episodes showing a Venda man discussing, with his wife, his wish to have a second and even a third wife.

Polygamy is legislated under the Customary Marriages Act. Over time, different generations have developed their own meanings of polygamy. Men have used culture to justify why they tend to date more than one woman at a time. I have become aware of women who feel the equality clause in the South African Constitution needs to protect their rights to marry more than one man too. While polygamy may be one of the practices that certain traditions within Africa have come to accept as culture, no in-depth research has been conducted about it and its prevalence in the minds of LGBTI people.

Interestingly, the final version of the Civil Union – Section 13 (2) – excludes civil unions from being recognized as marriages in terms of the Customary Marriages Act and thus excludes same-sex couples from contracting customary marriages. As such, the reference to husband, wife or spouse in the Customary Marriages Act does not include a civil union partner. This is possibly a result of the vocal opposition to same-sex marriage on the part of the National House of Traditional Leaders (NHTL) and the Congress of Traditional Leaders of South Africa (Contralesa), during the parliamentary deliberations on the Civil Union Bill.

This stark separation in law between civil unions and customary marriages serves to reinforce the idea that same sex relationships fall outside of African culture, customs and tradition, and undermines the recognition of same-sex relationships and practices in Africa. It also inhibits the need for further development of African customary traditions so as to embrace same-sex marriage.

According to the two local chiefs I spoke to, *divorce* is not sanctioned in 'African culture', or was not until recent Westernization made it possible. 'There was no room for divorce. If a man, over time, lost interest in you, got bored with you, he would be allowed to take [marry] a second and even a third wife. You would each have your own houses within the homestead for you and your children. You would stay right there and make your house a home for you and your children,' said Mncwabe. We live at a time when poverty, disease and the desire for independence contribute to divorces, argued Dlamini, Mkhize and Khumalo. For example, a dislike of independent thinking leads to abuse in a lot of relationships, there is power and dominance; in such cases women are not allowed an opinion or to exercise their own thoughts. Regarding finances, the man had control over everything; there was no concept of the equal distribution of wealth which we know and value today. All these contribute to divorce. How marriage is understood in 'African culture' has in some ways evolved. For example, the notion of divorce has developed over time and is now a practice that is more culturally acceptable.

The public hearings in Parliament on the Civil Union Bill were aimed at accessing public opinion on same-sex marriages and unions. From these hearings, it was clear that there were various traditional and cultural assumptions about and interpretations of marriage – an institution already under a lot of strain in our increasingly Westernized society. The basic premise that marriage takes place between a man and a woman, and that each has specific roles and obligations, has no place in a same-sex marriage (unless of course it is between two individuals who have assumed specific gender roles within a same-sex relationship). No-one has answers on what is culturally appropriate and acceptable when two people of the same sex marry. If two women want to marry each other, who is expected to pay lobola? If they have a child through artificial insemination, is it the woman who offers her egg who becomes 'the mother' or is it the one who offers her womb? In a case of two men, who pays lobola? If they decide to use the services of a surrogate mother to have children, is it the one whose sperm is used who becomes 'the father'? Sadly, the custodians of culture have not risen to the challenge of offering possible answers to these questions.

We are to be reminded that culture is not carved in stone and that it should serve to protect and promote the principles of *ubuntu*, which is essentially about humility and humanness. It is important to make use of cultural practices that take us forward, and discard those that undermine the core values of human rights.

The public hearings were aimed at affording citizens of the country the opportunity to engage each other on the issue of the proposed Civil Union Bill, to share and debate their views on the various aspects of the issue. Sadly these were rushed, disorganized and predominantly biased against same-sex marriages and LGBTI identities. People asked questions such as: 'How do they have sex with each other?'; 'How can these people be allowed to marry when they don't even know what commitment is?'; and 'Why is government promoting sin?' People made statements like 'Gays and lesbians cannot raise children – they will molest them'; 'A child needs the nurturing of the mother and the discipline of a father'; and 'Homosexuality – the Bible is very clear – is an abomination!' It was as if they were aimed at ridiculing and further stigmatizing the lesbian and gay community.

Turning to LGBTI community responses to the parliamentary public hearing in KZN, the Durban Lesbian and Gay Community and Health Centre (Durban Centre) and the Pietermaritzburg Gay and Lesbian Network regarded these hearings as chaotic, and put out a statement to that effect. In KZN the hearings were scheduled for Ulundi, and at the last minute were moved to Greytown. The public alerts on the change of venue were put out the night before. It is still unknown why crucial stakeholders were not informed about changes so they could mobilize communities to attend.

After the *Fourie* judgment in 2005, mini-conferences on same-sex marriage were convened by the Durban Centre (with the Treatment Action Campaign) in the Eastern Cape, primarily because these provinces are the homes of royal houses (Zulu and Xhosa), with kings who claim to be custodians of 'African culture' and tradition, and so that chiefs and headmen could participate in these debates. Unlike the public hearings, the mini-conferences on same-sex marriage seemed a good investment. They afforded community members a chance to engage with lesbian and gay people on a balanced scale. There were materials specifically developed for these mini-conferences that aimed at educating communities about lesbian and gay people, the Bill of Rights, and same-sex marriage. Parents, teachers and religious communities and leaders entered into dialogue with each other. While there were police at other meetings, there was no need to protect anyone against anyone else at these mini-conferences. Community members debated, argued, and protected each other throughout the processes. What was clear was that the opposition to same-sex marriages was largely due to the lack of understanding of human rights, of culture, of lesbian and gay people and their way of life and issues that affect them.

After the hearings in Parliament, the Civil Union Bill was signed into law by the Deputy President. Still, bodies such as Contralesa continued to voice their opposition to the legislation. In February 2007, two months after the legislation was passed, at Contralesa's National General Council meeting, Patekile Holomisa made it clear that the organization he leads does not support the Civil Union Act, and expressed the view that the Constitutional Court had been wrong. It seems that Contralesa has taken this position partly to gain publicity for itself. It utilizes the issue of same-sex marriage as a mobilizing tool and abuses its position in providing cultural leadership to promote hatred and to undermine the human-rights ethos envisaged in our constitutional democracy.

In a country where one in three marriages ends in divorce, and where a majority of households in many areas are headed by single women (and even single men), the conventional role of marriage and the structure of the family unit are undoubtedly under severe strain. The traditional view of marriage is also probably outdated. Whether or not this is desirable from a religious, social or even cultural point of view, the fact is that these trends are real and reflect a fundamental and probably permanent change in South African (and world) society. We need to understand that culture is not static, that it changes over time. It evolves, or it can even be changed very quickly. If the purpose of culture is to bind society together, and to nurture people within a community, then it needs to evolve. Culture is nothing without the people who enact it.

Looking at how the issue of same-sex marriage has been argued in our courts, we learn that the main debate was about how to claim individual rights to equality, to dignity and to freedom. In South Africa, we come from a history of being told whom to marry, where to live, where to work, and the identity of our sexual partners. This apartheid history is now gone, and we should not cling to its remnants. Marriage is perhaps one of the key tools LGBTI people can use to reclaim their personal power and legitimize their relationships.

For the majority of the people I spoke to, the traditional and cultural expectations of marriage have changed and continue to do so. Men never used to speak to or even touch their women in public. Now they are expected to talk about their feelings, tell her how he feels about her, and publicly display affection. For Khumalo and Ngobese, same-sex marriages are going to further challenge the role of men in raising children, questioning the validity of arguments made by anti-same-sex marriage institutions that a child needs a father and a mother (a male and female) as role models to be an emotionally, mentally and physically balanced individual and responsible adult.

Some conclusions
Same-sex marriage has indeed extended the definition of marriage and perhaps even challenged the way we ourselves think about marriage and culture. What is marriage, what it is about? What is culture, who constructs culture, based on what views, opinions, experiences, values and so on?

The passing of the Civil Union Act has further advanced our law in terms of understanding equality, dignity, freedom and unfair discrimination. A lot of gay and lesbian people are already in 'marriage-like' relationships, where there has been sharing of roles and responsibilities and expenses. Why should the law have to wait for society to understand this, to then provide these relationships, these families, the protection and regulation by law they deserve? Many in our society have still not really come to terms with the concepts of racism, xenophobia, sexism and other intolerances, but there is legislation protecting members of society from such abuses.

The contemporary cultural context of same-sex marriage in South Africa is that of legal regulation and protection – and cultural uncertainty. For African culture, LGBTI identities and same-sex marriage pose a lot of challenges, raising questions about definitions, meanings and processes. They challenge the concept of 'African' and ask the 'custodians of culture' to consider, debate, reconcile and pave a way forward on these and other matters related to fundamental human rights – privacy, equality, freedom and democracy.

We learned from Goodall and the chiefs that culture and identity are constructed and nurtured; that because these are not set in stone, they have changed with time, and continue to change. What the debate around same-sex marriage has done is further advance our understanding of marriage and family structures: that these are as diverse as people, and that, like every person, all deserve equal treatment, protection and regulation by the law as enshrined in the Bill of Rights of our Constitution. For society, the debate, the passing and the implementation of the Civil Union Act raises the need for urgent attention to community sensitization and education. The focus here should be on the Constitution, our values, morals, cultures, traditions and identities, and what these may mean for the achievement of equality, dignity, freedom and democracy in South Africa.

Notes

1 From the Zulu word for 'bride price', *ilobolo*; in the form 'lobola', the word is now deemed to have been absorbed into South African English. See *South African Concise Oxford Dictionary* (OUP, 1999)
2 http://en.wikipedia.org/wiki/Culture; see also Peter J Brown, Ronald L Barrett, and Mark B Padilla, 'Medical Anthropology: An Introduction to the Fields', in Brown (ed.), *Understanding and Applying Medical Anthropology* (Mayfield, 1998), 10-19
3 Ibid.
4 Ibid; see also Jane Goodall, *The Chimpanzees of Gombe: Patterns of Behavior* (Belknap Press of Harvard University Press, 1986)
5 Suzanne Leclerc-Madlala, 'What Prevents Prevention: An Overview of the Sociological and

Gender Context of HIV Prevention in Southern Africa', in *AIDS Legal Quarterly, Newsletter of the AIDS Legal Network*, November 2006

6 A term traditionally used to refer to the one cow set aside for the mother.

This essay also draws upon the following works:

Nonhlanhla Mkhize, 'Embracing and Resisting Change: Culture as a Source of Information in the context of HIV and AIDS', in *ALQ: A Publication of the AIDS Legal Network* (June 2007), 8-12

Nonhlanhla Mkhize, 'Who Are You to Say I Can't Marry? The Current Common-Law Definition of Marriage Violates My Right to Dignity', in *The Star*, 25 May 2005, and *The Mercury*, 31 May 2005. The article was part of the Gender Links Opinion and Commentary Service, which provides fresh views on everyday news.

Thanks

I would like to thank my interviewees: Mrs Makhosazane Mkhize and Mr Aron Mncwabe from Mpumalanga Township; Mr Xolani Dlamini from eNdwedwe; Ms Tholakele Hadebe, from KwaNongoma; Thabisile Khumalo from Umlazi and Senzo Ngobese from KwaMashu. I would also like to register my appreciation to the two local chiefs who allowed me time and space to engage this on this subject, and all the other individual community members who allowed me to quiz them and use their input here. Finally, Professor Leclerc-Madlala, Head of the School of Anthropology, University of KZN, for her input on defining culture, understanding African culture, tradition and customs.

'Now we have reached consensus'
Interview with Andries Nel

In the 1980s, Andries Nel was active in the National Union of South African Students (Nusas), South African Students' Press Union (Saspu), End Conscription Campaign (ECC), Students for a Democratic Society (SDS) at the universities of Cape Town and Pretoria and went on to work for Lawyers for Human Rights. As secretary of the African National Congress's Pretoria Central branch in the early 1990s, he was involved in the formation of the Gay and Lesbian Organization – Pretoria (GLO–P). In 1994 he was elected as a Member of Parliament for the ANC. Since 2002 he has served as Deputy Chief Whip of the ANC in Parliament. In this interview he talks about the parliamentary process around the Civil Union Act. He says that, for him, same-sex marriages were both a matter of principle as well as 'a personal issue' in that 'my youngest brother is gay'.

What is the ANC's current stance on gay and lesbian rights and how has it evolved over time?
The current stance, and I think it has been the stance of the ANC for quite some time, derives from the Freedom Charter – 'All shall be equal before the law and all shall enjoy equal human rights' – and places emphasis on the need for the dignity of all people to be protected. That standpoint goes back a long way, but obviously – like any policy position – it didn't materialize overnight. It is the result of a complex interplay of different factors, in the same way that ANC policies on non-racialism and non-sexism have a history of development.

Obviously, in any organization, the policy positions that the organization takes are not necessarily shared equally by each and every one of its members, but they will often defend that policy even when they have differences with it. When we say that there is a robust debate in the ANC we mean exactly that! The Civil Union Bill was a case in point. There is a long tradition within the ANC of taking issues, often very difficult issues, and tabling them before our members for discussion to a point of reaching an understanding and consensus. When the Civil Union Bill was first introduced in the Parliamentary Caucus there was a very heated discussion. By the end of that meeting it was clear that we were not quite at one on the issue, but we would be able to engage each other to find common ground, which then happened.

This took place after the Constitutional Court had ruled that Parliament had one year to address the discriminatory aspects of our marriage laws?
Yes. There was a delay in introducing legislation resulting from, among other things, the fact that marriage is strictly speaking the competency of the Department of Justice even though it is administered by the Department of Home Affairs. Between Justice and Home Affairs they had to work out who was going to draft the legislation and what it was going to say. That process took quite some time. We were chasing the 1 December 2006 deadline set by the Court. The point at which Parliament became involved was once that legislation was drafted and introduced. It didn't allow much time to have those internal discussions in our study groups and Caucus meetings, or in ANC branch structures. Once the Constitutional Court judgment was delivered, and we knew that the issue was on the agenda, there was no real discussion before the legislation was introduced. That really put a lot of pressure on the process. People were trying at that late stage to have a broad, consultative process. The issue was very raw, and very little preparatory groundwork had been done. The Constitutional Court ruling was fairly specific in what it said would be acceptable legislation. That placed many members of the Home Affairs committee in a dilemma. They had gone out in good faith to gather people's views, and had heard those views, and now they had to sit with the fact that, notwithstanding those views, they had to legislate in line with a court order.

Public participation is something the ANC is very committed to as a matter of principle. It is something we feel very passionate about and we are constantly looking at ways to expand and deepen public participation. The vast majority of our people don't have the necessary resources to come to Cape Town to make submissions, and that is why the approach followed by the Home Affairs committee, to go out and have hearings where people could make inputs, was an excellent one. On the Civil Union Bill, it was clear we had to hear people's views, but within the framework of the Constitution, and within the framework of a Constitutional Court order. So we created an opportunity for people to make submissions, and those submissions were listened to seriously. There was a lot of weighing of those inputs by the committee and by the ANC study group. That's why the process needed to be managed politically.

Did the Parliamentary hearings have any an impact on the drafting of the Bill?
Definitely. There were various versions of the Bill. There was the Bill as introduced by Home Affairs, that had gone through Cabinet. There was a version of the Bill as drafted by the state law advisors. Then there was the process of public hearings both at Parliament and as well as around the country. A series of modifications were made, including amendments to reflect the views expressed during public hearings.

Amending the Marriage Act directly was likely to stir up lots of resistance and emotion. The other issue that arose was the issue of priests being compelled to officiate at same-sex marriages. In the end, we debated the issues and decided to create a category of civil unions for both heterosexual and homosexual couples, because, for a variety of reasons, not everybody would necessarily want to enter something known as a marriage – which has particular religious connotations. We felt that we wanted to give people the option to choose how they would want to characterize their union and let that be open to everyone.

What about the issue of state officials, who officiate at heterosexual marriages, having an 'opt-out' clause, on the grounds of conscience, if they don't want to conduct same-sex marriages?

It was an important but not a central issue. We weren't happy with that compromise, but we said, 'Let it go ahead and we will see what happens, and if there is a problem we will have to come back to it.' Look, in principle it is wrong, but it doesn't appear to have caused any major problems thus far. We need to be clear that a state official who has objections needs to declare them upfront. That person would have to make it known immediately, so that the necessary arrangements are made. We couldn't let people be embarrassed, subjected to an assault on their dignity, when they are coming to have their marriage officiated.

The general point to be made is that democratic political processes are very often about people with different views and different needs and different aspirations trying to find solutions that can accommodate as many people as possible. But that process needs to be based on certain ground rules, certain underlying principles. We have a Constitution that spells out what those ground rules are. So, in matters like these, where a religious community has certain views, it is their right to make those known, but that can't be done at the expense of the ground rules – and those weigh very heavily on the side of human dignity.

One can't take for granted that everyone understands, accepts and supports everything in the Constitution, and the public hearings demonstrated a high level of homophobia. But, despite all the excitement that preceded the passing of the legislation, and the publicity that accompanied the first few same-sex marriages, things seem to have quietened down. However, one must be careful to not misinterpret that as consensus and support. I think there is still lot of work to be done.

There was a perception that in order to comply with the Constitutional Court's order, the ANC in Parliament had to force the Bill through, using the 'a three-line whip' to pull its own members into line.

The ANC's position all along has been that ANC Members of Parliament are, first and foremost, members of the ANC. As an ANC member you take an oath that you will defend and carry out ANC policy. The policy will be discussed vigorously and broadly, but once a decision has been taken all of us are expected to carry out and defend that decision irrespective of what your position was during the discussions that lead to the decision. We have consistently rejected the notion of a so-called 'free vote', or a 'vote of conscience'. We reject the notion that the implementation of organizational programmes, which have been mandated by the vast majority of South Africans, can be made contingent on the whims of individuals. That is not say it is not an issue that deserved to be dealt with utmost sensitivity, and we have always done that.

A lot was made in the media at the time the passing of the Civil Union Bill of the 'three-line whip'. A three-line whip is really less brutal and violent than it sounds. It is terminology that we have taken over from the British Parliament to designate the level of the seriousness of a vote or the need for the presence of Members in Parliament. A one-line whip means that ANC MPs are free to come and go as they please. A two-line whip means that ANC MPs are expected to be present unless given permission to be away. A three-line whip means that all ANC MPs are expected to be there and that no applications for leave will be considered. A three-line whip is normally called when a vote is serious and/or hotly contested, or in cases where a special majority is needed (such as constitutional amendments). We issued a three-line whip in the vote on the Civil Union Bill because it was hotly contested and because we had a Constitutional Court deadline upon us – we couldn't fail. The turn-out was overwhelming. I think it was probably one of the biggest majorities that we ever had for a piece of legislation.

In the run-up to the vote on the Civil Union Bill, there were a number of MPs who came to us and expressed misgivings. We discussed these and dealt with them in the same way that we have on similar occasions – we exercised discretion. But I must say those were few and far between. It bears testimony to the ANC's democratic culture of debate and decision-making. Some of the people who were most vehement in their opposition in that first Caucus meeting, who had good reasons to be absent, were there to vote. Through that process of political engagement around the issue everyone became convinced of the principle. It almost served as a mobilizing, rallying cry, that the ANC is not afraid to take difficult decisions. We have had our differences, we have had debates, and now we have reached consensus. I think Members of Parliament went to vote with enthusiasm. Obviously there were people even then who had misgivings, but it hasn't divided the organization in a way that some people feared it would.

'Counting the gay faces'
Interview with Glenn de Swardt

Glenn de Swardt is the manager of health and counselling services, and research, at Triangle Project, a Cape Town-based organization providing diverse, specialized services to LGBTI people. Triangle Project was actively involved in the same-sex marriage campaign.

What were the discussions that took place at the start of the same-sex marriage campaign?
I think one of the things that made many people that I spoke to in those days wary was the word 'marriage'. We have been socialized to think marriage equals wedding equals husband and wife equals white veil, bells, priest. So, marriage and religion had to be separated very carefully in our own heads, because that's where we came from as well. We started becoming more comfortable with marriage as a human right, and once people got their heads around that it was great. I think we all became more optimistic.

As an organization, we at Triangle Project discussed same-sex marriage on several occasions, just to see where we as individuals stood with it, where we as an organization stood with it. There was some discussion – what do we actually want? Do we want purely legal recognition? Do we want marriage? What is equal? Then we went on to: If it was there, would you want to get married? Is it an emulation of heterosexist society? Are we buying into a whole role structure? Should our relationships be more fluid? Would the concept of marriage add value to our relationships? Are our relationships actually ready for this? To what extent do we as a community respect our own relationships? Those were some of the discussions.

What about working with the media during the campaign?
I was active in interfacing with the media. I can only speak for myself. Every interaction with the media had to include separating the concept of marriage from wedding, religion, that kind of stuff – marriage in terms of heterosexist norms. How do you work out who's who? – that kind of primitive stuff. The media would also play off a religious voice, a conservative voice, and get your comment on that, which I found very unfair, because you weren't always given the space to unpack what the conservative voice was all about, from our perspective. So I don't think it was very easy or very friendly, not at all.

I think the media in South Africa have over the years been sensitized to issues around race – to some extent. I don't think that in those days they had even started to come terms with issues relating to sexual orientation or alternative sexual identities. I don't think we can necessarily blame them – I think their energies had been on shifting their ideologies and paradigms around other issues, women's issues and those kinds of things, and we were Flavour 42 that they just never got to.

Do you think there has been any shift in the media as result of the same-sex marriage process?
I personally do think so. We were quite vocal as an organization. I was shouting from the rooftops about how the media was addressing the issue, even the terminology they were using – like 'life' versus 'lifestyle', that kind of crap. Through these processes – our being angered, irritated, frustrated, and then tackling some of these issues and actively engaging with the media – I think they have become more sensitive. What did piss me off was the apathy of the community. They would phone and say, 'Have you seen this? Please deal with it' – and put the phone down. Write your own damn letter, start your own petition, go see your own Member of Parliament! I think with time we began to see, certainly in the *Cape Times* and the *Argus*, a more balanced perspective in terms of space allocated to different voices. The campaign is not over. It's ongoing, but we're more aware of it. And they're more aware that we're more aware of it. Quite a few publications have been taken to the press ombudsman. We are less reluctant to comment on the media.

What is your feeling about the apathy of the LGBTI community with regard to same-sex marriage?
People were getting excited about it and saying 'What can I do?' Many gay people were planning their weddings and talking honeymoon, the party, the hedonistic side, as opposed to the principle at stake, the human-rights issue. We went out of our way to get people to the public hearings, and when you expect 500 you get 50. I don't think we as a community actually take our rights very seriously. I think those of us who do take them seriously are seen as a bunch of nerds who get off on it – publicity types who rant and rave. Many people in the community also would like to think our lives are fabulous, 'So why are you shouting?' The apathy is pervasive. It's not just towards the same-sex-marriage campaign. If you look at the community's apathy around HIV and AIDS the silence is deafening. It's scary. I think it's kind of 'Let's sit back and wait. We'll carry on with our parties. If we don't get it we haven't lost anything.' That was the kind of mentality. I think the average queer person in South Africa hasn't had to fight for their rights. The battle has been fought by others. So they just enjoy the benefits, and let others get on with it. It's quite sad.

I saw far more, profoundly more, community support when we had a disaster such as the bombing of the Blah Bar [nine people were injured in a bomb blast at this gay venue in Cape Town on 6 November 1999], the Sizzlers massacre [nine men were killed in an attack on a gay massage parlour on 20 January 2003], the murder of two gay men last year. The murder of two lesbians last year got far less attention because they were two black women. With Sizzlers there was a huge collective mourning, horror, people were going there and putting flowers on the railing of the fence of the house. That got people going. We had people offering money, asking 'What can we do?', flying family members of the deceased down and paying for things. But not for the marriage campaign.

What about about the public hearings?
The Cape Town public hearings were held in the Woodstock town hall, which is a bright pink building. It looks like a pink Christmas cake. We had a strong protest there, outside, placards and so on. I remember watching people arrive. The whole thing was: Would Errol Naidoo be there or not? He's the leader of His People Church and very publicly opposed to same-sex marriage and homosexuality. And watching the Muslim people arriving, counting the gay faces that were present. It was three against one. What was very apparent was that the Parliamentary Portfolio Committee chairperson was totally insensitive to issues related to hate speech, human dignity, and people were able to stand up and really speak psychotic mumbojumbo. Their darkest, primal prejudices and rage were articulated in the sweet little candy-wrap of religion.

At times I also felt that gay people were silenced, that they were given less space. I remember feeling outraged when I saw that one of the committee members was reading a newspaper under the desk while all this stuff was flying around. Too few gay people – far too few. It was the usual faces, or prominent people. I remember an actor, a journalist, the Dean of Cape Town, Rowan Smith, people from IAM [Inclusive and Affirming Ministries] including Reverend Pieter Oberholzer [affiliated pastor of Good Hope Metropolitan Community Church], Judith Kotze [member of the NGK], Bishop David Russell [retired Anglican bishop], and Triangle Project certainly, about three or four of our volunteers, that was it. Amazing. There wasn't a collective statement made by Cape Town Pride, although Cape Town Pride was there. There should have been organizations making submissions, student groups, the Housewives' League of South Africa, the Spaniel Breeders' Association of the Western Cape. Where were they on this issue? We should be hearing more from the vegetarians, the trade unions. We never heard those voices. As a result the human-rights issue became a queer issue, and it became queer versus God. It's actually got nothing to do with the church, because we're not asking for religious rights.

The discussion should have been framed as a human-rights issue, not as a religious issue. The discussion should not have been allowed to stray. Everybody was exposed to arguments about the effect of same-sex parenting on children, the impact of same-sex marriage on the construct of the family, and moral decay. That should not have been allowed. It was irrelevant. We have passed that point already.

What about those gay and lesbian people who opposed the idea of marriage?
The space was there for anyone. But if I was a gay man and anti-marriage it would have been very difficult to go to a public hearing, where I'm hearing radical Christian and Muslim hate speech, and a few gay guys really trying to make their voices heard – I would feel like a traitor, like I was sabotaging the process. So I think those voices self-censored themselves for the collective. We have same-sex marriage now, but it is by choice. If you don't want it, that's fine. I was asked by the BBC if I wanted to get married. I said, 'No, definitely not.' So, they asked, why was I fighting for it? I said, 'Because I want the *option* to be able to get married.'

Was the protest outside Parliament a success?
I was impressed not by how many came, but by who came. The guy who came two hours from the Cape Flats to hold his placard – good for you. We had to get consent from the city, and that was a bit difficult. We couldn't have a large crowd, and they wanted to put us over the road, opposite Parliament. That kind of nonsense. I don't think we stopped traffic in Plein Street, but we certainly got a lot of media attention. There's always a flock of media types in that precinct hoping for something to happen, so we provided the entertainment. It wasn't just about the campaign. People who had never heard about Triangle Project were asking, 'Who are you and why are you doing this?' Not just in Cape Town, but nationally as well. That was good for organized queer culture in South Africa.

Putting it to Parliament:
The hearings and debates

Following the Constitutional Court decision in *Fourie*, in December 2005, a legislative process began that resulted in the passing of the Civil Union Act:
- On 1 August 2006 a Marriage Act Amendment Draft Bill is presented to the Portfolio Committee on Home Affairs by the Department of Home Affairs. It proposes a gender-neutral amendment to the Marriage Act. This draft Bill is, however, never to be officially tabled.
- On 31 August 2006 the Civil Union Bill (B26-2006) is introduced in the National Assembly (NA). This first draft of the Bill can be found at: www.info.gov.za/gazette/bills/2006/b26-06.pdf (all URLs last accessed 26 February 2008).
- In September and October 2006, hearings are held across the country for public consultation on the first draft Bill. A report on these hearings can be found at: www.pmg.org.za/docs/2006/061031hearings.htm.
- On 16-17 October, as part of the public consultation process, national stakeholder hearings are held by the NA's Portfolio Committee on Home Affairs (see section below for extracts of selected submissions)
- During October and November 2006 the Portfolio Committee on Home Affairs deliberates the first-draft Bill. The Bill is then amended significantly. The second version of the Civil Union Bill (B26B-2006) can be found at www.info.gov.za/gazette/bills/2006/b26b-06.pdf.
- On 14 November the Civil Union Bill is ratified by the NA and then referred to the National Council of Provinces (NCOP) – the second house of Parliament – for consideration.
- On 23-24 November the NCOP holds hearings on the Bill.
- On 28 November the final version of the Bill is passed by the NCOP.
- On 30 November the Civil Union Act is signed into law by the Deputy President and comes into effect immediately. The Civil Union Act (Act 17 of 2006) can be found at www.info.gov.za/gazette/acts/2006/a17-06.pdf.

Extracts from parliamentary submissions on the Civil Union Bill

On 16 and 17 October national stakeholder hearings were held by the National Assembly's Portfolio Committee on Home Affairs, in Parliament, on the first draft of the Civil Union Bill. Below are extracts from the written submissions of a number of organizations that made oral presentations to the Committee.

The first draft of the Civil Union Bill proposed the creation of a new legal category called a 'civil partnership' for same-sex couples only. Some stakeholders believed the Bill didn't go far enough and fell short of providing marriage to same-sex couples, and also by relegating same-sex relationships to a separate Act. Others believed that the Bill went too far in its legal provisions for same-sex relationships. This version of the Bill included a chapter on the legal recognition of domestic partnerships (registered and unregistered) for both same- and opposite-sex couples.

The extracts from submissions are given in the order and form in which they were presented to Parliament. Where submissions have been shortened, omissions are indicated by ellipses (...). The original footnotes, as contained in submissions, have been removed for the sake of brevity. The editors of this book have added some endnotes to clarify certain issues. For a full version of all these written submission go to www.pmg.org.za/viewminute.php?id=8331 and www.pmg.org.za/viewminute.php?id=8350.

Women's Legal Centre (WLC)

WLC welcomes the attempt by the legislature to recognise same sex relationships and domestic partnerships. These relationships were previously ignored and marginalized by our legal system, silently obliterated by the law, causing harm, suffering and stigma to partners in such relationships. ... The bill seeks to ensure a just resolution when domestic partnerships end. ...

The bill's introduction of a civil partnership rather than marriage for partners in same sex relationships creates precisely the separate but equal status that Judge Sachs cautions against. ... The discrimination is not only indirect – it is overt – if a gay person wishes to commit for life to their partner – they can only choose to enter into a civil partnership, not a marriage. This aspect of the bill perpetuates a caste like status and is constitutionally invidious. ...

Doctors for Life International and John Jackson Smyth[1]

... We support the submission made by others that the best way to deal with the contentious issue of so called 'same-sex marriage' is to pass a *constitutional amendment* defining marriage as between man and woman. We believe such a course has the support of the vast majority of South Africans. ...

... [W]e would remind Parliament that all rights in the Bill of Rights are subject to section 36 which provides for *limitation of rights* where it is reasonable and justifiable to do so in an open and *democratic society* taking into account all relevant factors. We submit that where a very substantial majority of our democratic society find any tampering with the meaning of the word 'marriage' to be repugnant, it should not be done.

Supplementary written submission by Doctors for Life International and John Jackson Smyth (dated 5 October 2006)

We understand that the following quotations from the [Constitutional Court] judgement [in *Fourie*] ... may be causing the Committee some anxiety:

(120) 'It is necessary, therefore, to make a declaration to the effect that the common law definition of marriage is inconsistent with the Constitution and invalid to the extent that it fails to provide to same-sex couples the *status* and benefits coupled with responsibilities which it accords to heterosexual couples' (italics added)

(122) 'Thus a legislative intervention which had the effect of enabling same-sex couples to enjoy the *status*, entitlements and responsibilities that heterosexual couples achieve through marriage, would without more override any discriminatory aspect from the common law definition standing on its own' (italics added) ...

'Status' is derived from the law. It is a legal word. For example, 'immigration status' , 'marital status', 'amateur status', all depend on hard legal facts, not on the perception in a lay person's mind. The term 'marital status' in section 9 of the Constitution is obviously a legal term. Status is conferred by the standing or status of the body creating it.

It follows that status does *not* necessarily depend on a title or name. For example a Monarch and President have different titles, but *equal status* as Heads of State. The chief executive officer of a school may be called either 'Head Teacher' or 'Principal'. The name does not affect status.

Both ['marital status' and 'civil union status'] arise as a result of Acts of Parliament ... The status of marriage depends upon the Marriage Act, 1961 passed by the Parliament of South Africa. The status of a civil union will depend upon an Act of Parliament passed by the same national Parliament. It will be signed into law by the State President of the Republic of South Africa. Perhaps that may give it a higher status than the Marriage Act which was signed into law by a Governor General! It will certainly not be less.

If Civil Union legislation were left to Provincial Parliaments, the status would perhaps be less than that of marriage. Since it will come from the national Parliament, it will provide a status equal to that of marriage. ...

South African Human Rights Commission (SAHRC)

… We live in a constitutional democracy in which the constitution is the supreme law of the land [Section 2 of the Constitution] and the constitutional court is embodied with the ultimate responsibility of deciding constitutional matters and giving effect to the rights that are enshrined in our constitution [Section 167 of the Constitution]. Once the constitutional court has spoken on a matter there is a need in our young and still fragile democracy to respect the court's decision even if we do not necessarily agree with it. In the matter at hand, it needs to be accepted that the constitutional court has delivered its decision and that the current laws that do not accommodate gay men and lesbians from marrying are inconsistent with our constitution. *Whilst everyone has the right to make their deeply held beliefs on the matter known this will not change the decision of the constitutional court.* …

It is not acceptable that merely because a decision is offensive to one's deeply held beliefs that the court's integrity is attacked and undermined. …

There appears to be a mistaken belief that majoritarianism will win the issue for the majority who do not support same-sex marriages. Within this milieu there is little substantive input on how parliament should give effect to the court's decision. …

It is undoubtedly exceedingly difficult for many people who find same-sex marriages offensive to accept the decision of the constitutional court. Accepting difference is a difficult issue, which we as a society need to grapple with. As a country that has experienced and lived through deep and intense pain occasioned by arbitrary discrimination we ought to be well practiced in identifying and recognizing the arbitrariness in the discrimination against people based on their sexual orientation. *We should learn from our past.* …

In many ways the current Civil Union Bill does not give effect in the commission's view to what the court intended. Rather, the Bill appears to give effect to what was argued by the State in opposition to the recognition of same-sex marriages. *This is undermining of the court and offensive to gay people.* …

Firstly, a separate system of union is created for same-sex couples. This gives effect to the offensive doctrine of *separate but equal*. The separate register that will be created to record civil unions further enforces this. …

Secondly, the Bill provides that the marriage officer must inquire whether the parties would 'prefer their civil partnership to be referred to as a civil partnership or a marriage *during the solemnization ceremony* ….' [Clause 11 (1), Civil Union Bill]. This creates the false impression that the two persons are being married when in fact they are being united through a civil union. *This is farcical and highly offensive to same-sex couples who wish to marry*. It is somewhat nonsensical that parties can during the saying of their vows refer to their being married when in terms of law they are partaking in a civil union ceremony.

Thirdly, marriage officers may refuse to solemnize a civil partnership on grounds of conscience [Clause 6 (1), Civil Union Bill]. *This leaves the door wide open for discrimination, offense and deep hurt to be caused towards same sex couples.* It cannot be accepted that whilst the freedom of conscience is protected in our Bill of Rights [Clause 15 (1)] that one's thoughts and beliefs can be acted upon in a manner that causes harm to others and violates their rights ...

The Civil Union Bill appears to be a grudging recognition of unions between same-sex couples. We should not advance equality grudgingly but rather willingly. ...

Intersex refers to persons with ambiguous genitalia and who are neither male nor female. The Marriage Act as it currently stands excludes such persons from marriage, as they are neither male nor female. The Civil Union Bill also excludes these people generally as it refers to two adult persons of the same-sex. Should the Civil Union Bill be passed *there would still be no provisions in our law for intersex persons to marry.* ... [See pages 268-273.]

The Civil Union Bill in its current form is not supported by the SAHRC. The Marriage Act should be amended to allow for all persons be they heterosexual, homosexual or intersex to marry. This should be provided for in gender and sex neutral language. Alternatively, parliament could fail to pass any legislation and allow the decision of the constitutional court to take its course. ...

There should be provision for another form of union outside of the traditional marriage, such as a domestic partnership that is open once again to everyone to participate in should they so wish.

Southern African Catholic Bishops' Conference

The Catholic Church teaches that 'homosexual acts are intrinsically disordered. They are contrary to the natural law. They close the sexual act to the gift of life. They do not proceed from a genuine affective and sexual complementarity. Under no circumstances can they be approved.' (Catechism of the Catholic Church, par. 2357. See also Romans 1:24–27; I Corinthians 6:10; I Timothy 1:10) While the Church says that homosexual ACTS are intrinsically evil, it does not say this about homosexual PERSONS. On the contrary, it states clearly that 'it is deplorable that homosexual persons have been and are the object of violent malice in word and action. Such treatment deserves condemnation from the Church's pastors wherever it occurs' (*Letter to the Bishops of the Catholic Church on the Pastoral Care of Homosexual Persons:* Congregation of the Doctrine of the Faith, October 1986).

... We contend that both the law of nature and Divine Revelation (and the constant teaching of the Church) make it clear that a homosexual union is in no way similar to marriage:

- marriage was given to us by God, is expressly willed by God and is compared by St Paul to the union of Christ and His Church; homosexual acts are against the natural law and are intrinsically disordered
- marriage of its very nature is ordained to the begetting and rearing of children; homosexual acts divorce the sexual act from procreation and the homosexual couple cannot cooperate with God to give new life
- man and woman were made by God in His image and as male and female they complement each other; this unique complementarity which makes conjugal love possible is absent in homosexual unions.

... [M]an-made laws cannot legitimize what is against the natural moral law. Civil law cannot make what is wrong right. ...

... [I]t would be wrong to redefine marriage for the sake of providing benefits to those who cannot rightly enter into marriage. Some of these benefits can be obtained in other ways. For example, any two individuals can agree to own property jointly or to choose a beneficiary for their will. These benefits could be extended by provisions that would not amount to a re-definition of marriage.

... [I]t is one thing to say that the state should not put unnecessary limits on individual freedom; it is something very different to say that the state should give legal recognition to a relationship that does not make a significant or positive contribution to the development of the human person in society.

... It is true that society has changed radically, but it is equally true that nothing can change the natural law or the revealed law of God. ...

Lesbian and Gay Equality Project[2]
... This submission considers the majority decision of the Constitutional Court to explain why the Bill does not give full and proper effect to the judgment. Both the majority decision of Justice Sachs and the minority decision of Justice O'Regan make it plain that Parliament's options are limited. In our view, the Constitutional Court's decision obliges Parliament to:
- Afford same-sex couples the right to get married (not 'civilly partnered'[3]);
- In terms of a law which does not apply only to same-sex couples; and
- Without imposing any conditions or limitations on same-sex couples that are not imposed on heterosexual couples who choose to get married in terms of the same law.

We do not believe that the Bill is capable of being amended to address these concerns. Given the fast-approaching deadline of 1 December 2006, we submit that there are only three realistic options open to Parliament at this late stage:[4]
- Enacting legislation along the lines of the Department of Home Affairs' Draft Marriage Amendment Bill of April 2006, which inserts a gender neutral definition of marriage into the Marriage Act, amends the marriage

formula to include the word 'spouse' and largely resembles the first choice identified in the SALRC [South African Law Reform Commission] report;
- Adopting the SALRC report recommendations regarding an amended Marriage Act and a new Orthodox Marriage Act; or
- Not legislating at all, thereby allowing the law to change automatically on 1 December 2006.

In our view, the third option appears to be the most pragmatic solution to adopt at this late stage in the process. ...

In our view, there is an urgent need for informed public debate on the issue [of domestic partnerships] and sufficient time for further consultation and consensus building on the complex issues related to the statutory recognition of domestic partnerships. The SALRC report, which appears to be the basis for this part of the Bill, has only just been published. Its reasoning and recommendations cannot be addressed within the proposed rushed timeframe.

... [T]he hearings have largely failed to address the fundamental issue at stake – how to give full and meaningful effect to the Constitutional Court decision – but have instead provided a space for the propagation of hate speech.

We are concerned that the Portfolio Committee on Home Affairs not only facilitated but indeed permitted presenter after presenter to infringe the prohibition of hate speech, as contemplated by section 10 of the Promotion of Equality and Prevention of Unfair Discrimination Act, 4 of 2000 ('the Equality Act'). ... In this regard we have lodged a formal complaint with Parliament. ...

The Inner Circle

It is important for us to bring to the attention of parliament that there are many diverse viewpoints on the issue of homosexuality and same-sex marriages within Islam and that the mainstream orthodox view is not the only one. ... [T]here are many different forms of Islam and many different interpretations of the Quran ... which parliament should be aware of. The Inner Circle is one such organization that holds a non-judgmental, non-sexist view on the issue and is bold enough to challenge the existing patriarchal interpretation of the scriptures.

The kind of arguments raised by the Muslim community and indeed many religious sects are mostly based on emotions, prejudice, predictions of a moral decay of society and a patriarchal interpretation of the scriptures. ...

In our research we also found that the Prophet Muhammad, may God's peace and blessings be upon him, never executed homosexuals, neither did he order them to be executed, nor did he banish any of them from Medina on the basis of sexual orientation. On the contrary, when a gay man ...[was] brought in front of the Prophet to be killed, the Prophet replied: 'I am forbidden to kill those who pray'.

Marriage in Islam is not a sacred union as many might want to believe ...

Instead, marriage in Islam is a social contract that binds two persons together ... allowing them to share in the personal and social benefits that goes with it. The minimum requirements of a marriage contract in Islam [are] similar to that of a business contract and [do] not stipulate that the parties engaging in such a contract should be of opposite sexes. In fact the terminologies used in such contracts are not gender specific.

The primary reason for marriage in Islam is also not for procreation. The latter is possible without a marriage contract ...

There are numerous examples in Islamic history of children being reared in homes where there is the absence of a mother or a father or both. In fact the Prophet Muhammad, may God's peace and blessings be upon him, himself was raised without a father and the nurturing of a biological mother for the most crucial part of his upbringing ...

The Inner Circle believes the argument that same-sex marriages will result into moral decay of society is weak, unfounded and a prediction void of facts. Moral decay affects every civilization and it is a consequence of ill-conduct and rule that has very little to do with sexuality and sexual orientation. ...

... The Inner Circle urges parliament to scrap the Civil Union Bill which is only perpetuating discrimination on the basis of sexual orientation and retarding the process of true equality for all South Africans. We propose that parliament grant equal marriages to all citizen[s] who wish to enter such a contract. Anything less is not equal. ...

Muslim Judicial Council
The Muslim Judicial Council objects to the proposed Civil Unions Bill.

Whilst recognizing the rights of individuals the Muslim Judicial Council hereby states that it disapproves of homosexual acts and holds it [sic] to be abominable. ...

It is most definitely a small minority who wishes to share the rights of marriage. Granting them their wish at the expense of the vast majority of South Africans can hardly be termed democratic. The Muslim Judicial Council is of the opinion that the spread of homosexuality and lesbianism will invite the anger of Allah, erode the family structure and expose young, innocent children to an unnatural lifestyle. ...

Christian Lawyers Association
... [The Constitutional Court judgment] clearly indicate[s] that the directive of the Court was that it is not the institution of marriage itself that is unconstitutional, but the fact that there is no manner in which homosexual couples

can have access to the status, benefits and entitlements that the institution of marriage provides to heterosexuals. ...

Our proposal then asks the fundamental question of what legitimate processes Parliament was obligated to follow in order to decide on whether to open up the institution of marriage or not. That is, how does Parliament ultimately decide on whether the appropriate remedy is to have a separate legislative framework or whether it is to open up the institution of marriage?

... [T]he answer to this question depends on the model that Parliament will ultimately decide to adopt for marriage in South Africa. ...

We argue that the traditional model understands marriage as a heterosexual social institution whose origins pre-date the State. ... all that the State did was to merely provide the formal legal recognition of an already existing institution. Conversely, the liberal and commitment model[s] perceive marriage as an institution that is formed as a result of two people desiring to formalise their love for each other, or two people desiring to be committed to each other.

We further argue that it is the traditional model that the State is obligated to protect and promote. ...

Furthermore, we argue that fidelity to our African cultural understanding of individual persons as first and foremost communal persons, dictate[s] that Parliament understand marriage not in the context of two people who love each other, but rather in the context of a social institution that has a common and shared public meaning. ...

Centre for Applied Legal Studies (CALS)

... **Registered and Unregistered Domestic Partnerships:** The Bill, while not a perfect formulation of ideal new laws for such partners, is an important step in providing for the recognition and protection of this category of family. ...

The Bill creates a new institution called a civil partnership. This appears to be a marriage in all but name. The question then is, 'Does the name matter?' CALS believes that there are important considerations of dignity involved in understanding why the name does matter. By telling couples of the same sex that they cannot use the same law and institution as heterosexual couples is saying to them that they are not equal, that their presence within marriage will somehow tarnish and infect the institution, and that they cannot describe their relationships in the same terms as others. All of these messages are insulting and hurtful. They are also unconstitutional. ...

... Our society is undergoing significant social change with a range of new forms of family operating alongside more traditional types. Our Constitution is clear about the need to accommodate a plurality of families ... Domestic partnerships should not be left outside of the coverage of our law ...

The Civil Union Bill presents Parliament with an opportunity to reshape the contours of family law in South Africa by endorsing legislation that acknowledges the reality of the millions of South Africans who live in permanent, intimate life partnerships but who do not get married (for a range of reasons). The complicating issue in this Bill is the creation of a civil partnership for gay and lesbian couples that purports to satisfy their desire to marry. The civil partnership fails to accommodate same sex couples who wish to marry and is instead perceived as segregationist and insulting. CALS calls on Parliament to refuse to endorse the sections of the Bill dealing with civil partnerships. Instead, legislation should be enacted that opens the institution of marriage to all couples, including those of the same sex.

We are aware that the issue of same sex marriage is highly contentious and has generated a lot of negative response from members of the public, some churches and some traditional leaders. While the space to air such concerns must be made available in the interests of openness and democracy in South Africa, a clear message must go out that the Constitution requires that gay and lesbian couples be treated equally and with dignity. Providing such couples with access to the marriage laws of our country will not derogate in any way from the rights of all others, even those who are morally opposed to homosexuality. We urge Parliament to take a clear and principled stand on this issue in the interests of human rights and democracy.

The Joint Working Group (JWG)[5]

Separate is never equal: The question as to whether Parliament will broaden the institution of marriage to include lesbian and gay people fundamentally tests its commitment to the transformation of South Africa. ...

Our Constitution represents a 'radical rupture' from a brutalizing past, toward a common humanity. Part of this journey has been the growing societal awareness of the humanity of lesbian and gay people. How far our society has come in rejecting its discriminatory past can be measured against the attitude it takes to the inclusion of lesbian and gay people within civil marriage. ...

In its judgment on same-sex marriage, the Constitutional Court made it clear that the status quo in terms of which lesbian and gay people are excluded from having the same status, rights and responsibilities as heterosexuals do in marriage is simply unacceptable. ...

Why the Civil Union Bill is objectionable: A civil partnership is effectively a *separate* institution from marriage. This is clearly evidenced by the fact that lesbian and gay people are required to register a civil partnership on a separate register to heterosexuals.

Our submission provides ten arguments as to why the Bill fails to meet the requirements of the Constitution:

1. Civil partnerships are inconsistent with the fundamental guarantee in the Constitution that prohibits discrimination on grounds of sexual orientation.
2. Creating two parallel institutions does not constitute equal treatment under our Constitution and amounts to a form of institutional segregation.
3. Civil partnerships exclusively applicable to same-sex couples are only legally acceptable in jurisdictions which have a lesser equality guarantee than SA.
4. Civil partnerships mark and stigmatize lesbian and gay people as 'other', second-class citizens and thus violate both the right and value of dignity in our Constitution.
5. Civil partnerships fail to respect the value of Ubuntu which requires that gay and lesbian people be affirmed as full members of the South African community.
6. Civil partnerships violate the fundamental freedom that should be afforded to same-sex couples to be able to choose to get married.
7. Civil partnerships do not respect the religious freedom of those lesbian or gay people who wish to be married; allowing same-sex couples to be married would not violate any religious group's freedom.
8. Civil partnerships conflict with the Constitutional Court's judgment in the *Fourie* case and would thus spark further litigation, and accordingly fail to resolve the status of same-sex relationships in South African law.
9. Civil partnerships would add to the administrative burden already borne by the Department of Home Affairs.
10. Civil partnerships are not in the best interests of the children of same-sex couples, nor do they adequately protect same-sex families. ...

Undoing a discriminatory past: Deliberations upon same-sex marriage must be sensitive to the history of stigma and marginalisation that has faced lesbian and gay people in South Africa ...

There is a great discrepancy between the Constitutional rights accorded lesbian and gay people, including the right to non-discrimination, and their lived reality. High levels of homophobia in South African society, and negative social attitudes towards sexual diversity make it difficult for same-sex couples to realize fully their constitutional rights to equality, dignity and privacy.

Original research conducted by OUT in conjunction with its partners in the JWG showed that LGBT people in both Gauteng and KwaZulu-Natal *suffer discrimination* in every arena of social life. The research revealed significant rates of victimisation among lesbian, gay and bisexual men and women in both provinces. Because they are stigmatised for their perceived sexual and/or gender 'deviance', lesbian and gay people are frequently targeted for sexual violence precisely because of their sexual and/or gender identity. ...

In light of the history and continued marginalisation of lesbian and gay people in South Africa, it is all the more important that the law in no way entrench attitudes towards gay and lesbian people that perpetuate marginalisation and discrimination.

Unfortunately, the Civil Union Bill, as it currently stands, continues the tradition of stigmatizing same sex relationships as second-class rather than treading a bold course towards a future where all relationships – whether homosexual or heterosexual – are treated with dignity and equal respect.

Recommendations

We welcome the fact that a large amount of thought has been dedicated to the Bill and to its provisions.

It must be stressed that we are not opposed to the Bill in its entirety. To the contrary, we welcome the introduction of domestic partnerships as a progressive step toward the regulation of relationships that previously fell outside the legal sphere. The key issue is that the law should offer recognition and protection to a wide range of families in our society because families take many shapes and sizes in our plural, and increasingly tolerant, context.

However, we cannot accept that the institution of civil partnerships adequately gives effect to the ruling of the Constitutional Court in *Fourie*. Moreover, we cannot accept the entrenchment of a second-class status in our law for lesbian and gay relationships.

Religious groups will likely challenge whatever decision Parliament takes. Their objection misses the point though. We live in a secular State where religion has to coexist alongside a society whose legal framework is located in the Constitution. What is a stake is not a limitation of religion or a dilution of the exclusive right of heterosexuals to marry. What is at stake is far more important: **it is about the inclusion of all people under a single legislative framework, the design of which was laid out by our Constitution.**

Many opponents of including lesbian and gay people within marriage are aware that their opposition runs contrary to the Constitution. They are thus calling for a constitutional amendment. Such calls should be seen for what they are: a threat to the very founding and structuring values of the Constitution, namely, equality, dignity and freedom. Parliament has been brave in choosing principle over populism on a number of key issues in our young democracy: it must be brave again on this issue.

In light of our submission that the only way in which truly to recognize lesbian and gay equality is to extend the laws relating to marriage to lesbian and gay people, we make the following recommendations:

• The current text of Chapter 2 of the Civil Union Bill be deleted;

- The Civil Union Bill should be renamed the 'Domestic Partnership Bill' and should provide for domestic partnerships for both lesbian/gay and straight people.
- A Marriage Act Amendment Draft Bill should be introduced to parliament as a separate Bill which provides for the inclusion of same-sex couples within marriage in both the common law and the Marriage Act. Such a Bill has already been drafted by the Department of Home Affairs and presented to the Home Affairs Portfolio Committee on 1 August 2006. This Bill also has the added advantage of curing certain pre-existing defects within the existing Marriage Act.

Parliament is now faced with a fundamental choice: *does it move South Africa forward into an era which respects human dignity, equality and freedom and categorically rejects apartheid philosophy, or does it continue to perpetuate values that seek to discriminate, stigmatize and dehumanize?*

We hope it will choose the former course and usher in a new era in South Africa. ...

Triangle Project

... For over a decade, the majority of South Africans, together with the international community, have been celebrating this country's having stepped out of a system of terrifyingly repressive social and sexual control. In the present climate of celebrating individual and collective freedoms for South Africans, it would indeed be a travesty of justice if 10-12% of its 'citizens' were again subjected to a lifetime of sexual control, policing and differentiated 'citizenship'. According to us, inclusive citizenship refers to the normalization of same-sex relationships; inclusive citizenship means that all citizens share the same rights, and not that groups differentiate[d] on the basis of sexual orientation should have different rights. According to constitutional provisions for the equity of all citizens irrespective of gender, race, class *and sexual orientation*, the citizens in a secular state such as ours have the rights to demand that the religious right does not hijack the agenda and change the discourse of rights into ... the rhetoric of sin and redemption. Triangle Project therefore applauds religious leaders such as Archbishop Emeritus Desmond Tutu of the Anglican Church and Reverend Moqoba of the Methodist Church who unequivocally support the right of same-sex couples.

Paranoia, hate speech and hate actions have increasingly been the source of the assault, rape and killing of young Black lesbians in our townships. Who can ever forget the killing of Zoliswa Nkonyana in February this year? Do we want to be remembered as a nation that is intolerant and homo-prejudiced? Do we want to be known as collective murderers because we wrongly believe that same-sex loving has been a colonial import? It was none other than Palesa Beverly Ditsie, a courageous

Black South African woman, who placed the right to same-sex sexual orientation firmly on the Beijing Platform of Action's Agenda in 1995. It was Simon Nkoli, a Black gay man, who is seem as the embodiment of the anti-apartheid struggle who tirelessly fought that gay rights be enshrined in the post-apartheid Constitution.

Thousands of citizens, as well as many beyond South Africa, know that allowing conservatives to derail the recognition of same-sex marriage would not only be a betrayal of the democracy that we have so long fought for; it would be a frightening reversion to the apartheid 'rights-for-different-groups' philosophy of a previous era.

South African Pagan Rights Association (Sapra)

... The Alliance wishes firstly to express its support for the equal recognition of same-sex marriages.

We are of the opinion that the current draft Civil Union Bill and the establishment of Civil Partnerships as separate but equal to Marriage, does not faithfully fulfill the criteria of the Constitutional Court's ruling on the unconstitutionality of the Marriage Act. ...

The Bill defines a 'civil partnership' as 'the union of two adult persons of the same sex', but fails to define 'marriage'. ...

By omitting to clearly redefine marriage as a union between heterosexual or same-sex partners, the existing and implied definition of marriage as a union between heterosexual partners only, remains unchanged and therefore unconstitutional. ...

It was with this right to equality and equal benefit for all in mind, that the South African Pagan Rights Alliance submitted a formal request to the Honourable Minister of Home Affairs to request an amendment of the Marriage Act. The Alliance requested the remove a discriminatory clause which prevented the Honourable Minister from recognizing Pagan candidates as religious marriage officers.

The Alliance notes that section 5 of the Civil Union Bill now permits the Honourable Minister to designate ministers of any religion or persons holding a responsible position in any designated religious institution, to be a religious marriage officer. South African Pagans welcome this important amendment. ...

Marriage Alliance of South Africa[6]

... We cannot in good conscience support or endorse this Bill. As explained below, the Bill seeks to legalise same-sex marriages, as well as certain other types of partnerships or unions. Our view is that whatever arrangements the State makes to recognise such partnerships or unions, it should not do so in a way that denigrates the institution of marriage and the family. Our view is that by recognising all sorts of other relationships, even for heterosexual couples, the Bill does exactly that: it undermines and devalues the institution of marriage. ...

... Parliament has not succeeded in this short time since the introduction of the Bill to equip the public to engage the contents of the Bill in any meaningful way, and has also failed to ensure adequate public participation given the importance of the Bill. ...

... [T]his Bill ought to be referred to the National House of Traditional Leaders in terms of section 18 (1) of the Traditional Leadership and Governance Framework Act 41 of 2003. ...

It should be clear that the Bill in its present form is fatally flawed. ... [I]t does nothing to protect the family as a foundational element of society, nor does it effectively regulate other kinds of relationships.

Rather than proceeding with this Bill, we believe Parliament has the moral and legal responsibility to adopt a constitutional amendment in which a marriage is defined as a voluntary union of a man and a woman. That would effectively protect marriage against any statutory or judicial challenge. ...

Nederduits-Gereformeerde Kerk (NGK) / Dutch Reformed Church (DRC)

... The DRC and other reformed churches support the principle of the equality and dignity of all people. ... Our Christian beliefs require us to recognize and defend the equivalent status of the Christian marriage in terms of our religiously and culturally diverse society. We would like to see that that which we regard as our right, also be available to all the citizens of our country.

... [F]undamental principles of equality of all people, regardless of sexual orientation, implies that relationships between people of the same sex (homosexual orientation) should also be addressed in this new Act. ... It was always clear that the Marriage Act could not simply be adjusted by amending a couple of words – although this may have been sufficient for the main concern of the case serving before the Constitutional Court. The complete rewriting of the act in terms of the diverse religious and cultural contexts and the history of South Africa is an urgent necessity. ...

South African Council of Churches

The historical context for developing viable options that recognize same sex unions or civil marriages lies within the confusion of church-state relations as well as faith and politics since time immemorial. ... It is within these parameters that currently the attempt at unraveling the discussion on civil unions, civil marriages and religious marriages takes place. ...

The SACC's Open Letter to the Portfolio Committees of Home Affairs and Justice, therefore, conveys two aspects that lie at the heart of this submission. First, it supports the Constitutional Court's decision and recommendations that parliament craft legislation that seeks to 'establish public norms that ... protect vulnerable people from unjust marginalization and abuse.' Second, also in line with the Constitutional Court judgment, is our concurrence that legislation so crafted ought not to interfere with the way in which faith communities recognize, celebrate or bless unions/marriages. Overall, our critique of the Civil Union Bill and recommendations to parliament are geared toward the fulfillment of the Constitutional Court's mandate, acknowledging its sovereignty over parliament. This we do despite knowledge of religious arguments that claim aspiration toward divine sovereignty which, in turn, seek to subvert the parliamentary decision-making process, by calling for an amendment to the Constitution. ...

... We argue that *the provisions in the CUB [Civil Union Bill] are precisely designed to project and differentiate between the legal status of same- and opposite-sex unions/partnerships*. It was in the same gist that provision of separate amenities and institutions under apartheid were designed specially to create the impression that 'separate development' provided equally for different population groups. We now know that those claims were mythical and fallacious ... [T]his piece of legislation not only projects inequality but is deeply and gratuitously offensive.

A further matter of concern that affects only same sex civil partnerships is the provision in section 6 of the CUB allowing a marriage officer, on grounds of conscientious objection, the ability to refuse to solemnize a civil partnership. ... This section will be construed to infer an unequal and discriminatory provision on same sex partnerships. ... Hardly anyone today would uphold any provisions for conscientious objection of a marriage officer who would refuse to solemnize a marriage on the grounds of race and/or culture. ...

The evolution of two different Acts (The Marriage Act and the proposed CUB) performing essentially the same function for two different groups of people, then, is blatant discrimination at worst and wasteful inefficiency at best. ...

Some will argue that since marriage is defined within the common law as a union between a man and a woman, one could not speak logically about 'same sex marriages'. They would argue the point that it would be semantically and linguistically proper to refer to such unions as 'partnerships', 'civil unions' or the like. They would argue that they are discriminating fairly on the grounds of language and definition. ... This resort to a definition to bolster discrimination may be a linguistic and semantic victory but ought not be allowed as a necessary and sufficient condition for denying gays and lesbians access to the legal, social, spiritual and psychological status long enjoyed by opposite sex couples. ... When we remove the religious veneer on these definitions the salient characteristics of marriage in contemporary society would be the promotion of a way of life based on mutual love, respect and loyalty. It also more contemporarily includes aspects such as public support, legal recognition of the personal, economic and propertied relations of the persons who volunteer to live in this union. These characteristics are by no means gender-specific. Indeed, the only characteristics which are gender specific are related to procreation. And maintaining these as key or sole characteristics of marriage are highly debatable and demeaning to those who might be unable for one reason or another to bear children. ...

The SACC's recommendation, under these circumstances, therefore, is to support the first option and simple recommendation of the Constitutional Court to amend the Marriage Act to include the word 'spouse' after 'husband'. We believe from a faith perspective that such an amendment would be 'generous', simple and illustrative of our commitment to advance the quest for genuine equality amidst our national diversity and difference. ...

Contralesa
[*The Civil Union Bill was also referred to the Congress of Traditional Leaders of South Africa (Contralesa), which presented its submission to the Portfolio Committee on Home Affairs on 24 October 2006*]
... The institution of Traditional Leadership is the sole and authentic voice of the overwhelming majority of the people of South Africa leaving [sic] in traditional communities. Although our government has tried to better their lives for more than a decade now ma[n]y of our communities have no basic services. For this reason and more although we appreciated the public hearings of this Committee many people would have liked to attend the public hearings but could not do so.

Due to the fact that they are fundamentally opposed to the idea of notion of a man marrying another man or a woman another woman as contemplated by the Bill before this Committee, we have been mandated to make this submission to our Parliament ...

We maintain that throughout Africa the indigenous people have had their traditions, cultures and languages invaded by foreign elements that have used force to disorient them and prevent them from utilizing their own traditional norms and values to maintain peace and order in their communities. Africa has paid a heavy price. Unfortunately as African majority governments have been voted into power using Eurocentric 'democratic' constitutions, they have generally refused to give recognition to their own traditional norms and values. The tragic consequences can be seen in the wars, strife and moral degeneration that are pervasive throughout the continent. Africans need access to systems of governance, particularly at the local community level which they know and understand. We appeal to the Parliament to set aside borrowed euro-centric thinking and approach this issues as Africans. It is a mater of greatest consequence to rural communities. Their wishes must not be ignored in what appears to be a determined effort to impose foreign ethical norms and values at any cost in South Africa. ...

Parliaments are known to have passed laws in order to achieve certain goals, only to find that, upon subjection to judicial scrutiny and interpretation, they bring about undesirable and unintended consequences. We submit that the Constitutional Assembly, which drafted and adopted the constitution, never contemplated that the provision prohibiting unfair discrimination against homosexuals could ever be construed as legalizing same-sex marriages. The judgment of the Constitutional Court is a classic case of an undesirable and unintended consequence. ...

We are reluctant to begin to outline the bases on which we assert that it is wrong to legalize same-sex marriages. There are things in life which do not merit justification for them to be valid. Opposition to same-sex marriage is one such thing. Same sex marriage is against nature, culture (all types of culture), religion and common sense, let alone decency. ...

In most African societies marriage is not just a matter for the two individuals concerned. Marriage is between two families, two clans, two tribes and even two nations. It is about the establishment of blood ties between the two entities through, among others, the birth of children. A same-sex marriage cannot bring about the birth of children. ...

The most worrying fact of all, though, is the seeming acceptance of this oddity to the extent that it appears to be a norm. There does not seem to be any attempts being made to help the afflicted to get remedy. The practitioners are having the field all to themselves, ready at a moment's whim to brand those who don't understand this oddity as being homophobic. For the record, we are not homophobic. We know and even respect some people who happen to be homosexual. We simply don't understand why there would be people who deem it appropriate that Parliament should be called upon to make a law to effectively say homosexuality is such a normal norm, that marriage as we have come to know it, should also include same-sex intimate relations. ...

We acknowledge that Gays and Lesbians are human beings and as such should [be] treated with human dignity. However to accord them rights to marry each other will offend and render useless the cultural norms and values which are also enshrined in the Constitution of the Republic of South Africa. ...

We objected to the certification of the Constitution on the basis that it is Eurocentric and will lead to undesirable consequences such as the Constitutional court judgement in question. The court's decision is in our view telling Parliament which passed our Constitution in 1996 to lie on the bed it has made for itself.

We consequently call upon our Parliament not to pass the Bill in question instead to amend the Constitution to sure the unintended consequences of extending the rights to marry same sex partners or to refer this matter to a National Referendum. ...

In our view no form or any amendment could ever cure such an objectionable and offensive piece of legislation. Like apartheid it can not be reformed. The only step that Parliament should take is for it to reject it in its entirety.

A letter of complaint about hate speech

During the public hearings on the Civil Union Bill, concerns were raised by LGBTI organizations and others about the homophobic hate speech that was expressed at the hearings. On 9 October, the Joint Working Group lodged a letter of compliant with Parliament on this issue. The letter was addressed to the Speaker, Baleka Mbete; the Honourable Deputy Minster of Home Affairs, Malusi Gigaba; and the Chair of Committees, Geoffrey Doidge.

Letter to Parliament
As the Joint Working Group, a national network of seventeen organizations working in the LGBT (lesbian, gay, bisexual and transgender) sector, we wish to express our serious concern about the manner and process by which the public hearings on the Civil Union Bill were conducted. ...

The concerns we wish to raise, based on our presence at the hearings held in Soweto, Polokwane, Welkom, Nelspriut, Rustenberg, New Hanover, Umtata and Upington, are as follows:
- At the outset of the hearings, no parameters for the discussions were set. ... The lack of parameters allowed numerous instances of hate speech, against lesbian and gay people, to be freely expressed. In these cases, no attempts were made by the Chair to curtail such speech and indicate that such speech was contrary to the Constitution.
- A climate of tolerance and respect was not created at the hearings, such that lesbian and gay individuals could safely and freely voice their views. To the contrary, allowing discriminatory comments from the floor resulted in lesbian and gay local community members being too fearful to express themselves at the hearings.
- The last minute rescheduling of the venue and/or times of the hearing in Limpopo and KwaZulu-Natal. This leads us to believe that there were interests to influence which constituencies were present at the hearings.

... In taking the public hearings to remote areas such as villages and rural areas, where there are no gay and lesbian organisations in operation, [the Portfolio Committee on Home Affairs] disadvantaged the potential for LGBT organisations and individuals to raise their concerns with the Bill. There are gay and lesbian people living in these areas, but they are understandably not publicly open about their sexual orientation; for them to come and speak at these hearings, in a climate of intolerance and without support, could pose a physical danger.

Parliament has the responsibility to conduct public hearings in a manner that embodies the principles of our Constitution and not to wittingly create a platform for victimization of citizens. In addition, parliament has a mandate to set the parameters for public discussions, within the context of constitutional values. This has not been the case in the hearings thus far.

Instead, the very tenets of equality and freedom, in relation to sexual orientation, were themselves up for debate at some of the hearings. ...

Based on the manner in which the public hearing process has been conducted, we question the ability of the Chair of the Committee who is tasked to facilitate a public participation process on the Bill, to take a non-partisan approach on the matter at hand. ...

We hereby request that parliament takes all necessary steps to ensure that our constitutional values are not compromised during the deliberations on the Civil Union Bill, and that a climate is created for equal and respectful participation by lesbian and gay individuals and organizations.

The Civil Union Bill is debated in the National Assembly

On 14 November 2006 a substantially amended version of the Civil Union Bill was debated in the National Assembly (NA) of the South African Parliament (available at www.info.gov.za/gazette/bills/2006/b26b-06.pdf).

The Bill was presented to the NA by the Minister of Home Affairs. All political parties had an opportunity to voice their position on the Bill. The Bill was passed by the NA (230 votes in favour, 41 against, and three abstentions). It was then referred to the second house of parliament – the National Council of Provinces (NCOP) – for consideration. Below are extracts from the debate in the NA on 14 November 2006 (from Revised Hansard).

Ms Nosiviwe Mapisa-Nqakula (Minister of Home Affairs, African National Congress)
... The process of debate on this Bill has been rigorous. The extensive media coverage on the debate on the Bill has resulted in the debate continuing in our homes, workplaces and communities throughout our country. One thing that came out of the debate has been an indication that people in all sections of our society feel very strongly about the issues being dealt with in this Bill. ... The challenge that we

shall continue to face has to do with the fact that when we attained our democracy, we sought to distinguish ourselves from an unjust painful past by declaring that: Never again shall it be that any South African will be discriminated against on the basis of colour, creed, culture and sex.

This House, in passing the Constitution in 1996, recognised the fact that our nation's commitment to this noble principle of equality should be the cornerstone of the society we want to build. In breaking with our past, therefore, we need to fight and resist all forms of discrimination and prejudice, including homophobia.... As far back as 1996, government itself recognised that the legal regime that regulates marriage in our country needs to be realigned with constitutional principles. It is for this reason that the Law Reform Commission started work on the review of the marriage legislation in the country. However, during that process, the definition of marriage in our current law faced a challenge within our courts. ... We've decided to reject the calls to amend the Constitution. Whilst we understand that the Constitution can be amended from time to time to deal with practical arrangements, we are cautious of an amendment to the Bill of Rights, as it is the bedrock on which our Constitution and our democracy is based. We also do not share the current view amongst others in our society that in order to recognise one of the rights in our Constitution, you need to take away another. Our Constitution clearly makes room for the right of people to be treated equally without a hierarchy including, as it is in this case, a situation where those rights are for a minority in our country. ... It is very important for members to appreciate that within the three spheres of government, Parliament should continue to be the one bearing the responsibility to pass legislation and not have the consequences of the judiciary performing this function on behalf of the legislature.

The principle of separation of powers therefore needs to be protected, and it is for this reason that we have chosen to adhere to the directive of the Constitutional Court, and not allow the Court itself to amend a piece of legislation.

The dynamic interface and respect for the different roles of the three spheres of governance will be a reflection of a healthy democracy.

Mr HP Chauke (Chairperson of the Portfolio Committee on Home Affairs, ANC)
... Let me start by taking this opportunity to outline the manner in which we have handled this Bill and that is that, when the Bill was tabled before Parliament, there were problems already around the constitutionality of the Bill. As we all know, the state law advisor found that there are problems within the Bill on which he could not give a clear report to Parliament on the constitutionality of the Bill with a number of recommendations that he made.[7] ... We then decided as a committee that we should embark on a programme of public hearings. It's normal procedure that on any Bill

that is before Parliament, we will have to have public hearings but we then extended the hearings to go around the country because of our understanding of the nature and the sensitivity of the matter that was before the committee. ...

One of the issues that came out [of the public hearings] was the issue of amending the Constitution. ...

The second view that came out of the public hearing was that of holding a referendum ... to test the will of the people. ...

The third thing that came out very strongly was that the Bill itself had in it a component that dealt with the issue of a civil union and the issue of domestic partnership. The majority of the people again felt that the issue of domestic partnership interfered with customary marriage and that it interfered generally with any relationship because what it was saying was that, like any relationship that you get into, it may be a registered or non-registered relationship, but automatically you would be covered by the law. Most of the people felt very strongly that it was not necessary for us to engage on that matter, especially a matter which was not quite urgent. We put it aside ... What was coming across, however, was the fourth point, which was the time allocated for Parliament to handle this matter because ... people felt very strongly that there was a need ... to have more time so as to allow more debate around the issue before us.

The last point obviously was the usage of the word 'marriage' in the Bill. People felt very strongly that, whatever it is that we want to do, we should not use the word 'marriage'. You know that there were a number of organisations and churches that marched to send their memorandums, who sent a number of submissions that were talking about the usage of the word 'marriage' itself. Other speakers will come who will address that part as to why we have opted to have 'marriage' in the Bill. ...

The biggest challenge ... is that we have to make sure that we meet the Constitutional Court judgment and, given the manner in which the Minister has elaborated on these issues, we have tried in fact to respond to that Constitutional Court judgment. We have removed the domestic partnership, as the people have said. We have looked at the Bill itself and said that to make it only for a specific group of people will not be correct. Why can't we open this Bill to allow not only same-sex partners but also each and every one? ...

Ms SV Kaylan (Democratic Alliance)
... A significant observation that emerged during the hearings is the extraordinary high level of homophobia and homoprejudice that exists in our country. While much of it is rooted in sheer ignorance, some of the views expressed were just pure vitriol and malice. On a personal note, during the public hearings I often had to sit on my hand and bite my tongue when outrageous and often provocative antigay comments were made. I would like to applaud the gay and lesbian group-

ings for standing their ground, often in the face of strong opposition, mockery and sarcasm. ... Five thousand eight hundred petitions, 637 written submissions and countless hearings later, we are here to vote on an amended version of the Civil Union Bill. It is quite unfortunate that the ANC pulled the amended version of this Bill out of the bottom drawer merely a day before voting in the committee. It is my considered opinion that the portfolio committee has misled the public in the hearings, because the version before us now is not the one presented during the hearings. I wonder how Judge Sachs will view the public participation clause he so expressly set out in the judgment. ... The Bill in front of us today is not purely a Civil Union Bill, but is in fact a second Marriage Act, merely couched in a different name in an effort to appease both sides and arrive at a middle-of-the-road solution. The essential difference is that the Marriage Act of 1961 allows for marriage between girls and boys. The Civil Union Bill of 2006 allows for the union or a marriage between boys and boys or girls and girls or girls and boys. To put it bluntly, the straight guys have two choices in respect of marriage, and the gay guys only have one option. ...

Parliament would do well to ask the Constitutional Court for an extension of time, so as to do justice to the task at hand and to rewrite the Marriage Act in the light of our democratic dispensation. ... The ideal is to have one Marriage Act for everyone. It is the only way to truly recognise the equality of all our people.

As a nation, we have a long way to go to eradicate discrimination on the grounds of sexual orientation. Some members of the DA are opposed in principle to the Bill as they are of the opinion that the Bill fails in terms of the equality clause of the Bill of Rights. The DA will allow a conscience and free vote on this Bill.

Ms I Mars (Inkatha Freedom Party)
... We as a party support strong moral values and the role of the family as the foundation pillar of society. We know that many colleagues across the political spectrum share this view. This, however, does not imply contempt of the Constitution or of the judgment of the court. Last week, and only last week, the ruling party presented the latest version of this Bill that is now before us. In all honesty, we have not been able to discuss it broadly enough, again, because of the shortage of time. ...

It would be the understatement of the year to say that the original Bill has caused tremendous controversy ... When the Portfolio Committee on Home Affairs took the Bill around the country in a comprehensive series of public hearings, it quickly became apparent that not only did it stir up emotions on all sides, it was also opposed by large sections of the communities on religious and moral grounds, as well as by the intended beneficiaries but for very different reasons. ...

This Bill is not supported by the IFP. I thank you.

Mr LW Greyling (Independent Democrats)

Madam Deputy Speaker, this is the tenth anniversary of our beloved Constitution. South Africans always mention with pride that ours is the most progressive constitution in the world. Unfortunately, however, the values of our society do not always match the progressive values of our Constitution. This has been particularly evident in the public hearings on this Bill, which some people have used as a platform to express some of the most deplorable and deep-seated prejudices. It is clear that we have a long way to go before we can build a truly tolerant society where all our divisions can be bridged. What has shocked the ID, however, has been the attitude of the ANC on this issue. Instead of showing true leadership, they chose to compromise on constitutional principles in an effort to appease both sides. Instead they have alienated both and drafted legislation that could be challenged in the Constitutional Court. In particular the clause that civil marriage officers can refuse to marry gay couples can certainly be seen to be discriminatory. Given our tragic history they should have also known that, as the South African Council of Churches stated, separate doesn't ever mean equal. As the ID upholds the Constitution and the values therein, we are left with no choice but to oppose the Civil Union Bill.

Reverend KRJ Meshoe (African Christian Democratic Party)

I believe this is the saddest day of the 12 years of our democratic Parliament when some members of this House, led by the ruling party, will be passing into law the Civil Union Bill which is opposed by the overwhelming majority of our people. ... Their views have, for all intent and purposes, been ignored and rejected. ...

The Civil Union Bill justifies immorality and by inference calls sexual perversion a legitimate alternative lifestyle that should be openly accepted. ... May I remind this House that rejecting God's house and despising His word will result in those doing it being given over to the consequences of their sins and divine wrath. ...

Adultery, sexual immorality and homosexuality are grave sins in God's sight since they are a transgression of His law and defile the marriage relationship between a man and a woman. ... While the ACDP appreciates that this Bill is an attempt to meet the Constitutional Court ruling, we nevertheless believe it has gone beyond what was required by the court.

Dr CP Mulder (Freedom Front)

This Bill that will make same-sex marriages possible is extremely controversial. Nobody wants it, not even the majority of the ANC caucus. The ANC had to resolve to compel all its members to vote for this Bill today and still it is being forced through.

... Why? Because the Word of God is not the highest authority in this country, but in fact the man-made Constitution is. ...

A constitution and its practical implications in law should take the values of the community it serves into account. Exercising rights should not go against the value system of society, because if it does, it estranges the constitution from the community. ...

The Christian community is against it. The Muslim community is against it. The traditional leaders are against it and yet it is still forced through.

Marriage is an institution created by God between a man and a woman. That is why God created Adam and Eve and not Adam and Steve. We will vote against this Bill for that reason.

Mr Mosiuoa Lekota (Minister of Defence, ANC)

Madam Chairperson, honourable members, I think it is important that we place the Bill in its proper historical context. The roots of this Bill lie in the pronouncements of our people over very many years and decades of struggle. In particular, the roots of this Bill lie in the declaration our people made at the Congress of the People in 1955. In the preamble of the Freedom Charter, our people declared, and I quote:

> Only a democratic state based on the will of all the people can secure to all their birthright without distinction of colour, race, sex or belief.

It was this declaration, amongst others, which guided us in drafting the present democratic national Constitution, hailed throughout the world as one of the most advanced at this time.

The Constitution itself does not prevaricate on this question, for it says so in Chapter 2, section 9, subsection 3. We ourselves declare to this House that:

> The state may not unfairly discriminate directly and indirectly against anyone on one or more grounds, including race, gender, sex, pregnancy, marital status, ethnic or social origin, colour, sexual orientation, age, disability, religion, conscience, belief, culture, language and birth.

What the Constitutional Court did was not to impose on us the task of making a new law. Rather, the Constitutional Court drew our attention to the fact that we have granted the right to all South African citizens to choose who to marry ...

The Constitutional Court reminded us that, in this regard, we have not as yet delivered in relation to those who prefer same-sex partners for life. They were not saying: Grant new rights. They said: You have already granted this right, but deliver on that right in relation to those who prefer same-sex partners. ...

The question before us, therefore, is not whether same-sex marriages or civil unions are right or not. That's not the question. The question is whether we suppress those in our society who prefer same-sex partners or not.

... Are we going to suppress this so-called minority, or are we going to let these people, like ourselves, enjoy the privilege of choosing who will be their life partners or not?

By the way, voting for this Bill is not advocating. We are not being asked to advocate same-sex marriages. We are being asked to grant this right ... you will continue to live your life as you choose, but let's grant the right to those who also must exercise the same right.

We have no need indeed to preserve for ourselves, purely because of the majority of our numbers, the exclusive right of marriage as recognisable in law, while we deny others the same right. Why would we want to do that? I take this opportunity to remind the House, to remind those who know, and inform those who do not know, that in the long and arduous struggle for democracy very many men and women of homosexual and lesbian orientation joined the ranks of the liberation and democratic forces. Some went into exile. ... others went into the prisons of the country with us. ... Some stood with us, ready to face death sentences. ...

Today, as we reap the fruits of that democracy, it is only right that they must be afforded similar space in the sunshine of our democracy. We do them no favour, but reward their efforts in the same way that our own efforts are being rewarded. I have to remind the House that, after all, culture is not static.

There was a time when voting was only for men. ... There was a time when society would not accept that women should vote. ...

This country cannot afford to continue to be a prisoner of the backward, timeworn prejudices which have no basis. The time has come that we as this society, as this Parliament, on behalf of our nation, must lead.

I therefore wish to urge members of the House to look past the prejudices of our time, and grant this right to those who have been pleading with us for so long now so that we may bequeath to succeeding generations a society democratic and more tolerant than the one that was handed down to us by those who preceded us. I thank you.

Dr EM Pheko (Pan African Congress)
Chairperson, the traditional institution of a union between a man and a woman for procreation must be protected. It cannot be equated with same-sex unions. Same-sex marriages are so repugnant that only four countries in the whole world have legalised them. Do we want our country to be the fifth in the world and the first in Africa to be in this mess? Which country in Africa will accept leadership from a country that suffers from Eurocentric eccentricity? Only those who have sold their souls to cultural imperialism will support this obscenity.

It is hypocritical in the extreme to talk of moral regeneration and the African Renaissance and then to turn around and surrender to this cultural aberration. It is no excuse that it is in the Constitution. It should never have been there in the first place.

The issues in the country are landlessness, inhumane squatting, unaffordable education, unemployment, lack of good health care and the eradication of poverty. These are the things that people fought for.

This Bill needed a national referendum if this Parliament were to respect the people of this country. ...

Advocate J de Lange (Deputy Minister for Justice and Constitutional Development, ANC)

I feel ashamed to be South African and to have experienced what people had to experience before the passing of this Bill, and about some of the things that were said in this House. If God is the God of love and you want to come and profess that God to us, then show us his loving face. ...

... [T]he ANC has very clearly stated its position on this. The Constitution is very clear; we are not doing any favours to gay people here. We are not giving them little pieces of goodwill. We are dealing here with what we decided upon at least 12 years ago when the equality clause was passed, which said we should not discriminate on the basis of sex, sexual orientation or marital status. That is what your Constitution says.

Today some of the people who helped pass that Constitution are sitting here with wide eyes saying: But we could never have meant that. What on earth do you think you meant if you said you are not going to discriminate on the basis of marital and on the basis of sexual orientation?

Regarding the [conscientious-objection clause] ... Let me remind you what Judge Sachs said on dealing with this issue about conscience. It says in paragraph 159:

> The principle of reasonable accommodation could be applied by the state to ensure that civil marriage officers who had sincere religious objections to officiating at same-sex marriages would not themselves be obliged to do so if this resulted in the violation of their conscience. ...

Now, we are told that the Constitutional Court will find that to be unconstitutional. I think the issue here is simply this. The Constitutional Court in its court order did two things. The substance of marriages is only dealt with in two places; in the common law, the definition of marriage and in the formula for marriage. In the rest of the Marriage Act it is just the procedures and processes of how you do that. ... Now, the issue for us in government was not whether we would allow this or not, but it was how to do it best.

Ms Nosiviwe Mapisa-Nqakula (Minister of Home Affairs, ANC)

Madam Chair, I just want to correct the fact that some people have made comments which I really think are not correct, and we need to set the record straight.

It is not true that we are dealing here with a new piece of legislation. I think what we are dealing with here is the same Bill which was presented before the portfolio committee or before Parliament. What has happened is that, on the basis of what has emerged from the public participation process and from the consultation with a variety of stakeholders, certain amendments have been made and that's what we are dealing with here. So, there is no new piece of legislation.

If I may touch on just two of those, most stakeholders actually made the point that there is a need to deal with the issue of domestic partnerships at a later date, because we had no constitutional deadline to meet. That has been removed from this piece of legislation.

The second issue was the issue of being separate but equal. In spite of trying our best to meet the two principles which were stated by the Constitutional Court and also to look at the rights, status, benefits and the responsibilities to give all those to same-sex couples in this particular piece of legislation, people still maintained that this was a separate but equal route. ...

... [W]e then had to actually make sure that this Bill did not only cater for same-sex couples but also for heterosexual couples who want to go the civil partnership route. That's what we have done here.

... [O]ne area which remains contentious, which I believe is still in the public discourse and there is a need to engage on, is the whole issue of marriage. There has been insistence on that from quite a number of stakeholders, that there should be no reference to marriage at all in this piece of legislation. ...

We believe we knew when we brought about this Civil Union Bill that this is not a matter society is going to agree on. That society is polarised. We are a divided society on this matter, but we have a responsibility of conducting continuous public education, of actually talking to people about the rights which have been provided by this very Constitution which we all passed in 1996, which we provided to all the people of South Africa. We now have a responsibility to deliver the promise contained, amongst others, in that Constitution and that Bill of Rights and that's what we are trying to provide here. ...

I think we all have a responsibility to step back, remove ourselves from the situation and look at the rights of a particular grouping of people here in this country, which does exist. It does exist and you cannot wish them away. There is no dustbin where you are going to collect a particular group of people and throw them into. We have a responsibility to society. Thank you.

The Civil Union Bill is debated in the National Council of Provinces

After the Bill was passed by the National Assembly, it was referred to the National Council of Provinces (NCOP) for consideration. The NCOP's Select Committee on Social Services called public hearings on 23 and 24 November 2006. On 28 November 2006 the NCOP passed the Bill (36 in favour, 11 against and one abstention). This was to be the version of the Civil Union Bill that would be signed into law by the Deputy President on the 30 November 2006.

A number of stakeholders made submissions in the NCOP, including the Joint Working Group (JWG), on behalf of the organized LGBTI sector.

The Joint Working Group (JWG)

... The JWG submission recognizes significant positive developments in the development of the Bill since it was first tabled in parliament.

• The Bill does not set up a separate institution solely for lesbian and gay people. Both heterosexual and same-sex couples may choose to marry in terms of the current Civil Union Bill.

• Lesbian and gay people have been unequivocally given the right to marry and will be able to achieve the same status that heterosexuals have in their marriages. The Bill allows same-sex couples to solemnise their relationships as marriages and have them recognized in law as such. In this way, lesbian and gay relationships are accorded the same status as heterosexual relationships.

Interestingly, the choice for same- and opposite-sex couples has been expanded by allowing them both to choose to enter into civil partnerships instead of marriages. Some people regardless of their sexual orientation do not wish to link themselves to the status, history and traditions of marriage. The Civil Union Bill gives all couples the opportunity to decide whether they want to form a marriage or a civil partnership whilst at the same time acquiring the same legal rights and responsibilities for their relationships.

Whilst welcoming the spirit of the Bill, the Joint Working Group still believed that there were a number of respects in which it could be improved.

Having various separate pieces of legislation dealing with marriage – including the Marriage Act, the Recognition of Customary Marriages Act and the Civil Union Bill – should be regarded as an interim measure only. There is no need or justification for so many separate pieces of legislation that effectively perform the same legal function.

In relation to the specific sections of the Bill, the JWG identified the following key problems:

Section 5 of the Bill will make it impossible for any minister or responsible person in a religious institution to solemnise marriages under this Bill where his or her religious institution has not made an application [in terms of Section 5 (1)] to be designated or has not been so designated despite having made such application [in terms of Section 5 (2)].

This will have a negative impact on many ministers of religion who wish to be marriage officers and who may decide to act against the dictates of the majority of the denomination of which they form part. Some religions may also not wish to take the step of being designated under the Civil Union Bill but may be happy for individual marriage officers to perform marriages in terms of the Civil Union Bill. Moreover, some individual ministers may wish to object to discriminatory policies of the denominations of which they are part and yet they will be precluded by the State from doing so. In this way, the State will prioritise the interests of religious authoritarian structures over those of the individual. This would violate the individual's constitutional rights to freedom of religion, belief and conscience referred to in the preamble of this Bill and thus would inappropriately silence debate and dissent within religious denominations.

Section 6 of the Bill is crafted in far wider terms than its counterpart in section 31 of the Marriage Act. In terms of section 6 of the Bill, any marriage officer may object on grounds of conscience to solemnising civil unions. By contrast, in terms of section 31 of the Marriage Act, only a minister of religion or a person holding a responsible position in a religious denomination or organisation may refuse to solemnize a marriage. Such a person may only refuse to perform a marriage on the basis that 'it would not conform to the rites, formularies, tenets, doctrines or discipline of his religious denomination or organisation'.

We have no objection to religious denominations only marrying people according to the dictates of their faith. We do, however, object strongly to allowing civil marriage officers to decide who they will marry and who they won't. This is particularly problematic when the basis for exercising conscience is limited to sexual orientation. ...

... [T]he message is reinforced that same-sex relationships merit different and unequal treatment to heterosexual relationships. Public officials, particularly magistrates, are required to honour and operationalise the Constitution. For this reason, we believe that this section may legitimate prejudice and is unconstitutional.

We believe that parliament has two choices here: either it restricts conscientious objection to religious marriage officers; or it allows civil marriage officers to object to marrying all couples that their religion does not allow them to marry. It cannot allow conscientious objection solely on the basis that parties to a marriage are of the same-sex.

The JWG also noted that Chapter 3 dealing with domestic partnerships had been severed from the Civil Union Bill.

It is critical that legislation – a Domestic Partnership Bill – be tabled in Parliament as a matter of urgency so as to ensure that vulnerable people who are, for whatever reason, unable to marry are able to gain legal protection for their relationships. However, we do not believe that domestic partnerships should be regulated in the same Bill as marriages or civil partnerships.

Ms JM Masilo (NCOP Select Committee on Social Services)
… the National Council of Province's Select Committee on Social Services rises to support the passing and enacting of the Civil Union Bill which was presented by the Department of Home Affairs to the committee on 21 November 2006. …

Significantly, Parliament's theme for this year 2006 is 'All shall have equal rights before the law'. Anything contrary to this fundamental principle is inhuman, as we have been reminded by Archbishop Desmond Tutu, our own reverend Nobel Peace Prize winner who is a Christian and an African. The Archbishop has always continued to publicly comment and to unapologetically acknowledge that homophobia or hating and discriminating against homosexuals is a crime against humanity and every bit unjust and evil as apartheid. …

As we all know, the current Marriage Act of 1961 does not even recognise marriages of other religions, and this is a blindly Christian bias. The Civil Union Bill thus facilitates for an enhanced constitutional right for all religious marriages. The Constitutional Court judgment sent a clear message that all South African adults have the right to choose their families and relationships while enjoying equal protection by the law. … The Civil Union Bill wisely shifts our paradigm to make us also understand that marriage is an expression of a dignified and solemn covenant between any two consenting adults irrespective of race, religious tradition or sexual orientation. … This Bill enables all capable consenting adults to express and share love and its manifold forms, meaning that gays and lesbians are also capable of constituting a family, including affection. They love the soul. …

This ANC-led government has and will also be lucid, transparent and consistent in embracing the Constitution of South Africa in its entirety. The People's Parliament will continue to respect the ruling of all courts, institutions of law. We will fulfil its mandate of making transformative legislation. …

Notes

1 Applications were made to the Constitutional Court, by Doctors For Life International and its legal representative Mr John Smyth, to be admitted as *amici curiae* in the *Fourie* case. They were granted leave to make written submissions and Smyth was authorized to address the Court orally.

2 The application of the Lesbian and Gay Equality Project for direct access to the Constitutional Court in the *Fourie* case was granted. The Court found it to be in the interests of justice for the *Fourie* and the *Equality Project* matters to be heard together. (See page 59 in this book.)

3 This applied only to civil marriage.

4 None of these options will preclude Parliament from considering other constitutionally permissible models at a later stage.

5 The Joint Working Group, representing the organized LGBTI sector, made both a lengthy written, and oral, submission to Parliament on the Civil Union Act. The version presented here is a summary version of the written submission that was made on behalf of the following organisations: Activate Wits, Behind the Mask, Durban Lesbian and Gay Community and Health Centre, Forum for the Empowerment of Women, Gay and Lesbian Archives, Gender DynamiX, Glorious Light Metropolitan Community Church, Good Hope Metropolitan Community Church, Hope and Unity Metropolitan Community Church, Jewish OutLook, LEGBO Northern Cape, Pietermaritzburg Gay and Lesbian Network, OUT LGBT Well-being, Out In Africa South African Gay and Lesbian Film Festival, Rainbow UCT, Triangle Project, UNISA Centre for Applied Psychology, XX/Y FLAME. The oral presentation made by the JWG to Parliament is available at http://www.exit.co.za/frmArticle.aspx?art=17 (last accessed 27 February 2008).

6 An application was made to the Constitutional Court by the Marriage Alliance, supported on affidavit by Cardinal Wilfred Napier of the South African Council of Bishops, to be admitted as *amicus curiae* in the *Fourie* case. The application, which included a request for the right to make both written and oral representations, was granted.

7 The state legal advisors refused to certify the Civil Union Bill, warning that is was unconstitutional.

3: FOR BETTER OR FOR WORSE
The Civil Union Act

The Civil Union Act:
Messy compromise or giant leap forward?

David Bilchitz with Melanie Judge

The Civil Union Act has famously provided the opportunity for same-sex couples to marry in South Africa. Yet it does so in the context of a piece of legislation that also allows couples to form a 'civil partnership' or a 'civil union'. What exactly are the differences between these terms and why does the Act create such a confusing array of relationship possibilities?

To understand the Civil Union Act, it is necessary to grasp that it was shaped by a range of social forces. Firstly, it represents the legislature's response to the Constitutional Court's finding in the *Fourie*[1] case that it had to enact a piece of legislation that provided same-sex couples with the same 'status, rights and responsibilities' for their relationships as heterosexual people have in marriage. The finding of the Court in many ways conditioned the debate that was to follow in the legislature, with various groups arguing for particular interpretations of this formula that would allow for the enactment of their desired remedy. Secondly, the Christian right and African traditionalists who recognized the constraints of the Constitution sought to promote a Bill which would prevent same-sex couples from 'marrying' but would allow them to form a 'civil partnership' that would provide same-sex couples with the same rights and responsibilities as heterosexual couples have. Thirdly, there were several submissions to Parliament that sought a constitutional amendment that would seek to protect marriage as an exclusively heterosexual institution. These voices – again largely from the religious right and African traditionalists – sought to deny any form of legislative recognition for same-sex relationships. Finally, gay and lesbian organizations, the human-rights community and the religious left sought an amendment to the existing Marriage Act (1961) that would have allowed same-sex couples to marry in terms of that Act.

What resulted from the public participation process in which these various forces were at play was an Act that did not repeal the Marriage Act but allowed both same- and opposite-sex couples to form a civil union which could take the form of either a marriage or a civil partnership. This essay will seek to investigate whether the resulting Act is an unsatisfactory compromise between these forces or whether it represents a genuine step forward for South African family law.

The initial Civil Union Bill

The Constitutional Court judgment in *Fourie* gave Parliament a year from 1 December 2005 to remedy the unconstitutionality of the existing marriage regime. The government did not act until July 2006. At this point, a flurry of activity began, with several different possibilities being proposed. The Department of Home Affairs first released a proposed Marriage Act Amendment Bill. It incorporated a gender-neutral amendment to the existing Marriage Act, which would have allowed same-sex couples to marry under that Act. However, this proposal was swiftly discarded, and later that month the Department of Home Affairs published the first draft of the Civil Union Bill.

The Bill was divided into two parts. Chapter 2 provided for the creation of civil partnerships for same-sex couples who wished their relationships to attract exactly the same legal rights and responsibilities as married heterosexual couples. Chapter 3 offered the opportunity for both same- and opposite-sex couples to form registered and unregistered domestic partnerships: such relationships would attract some legal consequences but generally offer fewer rights and responsibilities than a marriage or civil partnership. The focus of this discussion will be on Chapter 2, which involved the proposed creation of a new status or institution in South African law, the civil partnership. A civil partnership in terms of this Bill meant a 'voluntary union between two adult persons of the same sex that is solemnized and registered in accordance with the procedures prescribed in this Act to the exclusion, while it lasts, of all others'.[2] Only same-sex couples could have registered such a civil partnership, which had to be solemnized by a marriage officer.[3]

The initial Civil Union Bill would have created a personal law regime in South Africa with two related but central flaws: first, the Bill required same-sex relationships to be governed by a *separate* Act and institution (the civil partnership); secondly, the use of the term 'marriage' as designating a legal status would have remained the exclusive preserve of opposite-sex couples.[4] If all that was at stake was achieving the same rights and responsibilities for same-sex couples as opposite-sex couples already had in the law, then the initial Civil Union Bill would have achieved that aim.

Yet the Constitutional Court itself indicated the necessity to recognize that the exclusion of same-sex couples from the right to marry had an important symbolic content that served to entrench the inferiority of same-sex relationships: the exclusion 'represents a harsh if oblique statement by the law that same-sex couples are outsiders, and that their need for affirmation and protection of their intimate relations as human beings is somehow less than that of heterosexual couples ... It should be noted that the intangible damage to same-sex couples is as severe as the material deprivation.'[5] For this reason, presumably, the Court included in its finding of unconstitutionality that it was not only the rights and responsibilities of marriage that had to be accorded to same-sex couples but the same *status*.

To understand the problem with the initial Civil Union Bill, it is critical to understand the differences between 'civil partnerships' or 'civil unions' and 'marriage'. A civil partnership or union was proposed in several other countries as a way of granting same-sex relationships equal rights and responsibilities without using the term 'marriage' to describe such relationships.[6] But why is it necessary to avoid the use of 'marriage' to describe same-sex relationships? What importance can be attributed to the different locutions? In relation to a proposal by the Massachusetts legislature to assign 'civil unions' to same-sex couples and 'marriage' for opposite-sex couples, the majority in the *Goodridge* advisory opinion found that 'it is not the word "union" that incorporates a pejorative value judgment, but the distinction between the words "marriage" and "union".' The opinion continues: '[T]he dissimilitude between the terms "civil marriage" and "civil union" is not innocuous; it is a considered choice of language that reflects a demonstrable assigning of same-sex, largely homosexual, couples to second-class status.'[7] The *Goodridge* advisory opinion recognizes that the distinction between the two terms is suspect, for it contains within it a value judgment that would effectively entrench heterosexual supremacy: civil partnerships for gay and lesbian people but marriage for heterosexual people.[8]

These two institutions may thus be indistinguishable in terms of the legal rights they offer, yet nevertheless differ largely in terms of the social meanings and status they confer on a couple. Civil partnerships have been referred to as a 'pale shadow of marriage':[9] they come with none of the reputation, experience, position, influence, standing in the community, traditions and prestige of marriage.[10] Marriage has a long history, a particular status in society and a range of associated rituals. Marriage, for many, also has a religious and spiritual meaning. No other institution, particularly not one that is a recent creation of statute, has these attributes.

An amendment to the Marriage Act?
Since the difference between civil partnerships and marriage matters, the initial Civil Union Bill would have continued to relegate same-sex relationships to a lesser status and to prevent same-sex couples from having the choice to provide their relationships with the social meanings generally reserved for marriage. Consequently, during the parliamentary hearings on the Civil Union Bill in South Africa,[11] the organized lesbian and gay sector argued that no remedy other than allowing same-sex couples to be 'married' – both in word and substance – within the law would meet the requirements of the Constitution (as interpreted by the Constitutional Court in *Fourie*). Hence the solution favoured by many was simply to amend the Marriage Act to render it gender-neutral (the

words 'or spouse' would have been added into the marriage formula).[12] This was the remedy the Constitutional Court had stated would come into effect should Parliament fail to cure the constitutional defect within one year: in other words, its constitutionality was beyond doubt.[13] Such a remedy would have clearly embraced same-sex couples within the existing institution of marriage and rendered marriage for opposite- and same-sex couples equivalent in no uncertain terms.

This particular remedy, however, and its supporting reasoning, places in sharp focus what we wish to achieve as lesbian and gay people through the recognition of marriage rights for same-sex couples. If the right to marry is the only end goal, then perhaps an amendment to the Marriage Act would have been ideal. Yet many in the LGBTI community argue that the focus on marriage alone is predicated on a fundamentally conservative assumption: that same-sex couples should be admitted to equality provided that they are prepared to accommodate themselves to the 'ideal' of marriage set by heterosexuals.[14] This more radical perspective would contend that recognition of the right to marry may admit same-sex couples to respectability, but it does so while maintaining intact all the assumptions and features of the institution of marriage that have been oppressive to lesbian and gay people (as well as women and many others) over the ages. This model of relationship has, for instance, been centered on highly gendered constructions of male and female, and has served to maintain and perpetuate a particular set of gender relations, power structures and social and economic dynamics that are fundamentally unequal.[15] Apart from the problems relating to the connections of marriage to patriarchy, marriage has historically been tied to notions of possession, and its very status is said to dissuade and subordinate alternative relationship and familial forms.[16]

This perspective thus holds that same-sex couples should not only be admitted to equality on condition that they assimilate into a heterosexual institution;[17] rather, the very nature of what we regard as valuable forms of interpersonal relationships needs to be contested and reformulated in the light of lesbian and gay liberation.[18] Since no single model of relationship will cater to the needs of all individuals, the aim of law reform that extends recognition to same-sex couples should, it can be argued, not be concerned with marriage rights alone but rather seek to open a space, both in law and society, for different familial forms to be accorded equal respect and recognition.[19]

An amendment to the Marriage Act alone would have admitted same-sex couples to the institution of marriage without in any way challenging the dominance of this institution. A more creative and innovative legal solution would be necessary both to achieve status equality for same-sex couples while attaining wider social goals. We will argue in the next section that the Civil

Union Act that finally resulted from the public participation process, perhaps unintentionally, could provide an example of how to reconcile these disparate aims.

The Civil Union Act: Creating a range of relationship possibilities

After the oral and written submissions to Parliament,[20] the Minister of Home Affairs convened separate meetings with three main sectors: representatives of the lesbian and gay community,[21] representatives of various religious groups and representatives of the traditional leaders. These meetings appear to have been extremely important, because shortly thereafter a number of amendments were introduced to the initial Bill reflecting a number of the concerns expressed at these meetings. At the meeting with representatives of the organized lesbian and gay sector, the Minister explained the commitment of the government to equality for lesbian and gay people yet expressed her concern about the social divisiveness of recognizing full marriage for same-sex couples. The Constitution, she argued, was ahead of majority opinion in South Africa on homosexuality and, consequently, there was a need to create some compromise between the social forces at play. The lesbian and gay representatives, on the other hand, stressed the importance of having our full equality and dignity recognized in the law and that we were not to be relegated to a second-class status. The Minister was essentially presented with two bottom lines for the lesbian and gay community: same-sex couples should be able to have their relationships designated as 'marriages' in the law; and both opposite- and same-sex couples should be able to be married in the same Act.

Lobbying by the various groups continued after this meeting and a week later, we received a revised draft of the Bill. From our perspective, there are two central changes between the Civil Union Act and the original Bill: first, both same-sex and opposite-sex couples can form a civil union in terms of the new Act. This means that the Civil Union Act becomes an inclusive Act both for opposite-sex and same-sex couples rather than being a separate, exclusive Act only applicable to same-sex couples. Secondly, the law creates a relatively complex mixture of terms that can refer to different relationship forms with the same legal effect: the overarching category of the 'civil union' includes two relationship forms – 'marriage' and 'civil partnership' – between which one must choose. The legal consequences of a marriage both in terms of the Marriage Act and in terms of the common law apply to a civil union (and its two relationship forms).[22] This legal framework for personal relationships requires further scrutiny because it is not immediately obvious what the significance of these different terms is. The transformative possibilities of the Civil Union Act lie, in our view, precisely in the differences and similarities of the relationship forms it creates.

It is of central importance that the law allows same-sex couples to refer to their relationships as marriages, not just in the marriage formula at the time of their solemnization, but in terms of their actual designation in law. This means that the attempt to designate same-sex relationships as second-class by refusing the appellation of the term 'marriage' was not accepted by the legislature. The significance of this appellation can be appreciated when it is understood that only in five other jurisdictions around the world does the law expressly recognize that same-sex couples may form marriages.[23]

In addition, however, the Civil Union Act provides couples with a choice to create a 'civil partnership' as an alternative to marriage.[24] It is important to recognize that between the first draft of the Bill and the Act the meaning of a 'civil partnership' has fundamentally shifted. In the first draft of the Bill, a civil partnership was a new status or designation created in law solely for same-sex relationships while opposite-sex couples could only form a marriage. The regime was one of either/or and which designation one was given in the law depended upon the sex of one's partner.[25] This is how civil partnerships have generally been conceived of world-wide as alternative institutions providing legal rights and responsibilities for same-sex couples but avoiding the use of the term marriage to describe such relationships.[26]

In the Civil Union Act, however, a civil partnership is not a separate institution for same-sex couples. It is a status that two people of 18 years and older may decide to enter should they wish, irrespective of their sex or sexual orientation, which has the equivalent rights and responsibilities of a marriage in law.[27] It has no pejorative or exclusive meaning, but at first glance it is not clear on what basis it is distinguishable from a marriage. In our view, the choice between forming a civil partnership and a marriage has no legal consequences but provides the couples with an opportunity to decide on the personal and social meaning they wish to be attached to their relationship. Given that the connotations of a civil partnership are not yet clear in our society, this is an area of flux and creativity.

What then could lie behind the choice to designate one's relationship as a civil partnership rather than a marriage? Marriage has a particular history, a status in society and a range of associated rituals. For many, it also has a particular religious, spiritual and social meaning. Since we cannot simply create a status with the same historical resonances, the right to marry was critical for many people who wish their relationships to be associated with these meanings. Yet there are some who do not wish to associate their relationships with the institution of marriage, though they do wish to have the same legal rights and responsibilities emanating from their relationships. Some of these individuals see marriage as an oppressive institution linked to gender hierarchies; others see marriage as linked to notions of possession and property from which they wish to dissociate themselves. For these reasons and others, people may prefer to use the designation 'civil partnership' for their relationships rather than 'marriage'.

By giving both choices equal validity, the state effectively recognizes that the choice of social meanings should be an individual one, which should not be stigmatized in any way.[28] Whether intended or not, the law now opens up certain social possibilities that involve an interesting paradox: it is the very status and social meaning of marriage that, when provided as an equal option alongside civil partnerships, provides civil partnerships with a similar status; however, the creation of an equal alternative option to marriage also in some sense decentres marriage as the primary and privileged social option for committed interpersonal relationships.

This decentring of marriage occurs further through the use of the term 'civil union'. A civil union effectively becomes a general 'class' term for two possible forms in which the law will recognize and protect interpersonal relationships – a marriage or a civil partnership. This formula opens the door for the legislature to extend the notion of a 'civil union' even further to embrace a wide range of relationships, including registered or unregistered domestic partnerships, Islamic marriages and customary marriages. This could allow for the consolidation of personal law in South Africa within a broad class that is understood in and of itself to embrace diversity (both in social meanings and in legal consequences). In this way, marriage could become but one form of legal recognition a relationship can attain, with the notion of the 'civil union' becoming the class term to embrace a wide range of personal relationships within its ambit.[29]

In this respect, the Act has found a way to accomplish several goals at once: same-sex couples are enabled to marry and, if they wish, to embrace the social meanings attached to the institution of marriage. However, the legislation sets up a choice for both opposite-sex and same-sex couples to designate their relationships in a different way should they so wish. It also replaces 'marriage' as the central term protecting close interpersonal relationships with the notion of a 'civil union', rendering marriage simply one possible choice among others. On this reading, the Act represents a sophisticated piece of legislation that goes beyond purely including same-sex couples within the institution of marriage but also serves to create the foundations for a truly inclusive and diverse family law regime in South Africa.[30]

An unsatisfactory compromise?

Despite the possibilities the Civil Union Act opens up, there are several features of the new legal framework that it brought into being that constrain its ability to realize its potential. While the government responded to the representations and activism of the lesbian and gay organizations, it also appears to have listened in certain respects to representations from Christian-right groupings and African traditionalists. The government's attempt to compromise with these other groups resulted in certain features of the Act and the legal framework relating to marriage that threaten to undermine the advances made by the Civil Union Act in several important respects. These elements of the Act will now be analyzed, with brief proposals made for their reform.

The Marriage Act was not repealed

Perhaps one of the most problematic features of the current legal framework is the retention of the existing Marriage Act, which is reserved for heterosexuals alone and which was not repealed by the Civil Union Act. It is irrational that there be two pieces of legislation on the statute book that effectively perform the same function (at least for opposite-sex couples) and this feature of our current legal framework can only be explained as an attempt to appease those who do not want to have to marry under the same Act as same-sex couples.

The continued existence of the Marriage Act also could create several difficulties for transgendered people: should a transgendered person be married, in terms of the Marriage Act, to an individual who is of the opposite sex but then re-assigns their gender, such a person would be forced to divorce their spouse and re-marry under the Civil Union Act, even if neither party wishes to divorce. Such complications do not exist under the Civil Union Act, which is gender-neutral.

There are also a few provisions within the two Acts that are inconsistent with one another, which generally reflect the outdated nature of the Marriage Act. For instance, the Marriage Act distinguishes between the ages at which male and female minors may be married with parental consent: a male minor may be married at the age of 18 and a female minor at the age of 15.[31] Such distinctions are based upon highly contestable gendered assumptions and are, consequently, in our view constitutionally suspect. Moreover, this provision is inconsistent with the fact that the current age of consent in South African law for intercourse is 16. The Marriage Act thus allows minor females to be married at 15 but such persons are prohibited from consummating their marriages via sexual intercourse.[32] The Civil Union Act, on the other hand, does not distinguish between the ages at which men and women may marry.[33] The Marriage Act, until recently, only allowed marriages between persons of 21 years and older without parental consent.[34] The Civil Union Act, however, allows marriages to be conducted between persons of 18 years and older without parental consent.[35]

It also remains unclear whether there will be social distinctions between couples whose marriages are conducted under the Marriage Act and those married in terms of the Civil Union Act, though this seems unlikely. As more couples – both same-sex and opposite-sex – are married under the Civil Union

Act, and this becomes an act of choice (something that our activism needs to ensure), it seems that over time the archaic and gendered Marriage Act may well be repealed or fall into disuse. Nevertheless, its continued existence as an exclusively heterosexual Act is a symbolic affront to lesbian and gay people.

Conscientious objection for civil marriage officers

There are features of the Civil Union Act, however, that negatively affect same-sex couples in ways that go beyond the symbolic. Perhaps the most important of these is Section 6 of the Act, which allows civil marriage officers to object, on the basis of conscience, to the performance of civil unions between persons of the same sex. There are no good grounds to object to religious marriage officers only having to marry people according to the dictates of their faith. This would in fact appear to be an incidence of religious freedom as enshrined in Section 15 (1) of our Constitution.[36] Yet there are strong grounds on which to object to allowing civil marriage officers to decide who they will marry and who they will not marry, particularly if the basis for exercising their conscience is limited to sexual orientation.

The provision of a specific conscientious-objection clause relating to same-sex couples suggests that there is greater reason for civil marriage officers to object to solemnizing the unions of same-sex couples than to heterosexual couples: there is no clear reason why this should be so, unless the Act were entrenching the view that same-sex relationships are in some sense inherently more controversial than heterosexual relationships and thus not really equal in status and worth. To understand the insult inherent in this provision, consider whether the law, mindful of the controversial nature of interracial marriage for some in South Africa, should provide that civil marriage officers may conscientiously object to performing interracial marriages? The prohibition on interracial marriages was one of the most iniquitous laws of apartheid South Africa: should officers of the state be allowed to object to such provisions, they would be maintaining the injustice and oppression of the past rather than being forced – as public officials – to distance themselves from it. The same applies in connection with same-sex couples. Public officials should be required to uphold the law in an impartial manner and not cast judgment on people who approach them to fulfill an official function. For same-sex couples to be turned away by a civil marriage officer could be deeply insulting, hurtful and a violation of dignity. Public officials, particularly magistrates, are bound to honour and give effect to the principles enshrined in the Constitution. This section of the Civil Union Act may legitimate prejudice and is almost certainly unconstitutional: it should be replaced by an exemption only allowing religious marriage officers to refuse to marry those who do not conform with the tenets of their faith.

Reducing the scope of conscience for religious marriage officers

Section 6 of the Civil Union Act, discussed above, essentially creates an 'opt-out provision' for civil marriage officers. Section 5 creates an 'opt-in' provision for religious marriage officers. Thus, instead of automatically allowing religious marriage officers registered in terms of the Marriage Act to officiate at civil unions conducted in terms of the Civil Union Act, the Act requires denominations as well as individual marriage officers to opt in to the performance of civil unions. In order to do so, the religious denomination or organization in question must first apply to be designated by the Minister of Home Affairs to perform marriages in terms of the Civil Union Act.[37] The individual marriage officer must also apply in writing to be registered as a marriage officer in terms of the Civil Union Act.[38]

This raises a fundamental contradiction between the provisions relating to civil marriage officers and those relating to religious marriage officers. For civil marriage officers, the individual's freedom of conscience, belief or religion is prioritized over the state's duty to ensure the uniform application of the law. For religious marriage officers, however, the effect of the provisions is that their individual beliefs must give way to the discipline of the denomination: a religious denomination that fails to apply for a designation can prevent its ministers from solemnizing civil unions. This means that the state, in a violation of its supposed neutrality, effectively recognizes the view of the majority leadership of a denomination as opposed to minorities – even sizeable ones – within denominations. This will have a negative impact on many ministers of religion who wish to be marriage officers and may decide on the basis of their own faith convictions to act against the dictates of their denomination. It should be left to denominations to decide how to respond to marriage officers that do not perform marriages in accordance with the tenets of that denomination, or those who seek to revise those tenets in line with the diverse values reflected in their communities. It is neither necessary nor permissible for the law to constrain the social meanings that may develop within communities of faith and thus prevent the important and inevitable evolution of religion.

Same-sex customary marriages?

One of the last-minute changes to the Civil Union Act involved the exclusion of civil unions from being recognized as marriages in terms of the Customary Marriages Act.[39] Similarly, the reference to husband, wife or spouse in terms of the Customary Marriages Act does not include a civil union partner. This basically excludes same-sex couples from contracting customary marriages. Now, while it is debatable whether or not same-sex couples could have contracted marriages in terms of that Act anyhow,[40] the explicit exclusion in the Civil Union Act was a late addition that appears to have been a response by the legislature to the vocal opposition to same-sex marriage on the part of the National House of Traditional Leaders and the Congress of Traditional Leaders of South Africa.[41] The attempt to separate same-sex marriage from African custom and tradition conveys an exclusionary social message that seeks to marginalize and silence the multiple forms of same-sex relationships and practices that are present in Africa.[42] This statutory exclusion limits the capacity of individuals who may wish to express their same-sex identities through the celebration of African customary marriages.[43] It also constrains communities from developing African customary traditions further so as to include same-sex marriage. This exclusionary element of the statute should be removed as it inappropriately limits the manner in which African identities may be expressed and so undermines the extent to which the Act can embrace the diverse forms of interpersonal relationships that individuals may wish to enter.[44]

Same-sex life partnerships and domestic partnerships
A large number of South Africans live together in intimate relationships outside of marriage. At present the law provides little protection to partners within such relationships.[45] Arguably, same-sex couples are currently in a better position than opposite-sex couples in this regard as a result of the Constitutional Court's recognizing the notion of a same-sex life partnership.[46] Recognition of a same-sex life partnership was, however, based on the fact that same-sex couples could not get married: once same-sex couples can form marriages, it is arguable that those who are not married must be placed in the same position as heterosexuals who are not married. This may erode the notion of a 'same-sex life partnership' and thus mean that, in time, same-sex couples who are not married have very little legal protection. Given the recent introduction of the Civil Union Act, however, it is likely that, as a matter of fairness, courts will continue for an interim period to recognize 'same-sex life partnerships' in order to protect those same-sex couples who have not yet had an opportunity to marry.

There is thus a necessity, for both opposite- and same-sex couples, that domestic-partnership legislation be passed. When the legislature produced the final draft of the Civil Union Act, it removed Chapter 3 of the initial Bill that had dealt with both registered and unregistered domestic partnerships. There were certainly deficiencies in the proposed provisions, but it is nevertheless critical that legislation – a Domestic Partnership Act – be tabled in Parliament as a matter of urgency to address the current legal vacuum surrounding co-habiting partners. There are good reasons rooted in rights-based considerations to ensure that those who do not marry or form a civil partnership are able to gain some form of legal protection for their relationships. The legal rights and consequences of domestic partnerships may not be identical to those of marriages or civil partnerships but their recognition in law would again help expand the range of choices individuals would have as to the legal regime they wish to govern their relationships.

A giant leap forward?

The Civil Union Act arose out of a constitutional imperative but was also subject to a range of political pressures. The pressures of the Christian right and the traditional leaders failed to result in a legal framework in which same-sex relationships were relegated to a second-class status: this in itself is a major victory for lesbian and gay people. Yet their involvement in the process leaves a range of residual provisions in our law, which bespeak a legislature seeking a compromise between contending elements. While many of these compromises are unacceptable and must be challenged, they do not fundamentally alter the fact that the Civil Union Act represents a giant leap forward for South African family law. The transformative potential of the Act also goes beyond even what a pure amendment to the Marriage Act could have attained. The achievement of the Civil Union Act is that it serves to open up the social space for two important goals to be realized: the recognition of the equal status of same-sex relationships; and the potential decentring of marriage and the according of respect and recognition to a diverse range of familial forms. Continued activism, public engagement and education will be necessary to ensure that the Act's potential is indeed realized not only in law but in the wider social arena.

Notes

This article draws heavily upon an article co-authored by David Bilchitz and Melanie Judge, 'For Whom Does the Bell Toll? The Challenges and Possibilities the Civil Union Act Creates for Family Law in South Africa', *South African Journal on Human Rights* 23 (2007). Permission has been granted by the publisher to use sections of the original article. The adaptation of the article for this book, incorporation of additional material and changes in argumentative emphasis has been performed by David Bilchitz.

1 *Minister of Home Affairs and Another v Fourie and Another* 2005 (3) BCLR 355 (CC); 2006 (1) SA 524 (CC) (hereinafter referred to as '*Fourie*'); *Lesbian and Gay Equality Project and Others v Minister of Home Affairs and Others* 2006 (1) SA 524 (CC)
2 Civil Union Bill (B26-2006, 31 August 2006), Section 1, http://www.info.gov.za/gazette/bills/2006/b26-06.pdf (last accessed 17 January 2008)
3 Ibid., Section 4 (1)
4 The law allowed same-sex couples to refer to their relationship as a 'marriage' during the ceremony but the relationship would be registered and recognized in law as a 'civil partnership' irrespective of the couple's choice (see Sections 11 and 12 of the initial Bill).
5 *Fourie*, op. cit., paragraph 71
6 See, for instance, the regimes enacted in Vermont, Connecticut, New Jersey and New Hamp-

shire in the United States and the Civil Partnership Act (2004) in the United Kingdom. For an overview of different regimes in Europe, see William N Eskridge and Darren R Spedale, *Gay Marriage: For Better or for Worse? What We've Learned From the Evidence* (OUP, 2006).

7 See the Majority in the Goodridge Advisory Opinion 440 Mass. 1201; 802 NE 2d 565 at 14

8 For more detail in this regard see David Bilchitz and Melanie Judge, 'For Whom Does the Bell Toll? The Challenges and Possibilities the Civil Union Act Creates for Family Law in South Africa', *South African Journal on Human Rights* 23 (2007)

9 Barbara J Cox, 'But Why Not Marriage? An Essay on Vermont's Civil Unions Law, Same-Sex Marriage, and Separate But (Un)equal', *Vermont Law Review* 25:1 (2000), 130

10 Ibid.

11 See submission of the Joint Working Group to Parliament, drafted by OUT LGBT Well-being, found at www.pmg.org.za/docs/2006/061017out.pdf (last accessed 17 January 2008). See also pages 124-127 of this book.

12 As has been mentioned, such a draft was proposed by the Department of Home Affairs and then quickly withdrawn, though it was later denied that such a draft was ever formally proposed.

13 *Fourie*, op. cit., paragraph 159

14 Steven Seidman, *Beyond the Closet: The Transformation of Gay and Lesbian Life* (Routledge, 2002), argues that '[e]quality is not about extending equal rights to gays but only on the condition that we conform to dominant gender, sexual, familial and social norms' (118). See Pierre de Vos, 'Same-Sex Sexual Desire and the Re-imagining of the South African Family', *South African Journal on Human Rights* 20:179 (2004), 197, for similar arguments in the South African context.

15 These objections are discussed in Angelo Pantazis, 'An Argument for the Legal Recognition of Gay and Lesbian Marriage', *South African Law Journal* 114 (1997), 556, 567; Kerry Williams, '"I Do" or "We Won't": Legalising Same-Sex Marriage in South Africa', *South African Journal on Human Rights* 20 (2004), 32, 37; and Pierre de Vos, 'Same-Sex Marriage, the Right to Equality and the SA Constitution', *South African Public Law* 11 (1996), 355, 358.

16 See Paula Ettelbrick, 'Since When is Marriage a Path to Liberation?', in Andrew Sullivan (ed.), *Same-Sex Marriage, Pro and Con: A Reader* (Vintage, 1997), 122-128. There is also a line of thought within this more radical perspective that critiques marriage as upholding the importance of law in socially sanctioning and regulating interpersonal relationships. We do not deal with this latter critique as we are concerned in this chapter with the goals that a family law reform process should aim at. A discussion as to whether law should actually play any role in the regulation of interpersonal relationships is beyond the scope of this essay.

17 See, for instance, in this vein, Ruthann Robson, 'Assimilation, Marriage and Lesbian Liberation', *Temple Law Review* 709 (2002), 733ff

18 As early a work as Dennis Altman's *Homosexual Oppression and Liberation* (NYU Press, 1971, 1993) suggests that the goals of gay liberation are 'part of a much wider movement that is challenging the basic cultural norms of our advanced industrial, capitalist, and bureaucratic society and bringing about changes in individual consciousness and new identities and lifestyles' (244).

19 These theorists differ on whether the law should be invoked to recognize these relationships, some preferring a more *laissez-faire* model, others arguing for a law that embraces a wider range of diverse relationships. As has already been mentioned, we do not deal with the anarchic side of this critique. See Seidman, op. cit., 191. Marriage need not disappear, according to many of these theorists, but will become one form of socially valuable relationship among others. Nancy D Polikoff, *Beyond (Straight and Gay) Marriage: Valuing All Families Under the Law* (Beacon, forthcoming 2008), argues that the problem with the law is that it disadvantages all people in unmarried relationships and the remedy to this lies in 'drawing a different line'. This 'transformative vision' is also incorporated in an important statement signed by a range of signatories

interested in promoting family diversity in the United States ('Beyond Same-Sex Marriage: A New Strategic Vision for All Our Families and Relationships', www.beyondmarriage.org, last accessed 17 February 2008)

20 This submission was primarily authored by David Bilchitz and Kate Hofmeyr, with contributions from Melanie Judge, Fikile Vilakazi, Dawie Nel, Jonathan Swanepoel and Michael Yarborough. Beth Goldblatt and Sibongile Ndashe provided additional input. Fikile Vilakazi, David Bilchitz, Melanie Judge and Sebastian Matroos presented the Joint Working Group submission in Parliament.

21 Two representatives of the Equality Project (Jonathan Berger and Emily Craven) and two representatives of the Joint Working Group (Fikile Vilakazi and David Bilchitz) attended this meeting. The account provided of this meeting is from the first-hand recollection of David Bilchitz.

22 Section 13 of the Act

23 These jurisdictions are Canada, Spain, the Netherlands, Belgium and the state of Massachusetts in the United States.

24 In the Netherlands since 2001, couples also have a choice between forming a marriage and a 'registered partnership', two very similar legal institutions: see William N Eskridge, 'The Ideological Structure of the Same-Sex Marriage Debate (and Some Postmodern Arguments for Same-Sex Marriage)', in Robert Wintemute and Mads Andenaes (eds.), *Legal Recognition of Same-Sex Partnerships: A Study of National, European and International Law* (2001), 121

25 For instance, Section 3 (1) of the Civil Partnership Act 2004 in the United Kingdom (http://www.opsi.gov.uk/acts/acts2004/20040033.htm, last accessed 17 January 2008) provides that two people are not eligible to register as civil partners of each other if 'they are not of the same sex'.

26 The civil partnership regimes often differ in the extent to which they grant same-sex couples all the legal rights and responsibilities of marriage (see Eskridge and Spedale, op. cit., 87). We have argued that there are a range of reasons to object to a 'civil partnership regime' even if it grants all the legal rights and responsibilities of marriage to same-sex couples.

27 Perhaps the one area in which it may still differ from marriage will relate to the recognition of such partnerships by foreign countries: marriage may still be a more universally recognized form than a civil partnership. This difference, however, may be mitigated by the fact that generally countries that refuse to recognize same-sex marriages will often refuse to recognize same-sex civil partnerships. Where civil partnerships for same-sex couples exist overseas in the absence of full marriage for such couples, in general a same-sex marriage solemnized in South Africa will be recognized as a civil partnership in that jurisdiction. See, for instance, Schedule 20 of the Civil Partnership Act of the United Kingdom.

28 As with all legislation, determining the intention of the legislature is a matter of later construction and interpretation and is not dependent upon the drafter's actual intentions. The latter are notoriously difficult to determine, particularly where a piece of legislation is as contested as the Civil Union Act was. See in this regard Lourens du Plessis, *Re-interpretation of Statutes* (Butterworths, 2002), 94-96, 106-119. We do not assert that the drafters necessarily intended that the Act bear the interpretation provided above nor do I think that they were opposed to it; rather, we would argue that the meaning we provide to the Act offers the best possible construction of the Act.

29 The potential of the Civil Union Act accords with the view of De Vos, op. cit., and the proposal by Polikoff, op. cit., to adopt an approach that values all families with marriage as one option. It should be evident that the approach we advocate is importantly a non-hierarchical one that nevertheless provides for a range of legal possibilities for the recognition of relationships.

30 As discussed further below, the extent to which the Act is able to create meaningful social and

transformative change, in practice, will largely be determined by the extent to which heterosexual couples also enter into 'civil unions' – attesting to the truly inclusive potential of the Act – and the social meanings that will, over time, be attributed to the notions of 'civil union' and 'civil partnership'.

31 Section 26
32 Sexual intercourse is regarded as one of the elements of married life in our law. See *Dawood, Shalabi and Thomas v Minister of Home Affairs* 2000 (3) SA 936, paragraph 33.
33 It does not provide for minors marrying with parental consent but allows for marriages from 18 onwards.
34 Marriage Act, Section 24
35 Civil Union Act (Act 17 of 2006), Section 1
36 Constitution of the Republic of South Africa, 1996. Section 15 (1) provides that 'everyone has the right to freedom of conscience, religion, thought, belief and opinion'.
37 Civil Union Act, op. cit., Section 5 (1) and 5 (2)
38 Ibid., Section 5 (4)
39 Ibid., Section 13 (2)
40 Barbara Oomen, 'Traditional Woman-to-Woman Marriages and the Recognition of Customary Marriages Act', *Journal of Contemporary Roman-Dutch Law* 63 (2000), argues that given the acceptance of woman-to-woman marriage in many African customary traditions, such marriages could be recognized under that Act (274).
41 See Congress of Traditional Leaders of South Africa (Contralesa) submission to Parliament on the Civil Union Bill, found at www.pmg.org.za/docs/2006/061024contralesa.pdf (last accessed 17 January 2008). See excerpts from this submission on pages 131-132 of this book.
42 Oomen, for instance, discusses the institution of woman-to-woman marriages that, according to the research she cites, are generally not viewed as expressions of same-sex sexuality. They are contracted, she argues, for two principle reasons relating, first, to gendered constructions of powerful women as 'men' or, secondly, for the purpose of enabling a woman (perhaps as a result of being childless) to adopt the children of her female partner (276). See also Craig Lind, 'Politics, Partnership Rights and the Constitution in South Africa ... (and the Problem of Sexual Identity)', in Wintemute and Andenaes, op. cit., 291-293.
43 See Ruth Morgan and Saskia Wieringa (eds.), *Tommy Boys, Lesbian Men and Ancestral Wives: Female Same-Sex Practices in Africa* (Jacana, 2005), and Stephen O Murray and Will Roscoe (eds.), *Boy-Wives and Female Husbands: Studies in African Homosexualities* (Palgrave, 1998)
44 Incidentally and anecdotally, the Civil Union Act has in fact spurred on a questioning of traditional culture (and religions) and led to debates that entered the public sphere as to how the notion of lobola can be adapted to a same-sex context. It is hoped that some of the same-sex context will illuminate the essentially gendered and patriarchal nature of some of these practices and thus assist in the development of more egalitarian customs. See pages 97-104 and 249-247 in this book.
45 See *Volks v Robinson* 2005 (5) BCLR 446 (CC), paragraphs 65-67
46 See *National Coalition for Gay and Lesbian Equality v Minister of Home Affairs* 2000 (2) SA 1 (CC), paragraph 88. Such a partnership was recognized on the basis of factors that would generally have indicated the existence of a marriage-type relationship in the case of opposite-sex couples: the duration of the relationship as well as whether the couple lived together, shared living expenses, or had conducted a commitment ceremony (among other factors).

The achievement of equality and tolerance – how far have we travelled?

Jody Kollapen and Judith Cohen

> 'A democratic, universalistic, caring and aspirationally egalitarian society embraces everyone and accepts people for who they are. To penalize people for being who they are is profoundly disrespectful of the human personality and violatory of equality.' – Justice Albie Sachs in Fourie[1]

The passage of the Civil Union Bill has presented a formidable challenge to our fledgling democracy and our understandings of tolerance and acceptance of diversity. At times the debates were fierce and even often undermining of the Constitutional Court. The public hearings around the country were a callous foray in homophobia resulting in lesbian and gay groups feeling generally marginalized. Even at the parliamentary hearings, statements bordering on hate speech and most distasteful to gay and lesbian people were articulated and condoned by inaction. Despite the enormous negative public outcry, there were also many voices of reason and many of the debates demonstrated an in-depth understanding and acceptance of the Constitution and the values that our society is founded upon.

The South African Human Rights Commission (SAHRC), as an institution created in terms of the Constitution to support constitutional democracy and to protect human rights, observed with concern the many public debates, which reflected our society's response to the recognition of same-sex marriages. The Civil Union Bill was introduced into Parliament as a measure to comply with the Constitutional Court's ruling that the Marriage Act was inconsistent with the Constitution, as it did not permit same-sex couples to enjoy the status and the benefits coupled with the responsibilities it accorded to heterosexual couples (*Minister of Home Affairs and Another v Fourie and Another*). The Constitutional Court ordered that Parliament would be afforded one year to pass legislation that would cure the defects in the Marriage Act.[2] Furthermore, should Parliament fail to pass such legislation by 1 December 2006, the words 'or spouse' would be read in to the Marriage Act after the words 'wife / husband' in order to cure the defect.

There were two main groups that participated in the debates around the Bill. The one group was totally opposed to the Bill, relying very often on their religious beliefs and faith to support their arguments. This group argued that the notion of marriage could not be extended to same-sex couples. The other group supported same-sex marriages and even argued that the Bill did not go far enough in the spirit of equality in recognizing the rights of same-sex couples to marriage. The public hearings demonstrated that there was a great deal of public passion concerning the issue, and very few of the submissions expressed support for the Bill in the form in which it was presented. Some submissions felt that the Bill, which at that point provided for same-sex unions that would not be officially registered as 'marriages', did not go far enough in delivering on the right to equality and dignity and therefore did not comply with the Constitutional Court's order. On the other hand, those opposed to the Bill argued that any reference in the Bill to marriage would demean the institution of marriage and infringe upon their rights to religious freedom.

The Commission's objections to the Bill
The Commission's submissions did not support the Bill, because it did not in our view give effect to the Constitutional Court judgment and created a 'separate but equal' system reminiscent of apartheid. The presentation of the oral submission before the Parliamentary Portfolio Committee on Home Affairs and the engagement that flowed therefrom was robust. The Committee questioned the Commission about its role in educating the public generally about the issue. It was suggested that the objections to the Bill may well have been less vociferous if we, the SAHRC, been more effective in publicizing the Bill and educating the public on the human-rights implications of the Bill. As it stood, the initial Bill contained a number of provisions that, in the Commission's view, were discriminatory and offensive to gay and lesbian people. The Commission argued, on a number of grounds, that the Bill in its presented form would potentially contribute to the ongoing discrimination and stigmatization of gay and lesbian people.

Firstly, the Bill created a separate system of union for same-sex couples. This gave effect to the offensive doctrine of 'separate but equal'. The separate register that was intended for recording the civil unions further enforced this.[3] Labelling and recording a different system of union for homosexual and heterosexual persons provides a potential space for discrimination. Given that gay and lesbian people still experience enormous intolerance and discrimination in our society, creating a separate system of union would have merely contributed to their further stigmatization. A separate system would have been exclusionary rather than inclusionary. This runs contrary to the type of society that we are striving to create, in which everyone's dignity is respected and protected. The Bill failed to take into account that marriage is much more than simply the union between two people and that it also has social consequences.

Secondly, the Bill provided that the marriage officer must inquire whether the parties would 'prefer their civil partnership to be referred to as a civil partnership or a marriage during the solemnization ceremony'.[4] This would have created the public impression to those present that the two persons were being married, when in terms of law and the recording thereof they were being united by way of a civil union. This would have been farcical and highly offensive to same-sex couples who wanted to marry. It appeared somewhat nonsensical that during the taking of their vows parties could refer to their being married when in terms of law they were actually partaking in a civil-union ceremony.

Thirdly, the Bill provided that on grounds of conscience a marriage officer may refuse to solemnize a civil union.[5] This provision would potentially have left the door wide open for discrimination, offence and deep hurt to be caused to same-sex couples. It is unacceptable that, while freedom of conscience is protected in our Bill of Rights,[6] one's thoughts and beliefs can be acted upon in a manner that causes harm to others and violates their constitutionally protected rights to equality and dignity. In terms of law, marriage officers have a choice as to whether they want to become marriage officers. But this choice cannot be exercised in violation of another person's rights. Having made the choice they are required to discharge their obligations within the dictates of the Constitution. If it becomes untenable to continue as a marriage officer, then there is a choice to cease being a marriage officer rather than to withhold a service.

The finalization of the Bill

On 8 November 2006, during the final processing of the Bill within the National Assembly's Portfolio Committee on Home Affairs, and with the Constitutional Court's deadline fast approaching, members of the ruling ANC party tabled a proposal on the Bill. This proposal was debated within the Committee and was to become the final version of the Bill that was signed into law. This new Bill provided that both same-sex and mixed-sex couples were eligible to be joined in a civil partnership or be regarded as 'married' under the Act. Thus, whichever terminology the couple chose, it would be registered as such in the official government register. Further, the Bill provides a clause that government-employed marriage officers may refuse on grounds of conscience, religion and belief to solemnize a civil union between persons of the same sex provided they inform the Minister in writing thereof.[7] The Bill was hurriedly passed with reports that ANC Members of Parliament were told to vote in favour of the Bill. The final Civil Union Act is less than perfect; still, gay organizations appear to have embraced it. The debate and media interest generated by the Bill were more about tolerance and acceptance of gay and lesbian people within our society than the narrow issue of marriage. The debates provided an important opportunity to advance and exchange views about tolerance, diversity, equality and acceptance of difference. It also provided an opportunity to confront and challenge views that were discriminatory and homophobic.

Failure to show respect to the Constitutional Court

The Constitutional Court judgment and the Civil Union Bill caused a great deal of debate and anxiety within society. Considerable opposition came from religious groups who opposed the notion of same-sex marriage on the grounds that it went against the tenets of their religious belief system entrenched over thousands of years. There was a clear conflict between deeply held religious beliefs and the interpretation of our Bill of Rights by the Constitutional Court.

Many religious groups failed or simply refused to acknowledge that we live in a constitutional democracy in which the Constitution is the supreme law of the land.[8] This is the constitutional model that we have chosen. Central to the Constitution is the Bill of Rights, which emphasizes the constitutional values of equality and dignity. There cannot be a conditional commitment to equality, otherwise some would be more equal than others. The commitment to equality requires that we move beyond many of the prejudices and stereotypes we have constructed and nurtured in the past. The Constitutional Court is embodied with the ultimate responsibility of deciding constitutional matters and giving effect to the rights that are enshrined in our Constitution.[9] The system may not be perfect, but at the very least we must respect it and show fidelity to it. Those who are not happy with the model must use the constitutional mechanisms available to seek to change it. The Constitutional Court had ventilated the same-sex marriage issue fully and delivered its considered decision. The matter had also been fully ventilated in both the High Court and the Supreme Court of Appeal (SCA). In the former court, the court was of the view that the issue of discrimination had not been fully placed before the court. In the latter case, the SCA found that the Marriage Act is discriminatory towards gay people.[10]

There appeared however an unwillingness or inability by some to accept and understand that although everyone has the right to make their deeply held beliefs on the matter known, that this will not change the decision of the Constitutional Court. Some went as far as to attack the integrity of the Court and argued that it had overstepped its jurisdiction as its decision did not reflect the constitutional drafters' intentions. In the view of the SAHRC, it was not acceptable that merely because a decision was offensive to some people's deeply held beliefs that irresponsible statements were made that undermined the Constitutional Court.

The public hearing process – a foray in homophobia

Extensive measures were taken to enhance and enrich public participation and comment on the Bill, as is evident by the many country-wide public hearings that were organized in the latter part of 2006.[11] Much of the input at the public hearings appeared to focus on general opposition to same-sex marriages, with the incorrectly held belief that the more opposition there was to the recognition of same-sex marriages the greater the likelihood there would be of convincing Parliament not to give effect to the proposed legislative changes. Clearly, it was thought that crude majoritarianism and simple loudness would win the issue for those who did not support same-sex marriages. Parliament was faced with the task of giving effect to the Constitutional Court's decision, although the public hearings failed to give any substantive input as to how Parliament should do so. Public participation did not substantively address the content of the legislation.

Within the debates, it appeared to be almost forgotten that marriage is an institution recognized by the state in South Africa. Marriage, in terms of the Marriage Act, is a civil act, not a religious act. The separation of church and state has long been in effect. All civil acts and legislation must comply with the Constitution, the supreme law of the land. As the Constitutional Court stated, the Marriage Act and the common-law definition of marriage were in conflict with the Constitution and violated the rights enshrined in our Bill of Rights. It was therefore incumbent on Parliament to make the necessary legislative changes in order to ensure that the civil institution of marriage would come in line with the values and rights enshrined in the Constitution.

We live in an ever-changing and fast-changing society. Many of the social mores and practices of the past have been changed or discarded. Some would argue that these changes are for the better while others would argue that they are for the worse. Living in a constitutional democracy we need to re-examine many of our long-held beliefs and re-evaluate whether these are in line with our constitutional values of equality, dignity and the advancement of human rights and freedoms. Justice Albie Sachs, in his judgment in *Fourie*, was alive to this and pointed out how over time many social mores and practices have changed. What was once considered acceptable is no longer. He said:

> Slavery lasted for a century and a half in this country, colonialism for twice as long, the prohibition of interracial marriage for even longer, and overt male domination for millennia. All were based on apparently self-evident biological and social facts; all were once sanctioned by religion and imposed by law, the first two are today regarded with total disdain, and the third with varying degrees of denial, shame or embarrassment.[12]

So too will discrimination against persons based on their sexual orientation become recognized as such. Gay and lesbian people will eventually be accepted as full citizens in a society in which they can reach their full potential and be treated equally and with dignity.

It is undoubtedly exceedingly difficult for those who find same-sex marriages offensive to accept the decision of the Constitutional Court. The Court is asking that everyone in society accept difference. As a country that has experienced and lived through deep and intense pain occasioned by discrimination, we ought to be well-practised in identifying and recognizing the injustice of discrimination against people based on their sexual orientation. There is a need for our society to transport the lessons of prejudice and discrimination from the past into the present in order to demonstrate the capacity to learn from our past.

Few South Africans can argue that there have not been increased levels of tolerance of gay and lesbian people during the past 13 years of democracy. Much of this change has been preceded by catalytic court decisions. Many successful non-discrimination cases have been brought before our courts and progress has been made in pushing back prejudice. Our challenge is to be an open society in which everyone is respected. We are still learning to accommodate difference. As Justice Sachs said:

> The hallmark of an open and democratic society is the capacity to accommodate and manage difference of intensely held world views and lifestyles in a reasonable and fair manner. The objective of the Constitution is to allow different concepts about human existence to inhabit the same public realm, and to do so in a manner that is not mutually destructive and that at the same time enables government to function in a way that shows equal concern and respect for all.[13]

An indicator for equality

The passing of the Civil Union Act is a significant indicator for the recognition of equality in South Africa. In all societies contestation about rights is inevitable. Thus we need to assess the extent to which our society has emerged from this contestation energized and committed to our constitutional democracy. This will only happen if we conduct the debate within the terms of the constitutional commitment to dignity. Debates that are conducted in a manner which do not respect the dignity of everyone will detract from the potential that these critical debates can play in transforming our society and ensuring a commitment to equality and freedom.

The passage of the Civil Union Bill was characterized as a grudging recognition of unions between same-sex couples. Equality should not be advanced grudgingly; rather, it should be advanced willingly in a manner that affords dignity to everyone. The initial Bill placed before Parliament indicated a minimalist approach towards advancing equality, while the second, final version of the Bill went a lot further in adhering to the spirit of the Constitutional Court judgment. The State should take the lead in advancing equality and should do so generously, particularly when the Constitutional Court has granted the opportunity to the legislature to do so. This would be in line with the spirit of our Constitution.

South Africa has experienced rapid transformation, which has resulted in a Constitution that embodies noble aspirations and values. This has consequently created a gap between the commitments of our Constitution and the views and lived realities of those who live in our democracy. This gulf was evident in the discourse that accompanied the Civil Union Act. While we can be critical of the intolerance and callous indifference displayed by many during the process, we also need to understand the challenges of bridging the enormous gaps between the views held by a large proportion of our society and the ideals and aspirations of our Constitution. As we build our constitutional democracy and create a culture of human rights, we need to understand that at times there is still a lack of knowledge about rights and that offensive utterances are not always a case of showing disrespect but rather a lack of knowledge. As we journey towards achieving a society that reflects our constitutional aspirations, we need to ensure that everyone walks this journey together, and that entrenched prejudices are obviated.

The Civil Union Act will not in itself lower levels of intolerance and homophobia in our society. But the process of legislative change has provided an opportunity for many people to reflect on their values and understandings of equality. There is still a long way that we as South Africans need to travel in order to achieve a culture of human rights in which the values of our Constitution are reflected in the lived realities of people's experiences. During apartheid we experienced discrimination on the basis of race. It appears that not everyone has taken the lessons that can be learnt from this experience and transported them into our new democratic realities.

Notes

1 *Minister of Home Affairs and Another v Fourie and Another* 2005 (3) BCLR 355 (CC); 2006 (1) SA 524 (CC) (hereinafter referred to as '*Fourie*'), paragraph 60
2 Justice Kate O'Regan did not agree with the majority judgment in this regard and argued instead that the Court should merely read in the relevant words to the Marriage Act and thereby immediately remedy the discrimination. (See pages 68-69 of this book.)
3 Civil Union Bill (B26-2006), Section 12 (5)
4 Ibid., Section 11 (1)
5 Ibid., Section 6 (1)
6 Section 15 (1) of the South African Bill of Rights states: 'Everyone has the right to freedom of conscience, religion, thought, belief and opinion.'
7 Civil Union Act (Act 17 of 2006), Section 6
8 The Constitution of the Republic of South Africa (1996), Section 2
9 Ibid., Section 167
10 *Fourie and Another v Minister of Home Affairs and Another* (the Lesbian and Gay Equality Project intervening as *amicus curiae*), case number 17280/02, handed down on 18 October 2002. Unreported. This matter was held in the Pretoria High Court. *Fourie and Another v Minister of Home Affairs and Another* 2005 (3) SA 429 (SCA); 2005 (3) BCLR 241 (SCA).
11 See http://www.pmg.org.za/docs/2006/061031hearings.htm (last accessed 13 December 2007)
12 *Fourie*, op. cit., paragraph 74
13 Ibid., paragraph 95

The Civil Union Act:
More of the same

Elsje Bonthuys

With the enactment of the Civil Union Act in 2006, South Africa found itself in the company of countries such as Canada, Belgium, Spain, Denmark and the Netherlands in permitting same-sex couples to enter into marriage or an equivalent institution. Much was made of the fact that South Africa was the first African country, and also the first country outside of Europe and North America, to do this.

The unspoken subtext of much of the praise for South Africa was that other African, Asian and South American societies are prevented from doing the same by conservative religious or cultural beliefs which are hostile to same-sex relationships in general, and strongly opposed to same-sex marriage in particular. South Africa was lauded as an example of what a 'third world' country could achieve when guided by a strong Bill of Rights and a commitment to the rule of law. This view draws upon the dichotomy between culture (or religion), on the one hand, and equality and human rights, on the other hand, which is so familiar to lawyers in debates about gender equality versus culture and religion.[1] The juxtaposition of equality with culture/religion implies that the achievement of constitutional equality depends upon the eradication of discriminatory cultural and religious beliefs and practices. In other words, societies must choose either to protect culture or to achieve human rights by relying on law and constitutionalism.

Among lesbian and gay groups, the recognition of same-sex marriage is regarded as reason for celebration, even by those who consider it as only a symbolic victory. They usually perceive the Civil Union Act as the successful culmination of the struggle for inclusion of same-sex couples into a 'two-tier hierarchy of monogamous intimate partnerships: married and not married'.[2] However, this dual classification of relationships as either marriage or non-marriage is not an accurate description of South African legal or social reality. Like other former colonies, we have a dual legal system with colonial law existing alongside, but usually taking precedence over, indigenous legal systems. As a result, there are different forms of marriage, which attract different levels of legal recognition. Islamic religious marriages, for instance, have very few legal consequences, unless the couple also marry each other in terms of the civil law. Customary marriages, concluded by African people, received limited legal recognition since colonial times, but even after receiving full recognition by way of the Recognition of

Customary Marriages Act (Act 120 of 1998), their status is still somewhat lower than that of civil marriages.[3] Civil marriages, conducted by religious officials or civil servants, derive from the legal system introduced by the Dutch and British colonial powers and have always been privileged over other forms of marriage in South African law. This privilege is obviously associated with the political, social and economic power of the colonial government as, conversely, the lack of recognition of African customary and Muslim marriages reflects the lower racial, cultural and religious status of the people who conclude these kinds of marriages. Clearly, therefore, same-sex couples have not merely been granted access to the institution of 'marriage' – they have been allowed to conduct a particular kind of marriage, which is inevitably associated with particular racial, religious and cultural factors and a particular legal status.

My project in this paper is twofold. First, I aim to show that the dichotomy between culture and equality for same-sex couples is not necessarily true, at least in respect of indigenous Southern African culture. Drawing on social-science literature I describe how African customary law can accommodate a wide variety of same-sex relationships and institutionalize them without threatening the social structures of traditional African societies and of contemporary urban township life. By modelling the Civil Union Act on civil marriage, however, the legislature has ignored the rich and varied possibilities for recognizing same-sex families presented by customary law and opted instead for simply expanding the scope of civil marriage. Delinking the Civil Union Act from customary marriage may have been a deliberate placatory response to traditional leaders' vociferous opposition to same-sex marriage. However, given the history of the Act, it appears simply not to have occurred to the legislature to consider recognition of customary marriages as part of customary law.

My second aim is to show that, by modelling itself on *civil* and not *customary* marriage, the Civil Union Act depends upon a certain 'Westernized' form of lesbian and gay identity that excludes many African people who have sexual relationships with others of the same sex. These excluded African practices and identities may be more radical and have more potential for liberating us from the binary categories that currently describe and define sex, gender and sexual orientation. I approach this project by way of two questions. First, I examine what kind of marriage same-sex partners have been admitted to. Second, I investigate who the lesbian women and gay men are who have been permitted to conclude civil unions.

Which kind of marriage can same-sex couples enter into?

Section 13 (1) of the Civil Union Act determines that '[t]he legal consequences of a marriage contemplated in the Marriage Act apply, with such changes as may be required by the context, to a civil union', while several provisions of the Act simply replicate those of the Marriage Act. It is therefore clear from the wording of the Civil Union Act, and in particular, its duplication of the requirements and consequences of the Marriage Act, that same-sex couples have been admitted to the companionate, voluntary, monogamous civil marriage based on Judaeo-Christian moral values as represented by the Marriage Act and not to any of the other forms of marriage which exist in South African society and law. This re-affirms the paramount status of civil marriage and strengthens its position as the template and ideal towards which all other relationships should aspire.[4]

Yet the failure to even consider the integration of same-sex couples into other forms of marriage also reinforces the dichotomy to which I have referred, between culture and religion, on the one hand, and modernity and progress on the other hand. The Recognition of Customary Marriages Act, the legal vehicle for giving official recognition to customary marriages, seems not to contemplate a customary marriage between spouses of the same sex. In electing civil marriage as the only form in which same-sex relationships can be celebrated, the Civil Union Act implies that civil law is capable of changing to accommodate the demands of modern society and the dictates of our progressive Constitution, but that the law associated with racial and religious 'others' cannot do the same.[5] This view is underpinned by a belief that African and Muslim communities are too conservative to tolerate radical change or 'modern' ideas like equality for same-sex couples.

There is little or no material available on the acceptance and formal recognition of same-sex relationships within South African Jewish, Hindu, Muslim and 'black' communities. However, an emerging body of social-science evidence (largely ignored or unknown in legal circles) clearly illustrates that customary law and African communities in Southern Africa accepted and accommodated same-sex relationships, both in the past and at present. In this part of the essay I show instances of this tolerance and accommodation. But this does not imply that all African communities are equally tolerant or that there are any ethnic groups that completely and openly accept all forms of same-sex relationships. Nevertheless, some cultures have created spaces within which certain forms of same-sex activity is allowed, or sometimes simply ignored. Whether or not a particular same-sex couple will be allowed openly to have a sexual relationship is determined by the interaction between a range of factors, such as their particular cultures, Christian beliefs by family and community members (often opposed to allowing same-sex activity), or whether they are in an urban or rural setting and their ability to provide financially for themselves and for others.[6]

It is a little-advertised fact that customary law in many Southern African societies has long allowed marriages between women. These marriages are not experienced as disruptive in the African communities that have institutionalized them within the socially accepted patterns of marriage.[7] Often these marriages were concluded by older widows whose husbands had died childless. The widow then marries another woman (the 'wife') who is expected to have sexual intercourse with a designated man in order to bear children. The children from the marriage will then be regarded as the children of the deceased man, thus raising children for the deceased man's household.[8] Although it is generally asserted that these woman-to-woman marriages do not entail sexual relationships between the female spouses, they nevertheless provide a well-known example of socially acceptable and legally integrated same-sex marriage.[9]

Another form accepted in customary law and in African communities is the so-called 'independent' woman-to-woman marriage where the motivation is not to raise offspring for a particular man but to found a homestead and consolidate the status and wealth of an influential woman. Children born to the 'wives' would be considered to belong to the families of the 'female husbands' and, again, it is generally assumed that no sexual relations take place between the spouses, although, in fact, they may.[10] The best-known example in South Africa is the Rain Queen of the Balobedu (Lovedu), who usually marries many wives and has many children.

In addition, it is also considered acceptable for female traditional healers (sangomas) to marry so-called 'ancestral wives'. The ancestral spirits who assist the sangomas choose or approve of ancestral wives for both male and female sangomas. The functions of these wives are to assist the sangomas in their healing ceremonies and practices, and it was generally thought that no sexual relations took place between the female sangomas and their wives. Yet recent evidence indicates that, at least in some of these marriages, the women do have sex with one another, although researchers and community members often assume that, because there is no heterosexual penetration, no sex takes place.[11] This very patriarchal and heterosexist definition of sex may also explain the popular belief that there is no sex involved in other forms of woman-to-woman marriages.

There is also evidence of marriages between African men, but the sexual nature of these relationships is often more visible than in the case of women married to other women. Marc Epprecht gives examples of early 20th-century marriages between Zimbabwean men who have lost their access to land, in which younger men fulfilled the sexual and household roles of women while the older men provided financially.[12] Similar relationships were found in South African mining compounds when older migrant workers, who were involved in customary marriages to women in the rural areas, also married and had sex with younger men at the mines. The younger 'wives' would also perform household chores like cooking, cleaning and mending clothes and sometimes they would dress as women and adopt typically feminine forms of behaviour.[13] Mine marriages are no longer prevalent, possibly because the demise of apartheid has allowed rural wives and children to join their husbands in the areas where they work. Finally, Ronald Louw describes how, in the 1950s and 1960s, gay marriages were publicly celebrated in the African township of Mkhumbane in Natal.[14]

Although these same-sex marriages are not widespread or numerous in African communities, and although many of the woman-to-woman marriages may not have included sex, they nevertheless demonstrate that the customary concept of marriage was flexible enough to accept and accommodate different family formations long before the Civil Union Act – at a time when civil-law marriage absolutely required monogamy and sex-specificity. In fact, upon closer inspection it seems that it is not African marriage that is the more conservative and less adaptable institution, but civil marriage.

Which lesbian women and gay men?

At the same time as allowing certain same-sex couples access to the marriage-like institution of civil partnerships, the Civil Union Act has inevitably excluded other same-sex and opposite-sex couples from the benefits it bestows.[15] In this section I ask who those excluded same-sex couples are and, in particular, what their racial, cultural and social characteristics are.

Pierre de Vos has noted that the same-sex couples who have been successful in challenging discrimination based on sexual orientation in the Constitutional Court are characterized by their similarity to middle-class heterosexual couples in their behaviour, views and the division of labour within their relationships.[16] It seems, therefore, that the same-sex couples who are permitted entry into the institution of marriage or civil partnerships are sophisticated, openly live together with their partners and have access to medical aid and pension funds – in short, urban middle-class people who have the social and economic wherewithal to flout the norms of their families and their religious and cultural communities. They identify themselves as irrevocably and immutably gay or lesbian, and assert their rights to have their sexual relationships publicly acknowledged, as well as their rights to engage in permanent and exclusive relationships with people of their own sex.

Contrasting with this self-conscious, immutable gay or lesbian identity, literature on African same-sex relationships shows more complex patterns of behaviour. Although there are African people who identify themselves as lesbian or gay in the 'modern' sense, they represent an urban, often middle-class fragment of those who engage in sex with others of the same sex.

Both among people who engage in same-sex activity and members of African communities, there is a belief that people who have sex with others of the same sex are in fact members of the opposite sex or even biologically intersexed. For instance, Elizabeth Khaxas and Saskia Wieringa note how, in the Damara community of Namibia, long-standing relationships between women in which one partner adopts masculine behaviour, clothing and social roles are accepted. These 'masculine' women don't identify as lesbians. Instead they feel that 'it may have to do with hormones, or maybe with having both male and female genitals, hermaphrodites' and they sometimes believe that they can have a role in their partners' conceiving children.[17] In effect, they explain their sexuality and define themselves in terms of bodily sex or gender identity, rather than as having a distinctive sexual orientation.[18]

In other contexts the identity of being gay is reserved for men who adopt a passive role in sexual encounters with other men. It is accepted that, in time, men may change from being gay (being the passive sexual partner) to being heterosexual (becoming the active partner). For instance, Hugh McLean and Linda Ngcobo studied men who have sex with men in the African townships around Johannesburg in the 1990s and found that active, and usually older partners (*injonga*), were often regarded as heterosexual by community members and themselves. The younger partners (*skesana*), who adopted feminine behaviour and sometimes dressed as women, were regarded as gay, but there was evidence that this was tolerated because of a belief that they were intersexed ('hermaphrodites'). However, when they became older, the typically feminine *skesana*s may themselves have adopted the male behaviour and roles of *injonga*s in their own relationships with younger men.[19] In the mine marriages discussed above, the younger 'wives' would sometimes terminate the relationships once they themselves had acquired sufficient economic resources and status and some of them would, in turn, take younger male 'wives'.[20]

Community tolerance is often based upon a belief that those who practise same-sex relations are intersexed and therefore cannot be held responsible for their biological urges.[21] Other studies suggest that community disapproval of same-sex relationships is not necessarily directed at the sexual activities themselves, but at the failure to procreate. Many people who are involved in same-sex relationships are therefore also married or also have sexual relationships with people of the opposite sex and define themselves as bisexual, rather than lesbian or gay.[22]

Nevertheless, it seems that many women who have sex with other women do not openly identify themselves as lesbian, bisexual or intersexed. Instead, they simply remain silent about their sexual activities, because silence opens up spaces for community tolerance of their relationships.[23] Ruth Morgan and Saskia Wieringa remark of these women that 'silence isolates, but also protects them'.[24] One of the most interesting examples of this is Kendall's description of ritualized female friendships, which often also involved a lot of sexual activity, in Lesotho between 1992 and 1994. Neither the women themselves nor other community members saw these relationships as lesbian, because what the female friends did together was not regarded as sex. Instead, sex was seen as heterosexual penetrative acts that could result in procreation. As long as the women continued to perform their wifely duties and procreated within heterosexual marriage, it seems that same-sex friendships involving physical intimacy were not experienced as a threat to the social order. Husbands and other community members were aware of the relationships and even joined in celebrating 'anniversaries'.[25] A similar, but older phenomenon was the *oumapanga* relationships in late 19th-century Namibia. They were ritualized friendships between women, or between men, which sometimes involved same-sex activities, but which were socially accepted.[26] It is interesting to note that these relationships tended to disappear when people came into contact with Westernized notions of sexuality, and, in the case of the *oumapanga* relationships, with Christian missionaries who strongly disapproved of them.

The kinds of lesbian and gay couples for whom the Civil Union Act caters identify themselves as lesbian or gay. They profess to have a fixed and exclusively lesbian or gay sexual orientation, which they cannot change. They demand that their (monogamous) relationships should be publicly acknowledged and they are often financially independent from other family members. Many African people who are involved in same-sex relationships do not fit this profile. Often their same-sex activities coincide with heterosexual relationships or are associated with particular life stages, to be abandoned later on.[27] More importantly, they do not necessarily identify themselves as exclusively lesbian or gay, but often take on the gender identity of the opposite sex, as transsexuals do. Members of this latter group perceive their relationships to be heterosexual and this is also sometimes accepted by community and family members. The Civil Union Act fails to reflect a perception or understanding of the complexities and nuances of same-sex relationships in African communities. It also posits an inherent and fixed gay or lesbian identity that may be more essentialist and less progressive than the fluid sexual practices in African communities.

At the same time, it needs to be pointed out that these kinds of same-sex practices are not exclusive to African people. Many white and 'Westernized' people have same-sex relationships that coincide with heterosexual relationships, while people other than Africans may only have same-sex relationships at particular stages of their lives and so forth. The Civil Union Act's exclusion of African people who have sexual relationships with others of the same sex points to the wider problem that the legislation ignores and excludes those same-sex sexual practices which do not neatly mirror heterosexual relationships.

Conclusion

In criticizing the Civil Union Act, I am not implying that same-sex marriage should not have been legalized, nor am I arguing that customary law is absolutely superior to civil law in its way of dealing with same-sex relationships. In fact, both systems of law are deeply rooted in patriarchy and it is clear that the recognition of same-sex marriage in African societies often serves to preserve the gendered status quo. For instance, accepting the marriages of female sangomas to ancestral wives serves the spiritual interests of other community members and probably proceeds from an inability to conceive that 'ancestral husbands' could serve the supporting roles generally reserved for women. Women's marriages to other women are also accepted when they perpetuate the lineages of deceased men, and when they serve the purpose of consolidating wealth and power. The community does not recognize these relationships as sexual, and some instances community acceptance is premised on the parties' adhering to stereotypical gender roles, or because they continue to procreate within opposite-sex relationships and thus satisfy community norms. We could say that same-sex activity is tolerated in customary law and in African communities to a greater extent than in the civil law, but that this tolerance is limited by the implicit understanding that such relationships should not question or undermine patriarchal gender roles and heterosexual family structures.

Nevertheless, the popular and legal perception of customary law as static and unable to accommodate changing family structures is inaccurate. Subject to the limits described above, it is customary law and not civil law that has proved to be more malleable and more responsive to same-sex relationships. Indeed, as we see from Kendall's study and the *oumapanga* relationships, the imposition of colonial lifestyles and sexual norms may diminish or eliminate the spaces for such relationships that had existed in more 'traditional' societies. Customary law as practised by African communities in Southern Africa contained a relatively wide array of mechanisms and forms for accommodating same-sex relationships, for incorporating them into the social fabric and sometimes even valuing them by the community. In forgoing the opportunity to engage with these mechanisms, the Civil Union Act is somewhat impoverished and disappointing. Instead of drawing upon the customary examples to imagine richer concepts and more sophisticated forms of legalization, the legislature has simply ignored the customary law and extended the civil law of marriage to same-sex couples.

Returning to the failure of countries outside of Europe and North America to recognize same-sex marriage, I argue that this may not simply be the result of religious or cultural conservatism. Indeed, it may well be that, as in South Africa, such marriages already exist within certain religious and cultural communities. Perhaps it is time for us to turn our attention more closely to the ways in which same-sex relationships are and have been tolerated in other South African communities and in similar communities in other countries. We may find novel and interesting possibilities for broadening the scope of social inclusion, not just of same-sex families, but of all 'non-traditional' family formations.

On a less optimistic note, however, we must remember that the Recognition of Customary Marriages Act contains no provisions allowing customary marriage between same-sex couples, despite the evidence that customary societies tolerated and institutionalized such relationships. Morgan and Wieringa tell of an incident during the process of re-drafting the marriage law in Benin in

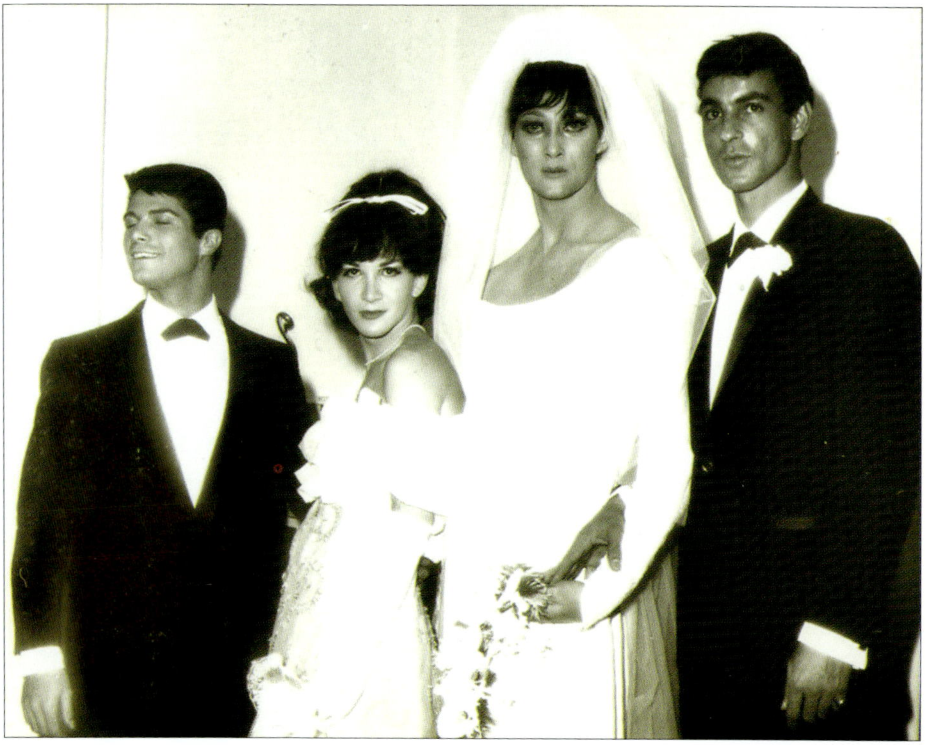

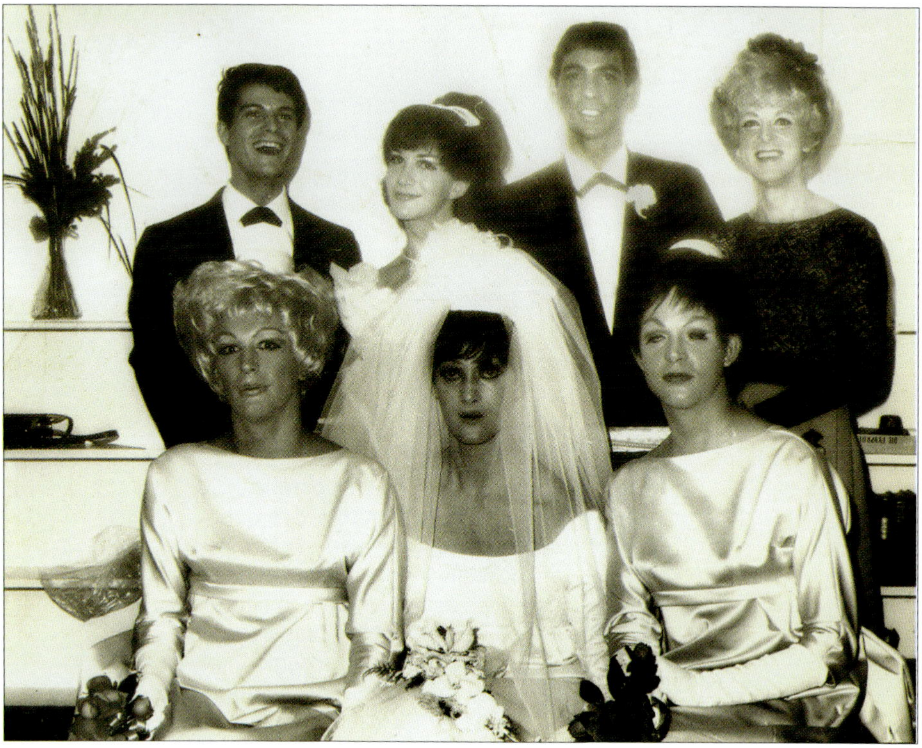

The prehistory of gay marriage: 'Camp' – and partly parodic – gay weddings took place in the 1960s and 1970s in South Africa, with some participants in drag. These pictures were given to GALA by Michele Bruno (standing, centre).

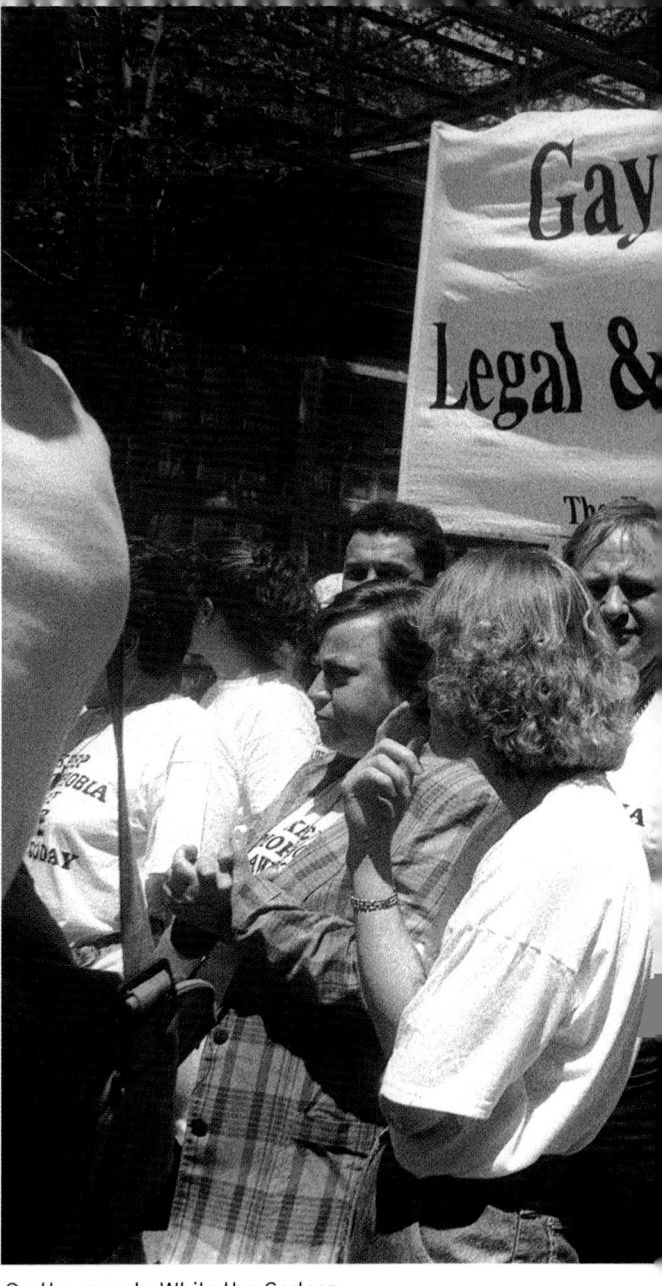

On the march: While the Codesa negotiations for a democratic dispensation in South Africa were taking place in the early 1990s, gay and lesbian people were marching in ever-increasing numbers to demand the guarantee of their human rights – including the legal recognition of same-sex marriages. This photograph is from the 1993 lesbian and gay Pride march in Johannesburg.

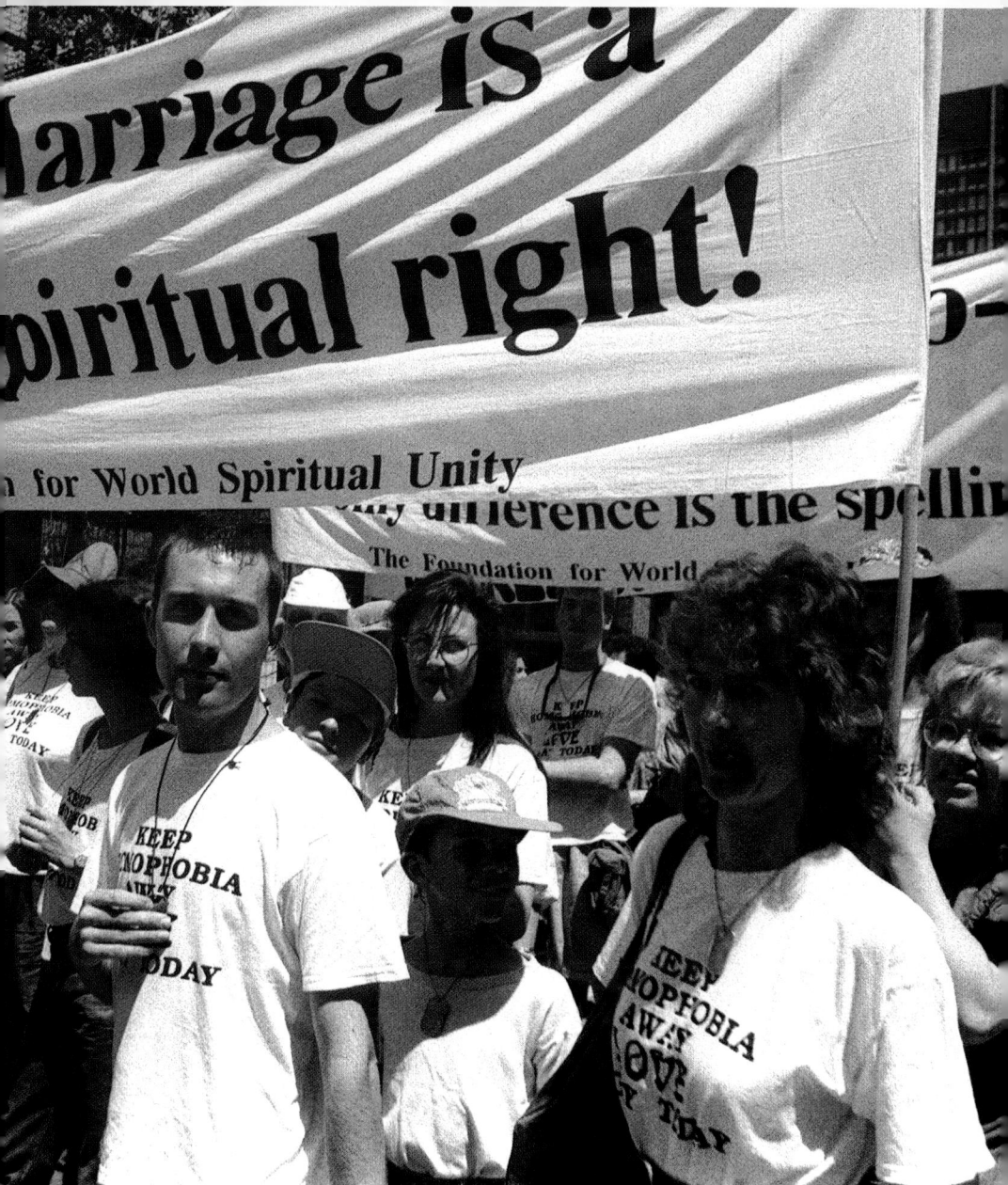

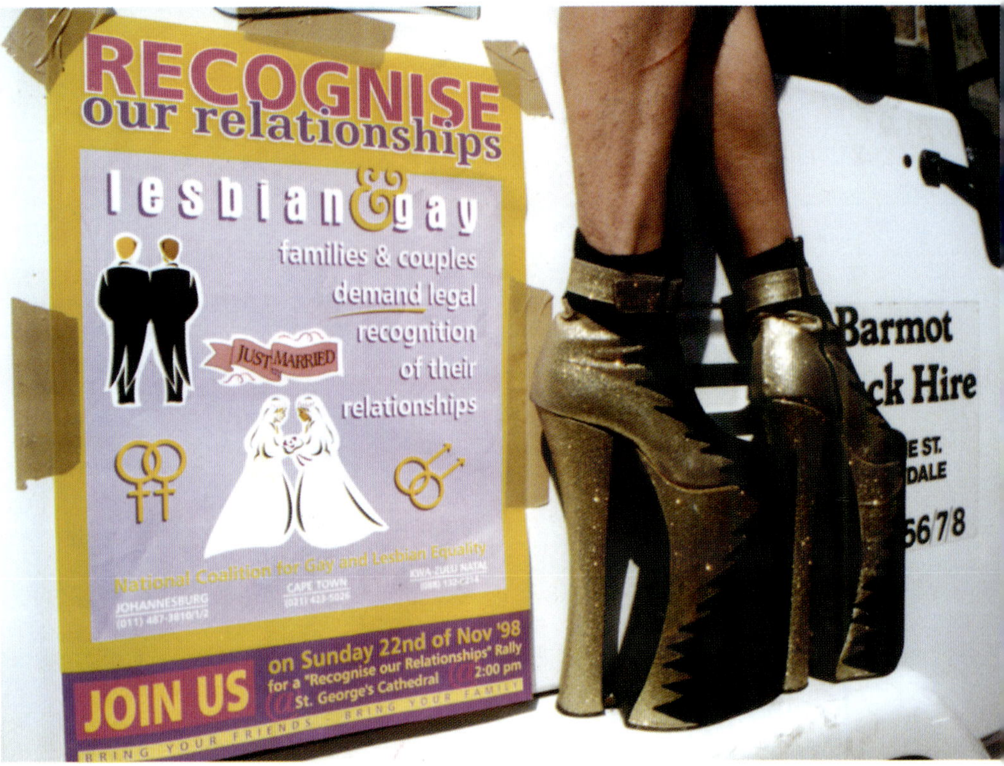

Putting our foot down: The theme of the 1998 gay and lesbian Pride parade in Johannesburg was 'Recognise Our Relationships', as this poster produced by the National Coalition for Gay and Lesbian Equality (NCGLE) shows. The legs alongside belong to performance artist Steven Cohen. Below, the newsletter of the Lesbian and Gay Equality Project (1998) focuses on the 'Recognise Our Relationships' campaign, and highlights the 'Polmed' victory.

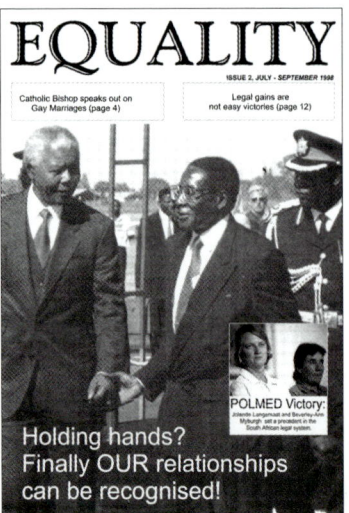

Down the rainbow aisle: opposite page, top, Sibongile Malaza (left) and Pretty Rabiama were the first couple to get married at the Hope and Unity Metropolitan Community Church (HUMCC) in Johannesburg in 1995. The couple was married by Reverend Tsietsi Thandekiso (far right), the founder of the church. Since its inception in 1994, the HUMCC has provided a safe environment for black gay men and lesbian women to express their Christianity and has blessed numerous same-sex marriages. Opposite, below, Polly Motene (left) and Robert Poswayo (right) held a public wedding celebration in Soweto in 1997. 'I was nervous about what the reaction of the community might be,' said Polly. 'I wore a suit because I wanted the community to see this man-to-man wedding,' he told The Star

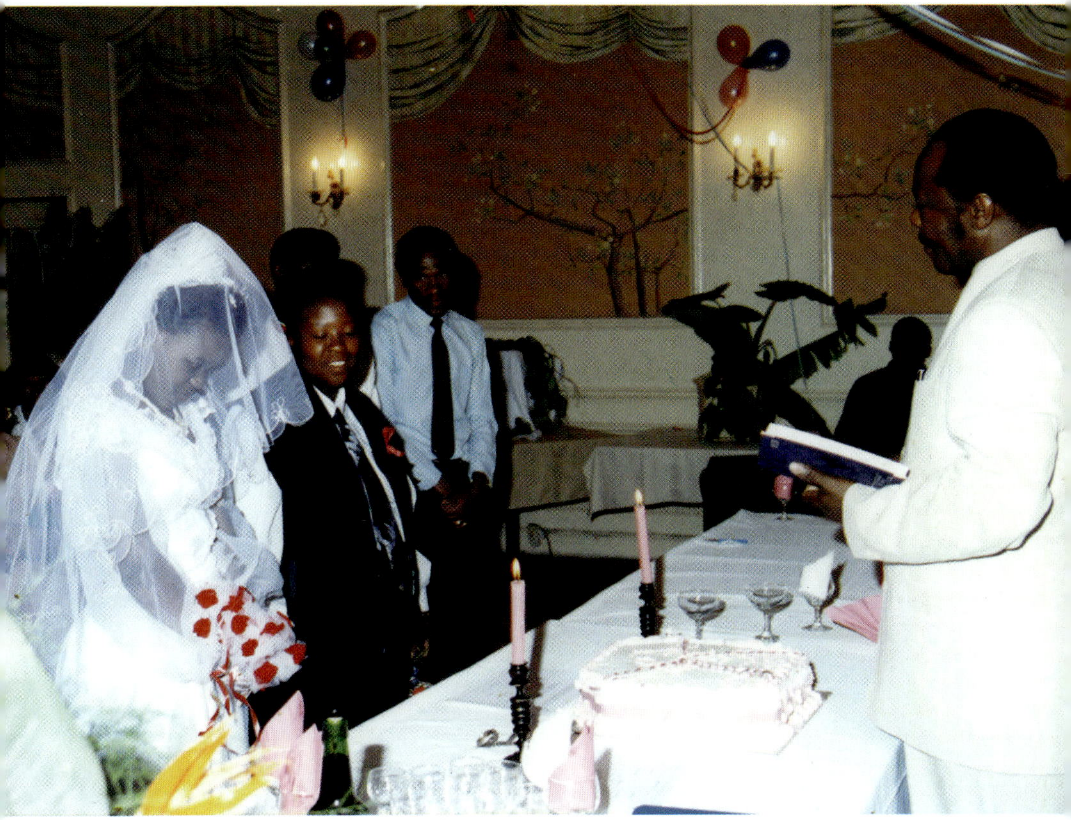

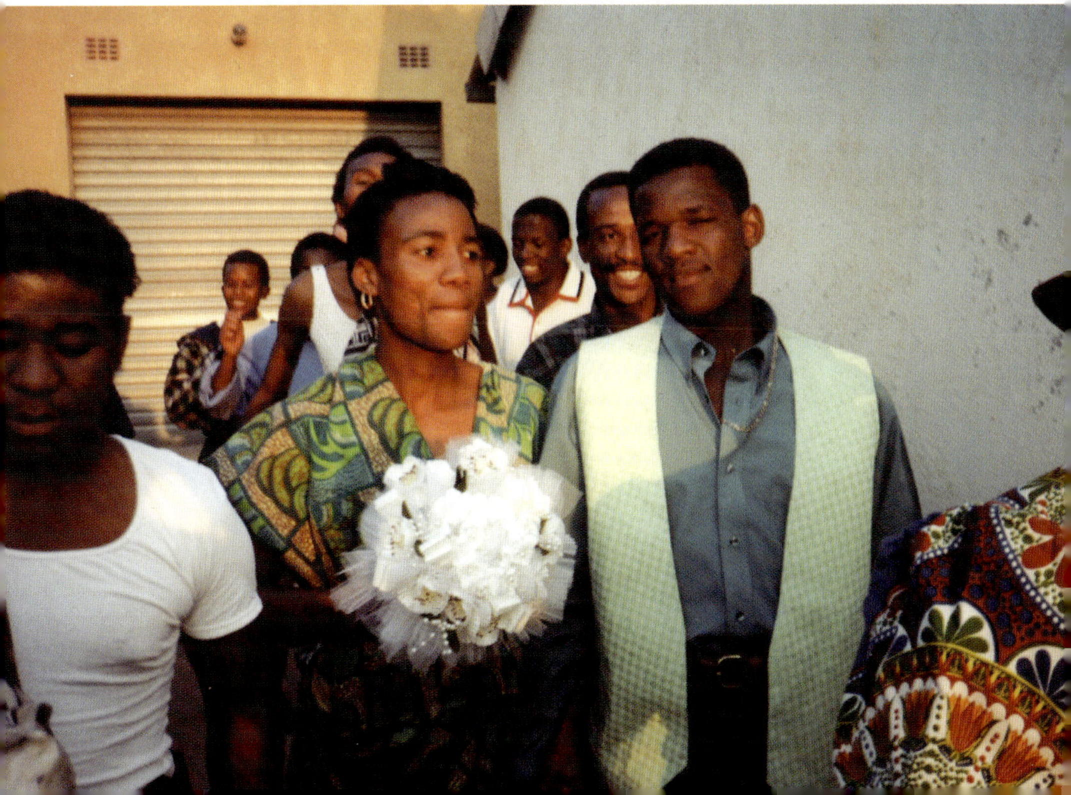

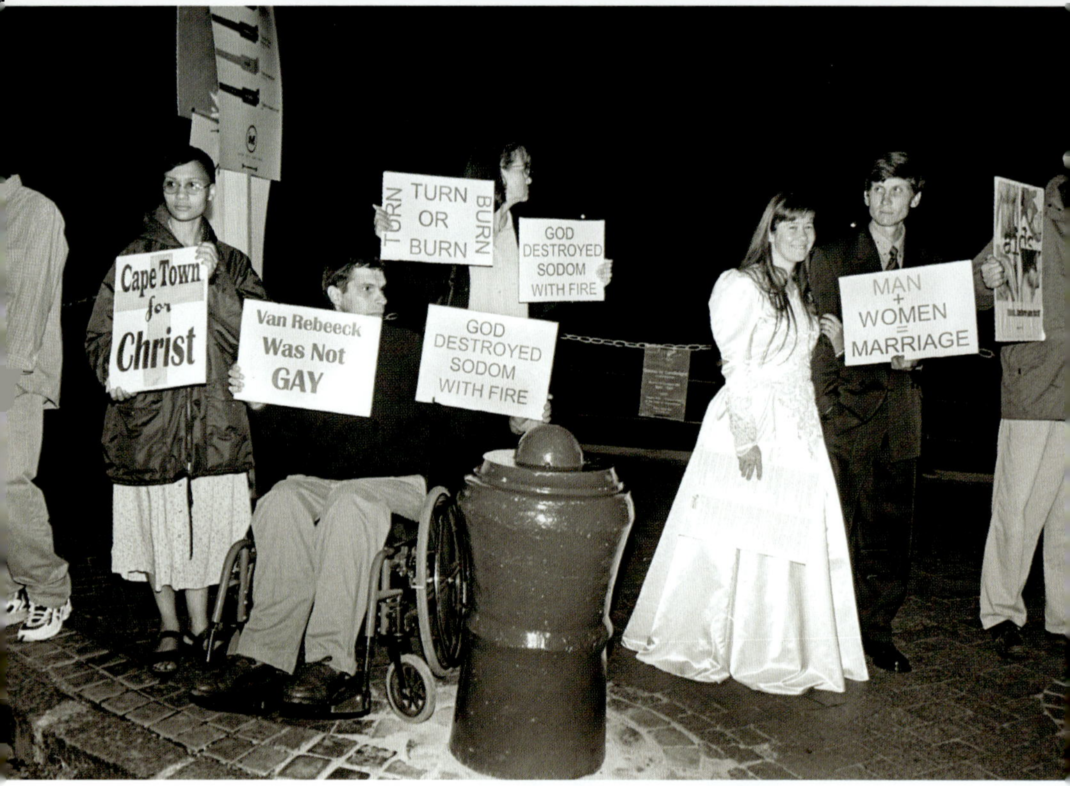

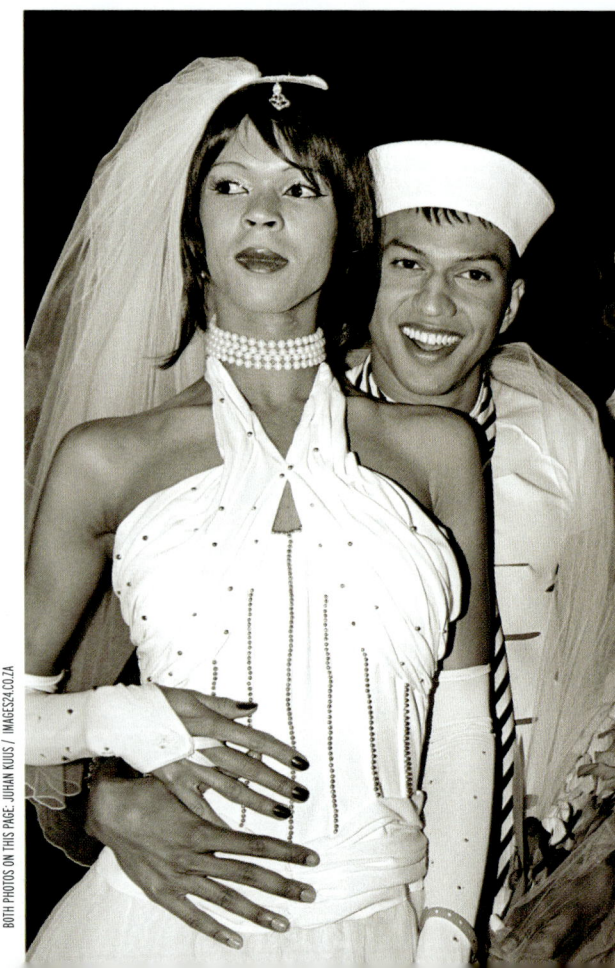

Not just fancy dress: The Mother City Queer Project (MCQP) is an annual 'queer' fancy-dress party in Cape Town that has taken place since 1994. The theme in 2002 was 'The Wedding' and revellers came dressed accordingly (right). Conservative Christians protested outside the event (above), which was held at the Castle of Good Hope in Cape Town on 14 December 2002.

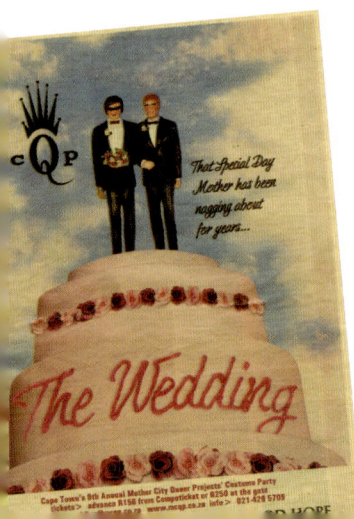

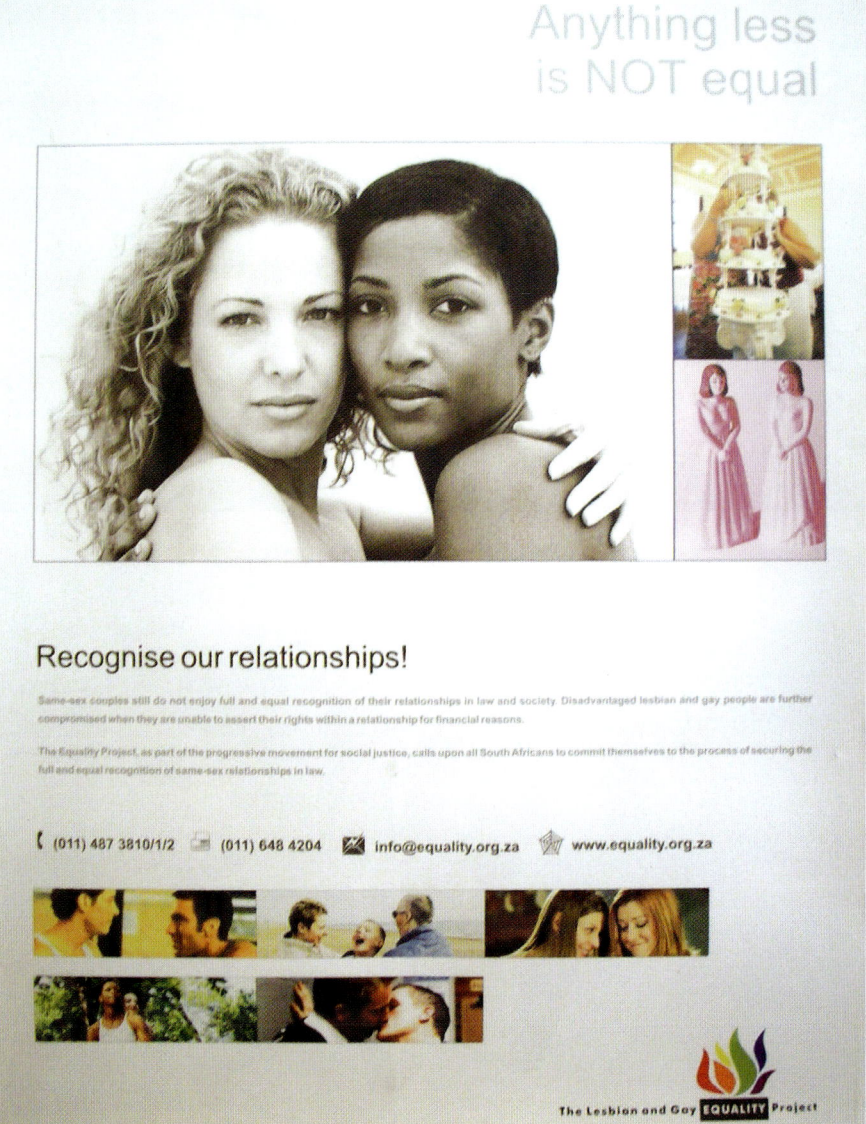

Campaign trail: A 2004 Lesbian and Gay Equality Project poster in support of the right of same-sex couples to marry

IMAGES24.CO.ZA / RAPPORT / ANTOINE DE RAS

SIDDIQUE DAVIDS / BEELD / IMAGES24.CO.ZA

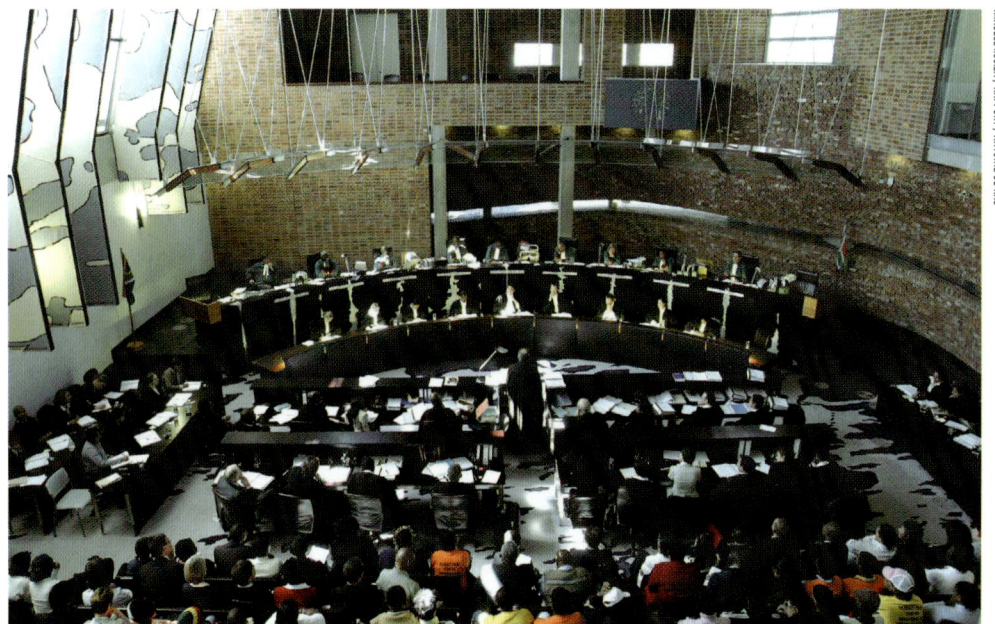

Going a-courting: On 14 May 2005 the Constitutional Court hearing on same-sex marriage was held. Above, the inside of the court that day, with the judges and members of the public in the gallery. Below, Cecilia Bonthuys (left) and the late Marié Fourie (centre), the lesbian couple who challenged the common-law definition of marriage. Dominee André Muller (right) was there to support them. (See page 48.)

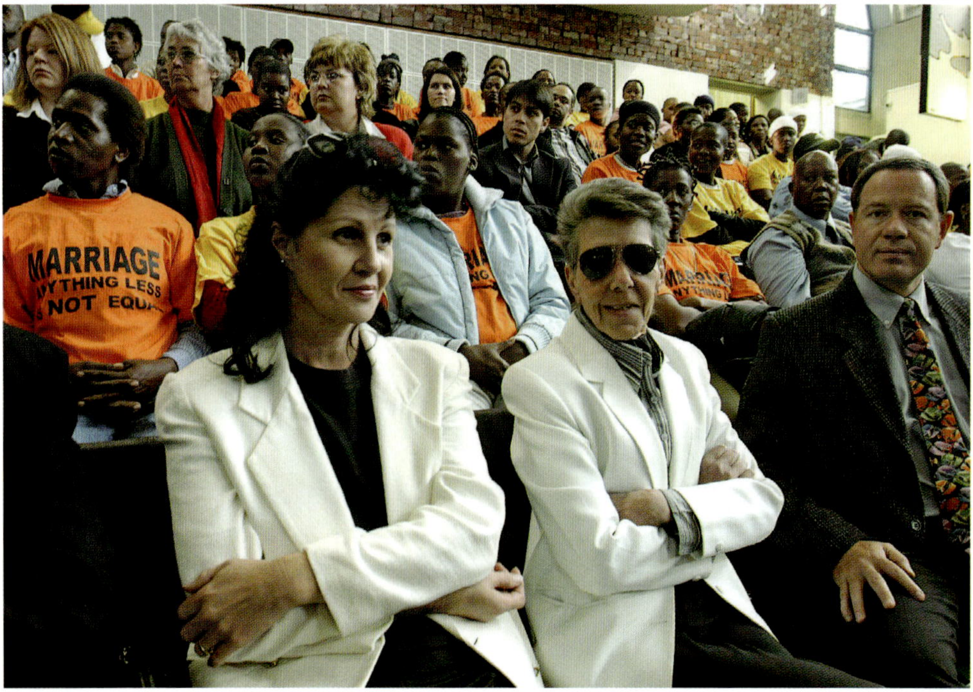

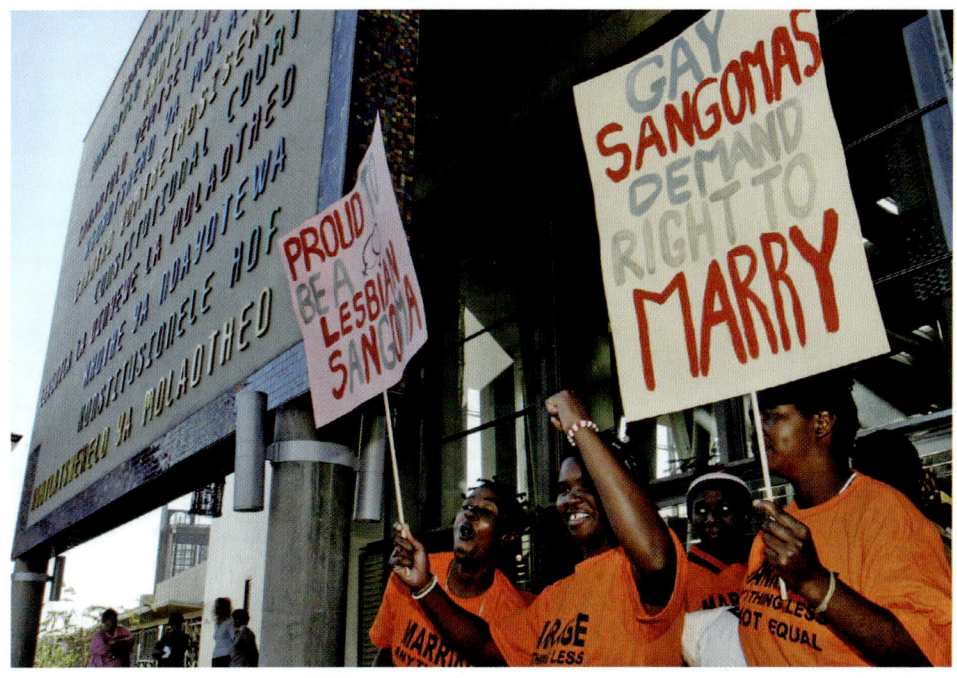
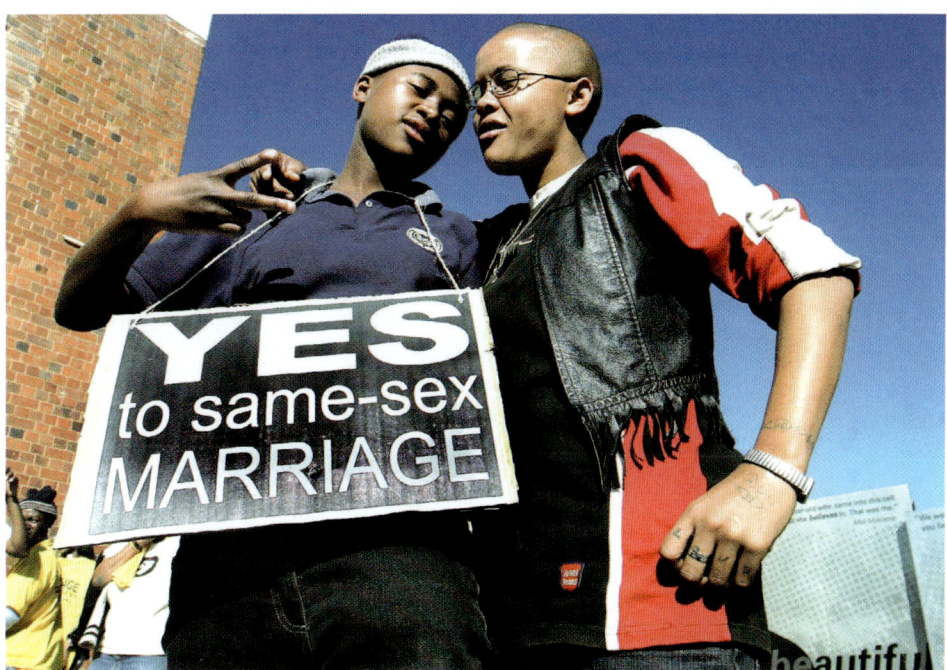

What do we want? Outside the Constitutional Court on 14 May 2005, a group of sangomas (above) and lesbian activists (below) say 'yes' to same-sex marriage.

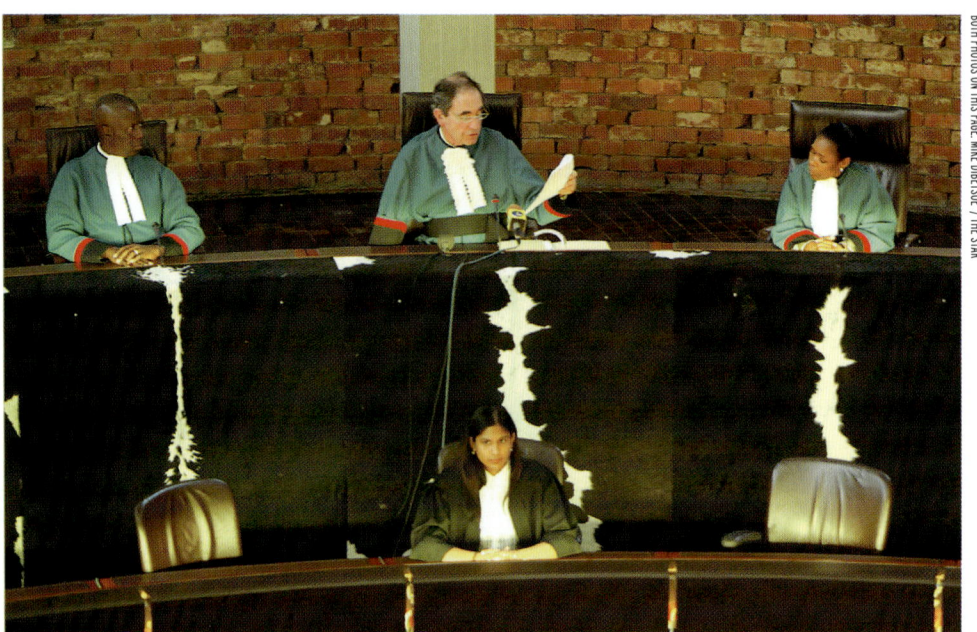

Judgment day: On 1 December 2005, Justice Albie Sachs (above, centre) delivered the Constitutional Court's judgment in *Fourie*, which, a year later, would lead to the promulgation of the Civil Union Act.
Below, former Lesbian and Gay Equality Project director Carrie Shelver (left) and the late Azu Udogu (right), an immigrant from Nigeria, at the Constitutional Court following the Sachs judgment. 'In Nigeria,' said Azu, 'I was harassed, I was arrested by the police. I came to South Africa so I could live free from that. Now I can marry my man!'

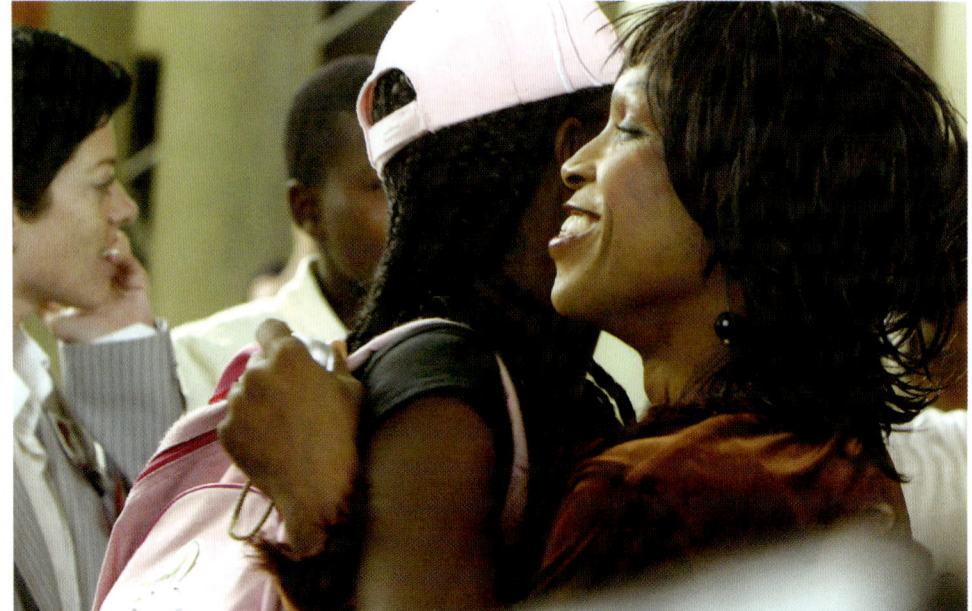

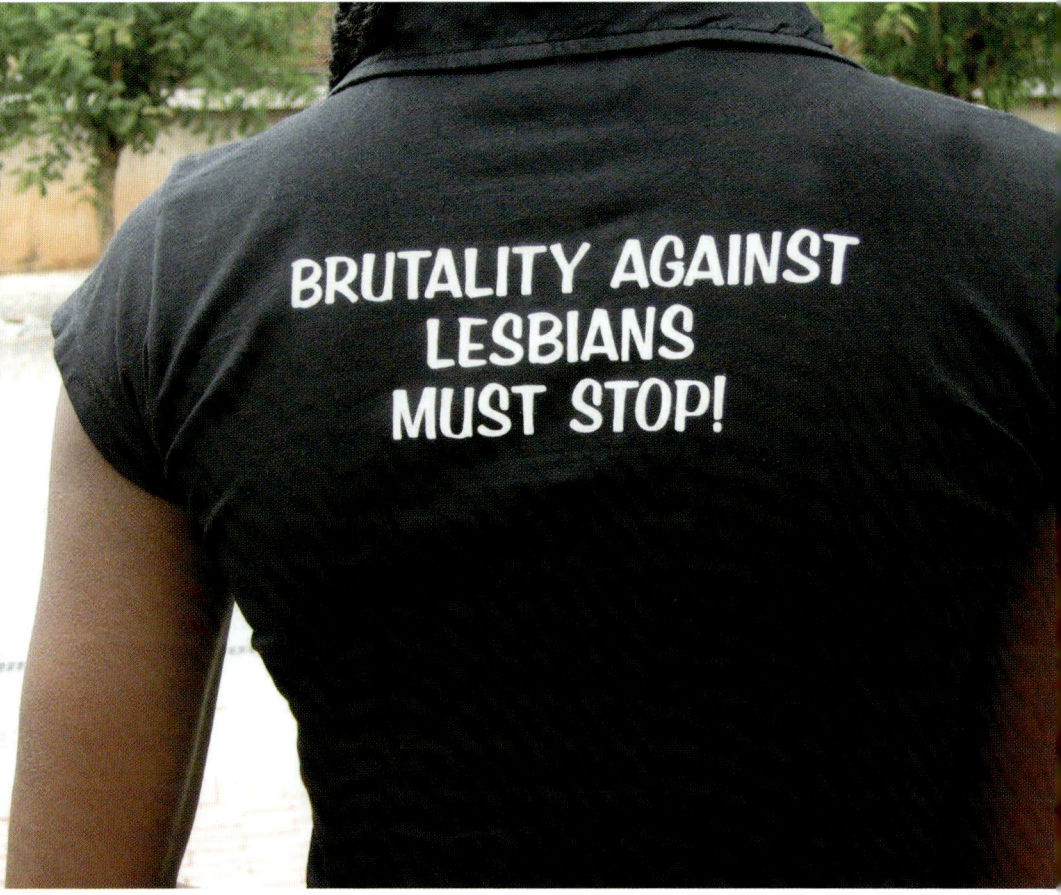

Stop the hate: A teeshirt, worn at the Court on the day of the Sachs judgment, reminds us of the ongoing attacks on black lesbian women, despite constitutional protections.

JAMES OATWAY / SUNDAY TIMES

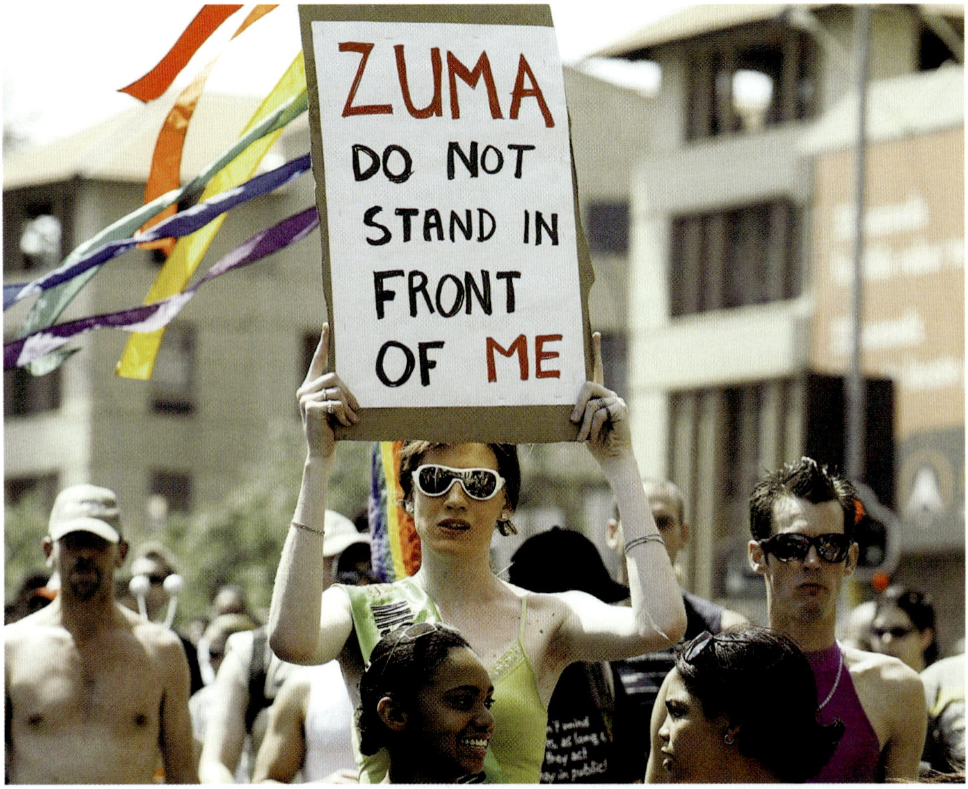

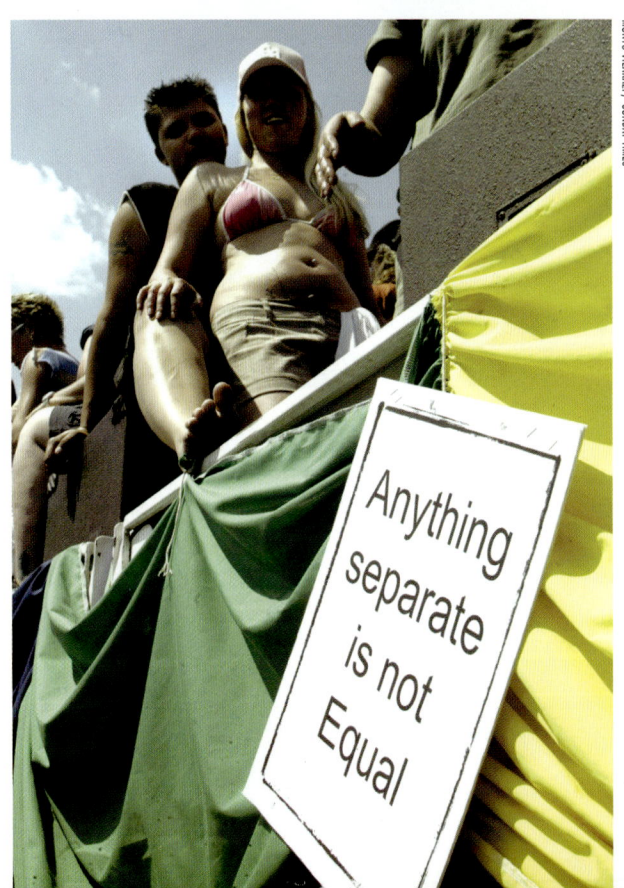

Can't stand it: Addressing crowds attending Heritage day celebrations on 24 September 2006, the then ANC deputy president, Jacob Zuma, said: 'When I was growing up, *ungqingili* [homosexuals] could not stand in front of me.' At that year's gay and lesbian Pride parade in Johannesburg, above, a marcher displays a response to Zuma.

At the same parade (right), participants react to the draft Civil Union Bill, which was open for pubic debate at the time. The Bill proposed a separate Act for same-sex couples.

MUNTU VILAKAZI / SUNDAY TIMES

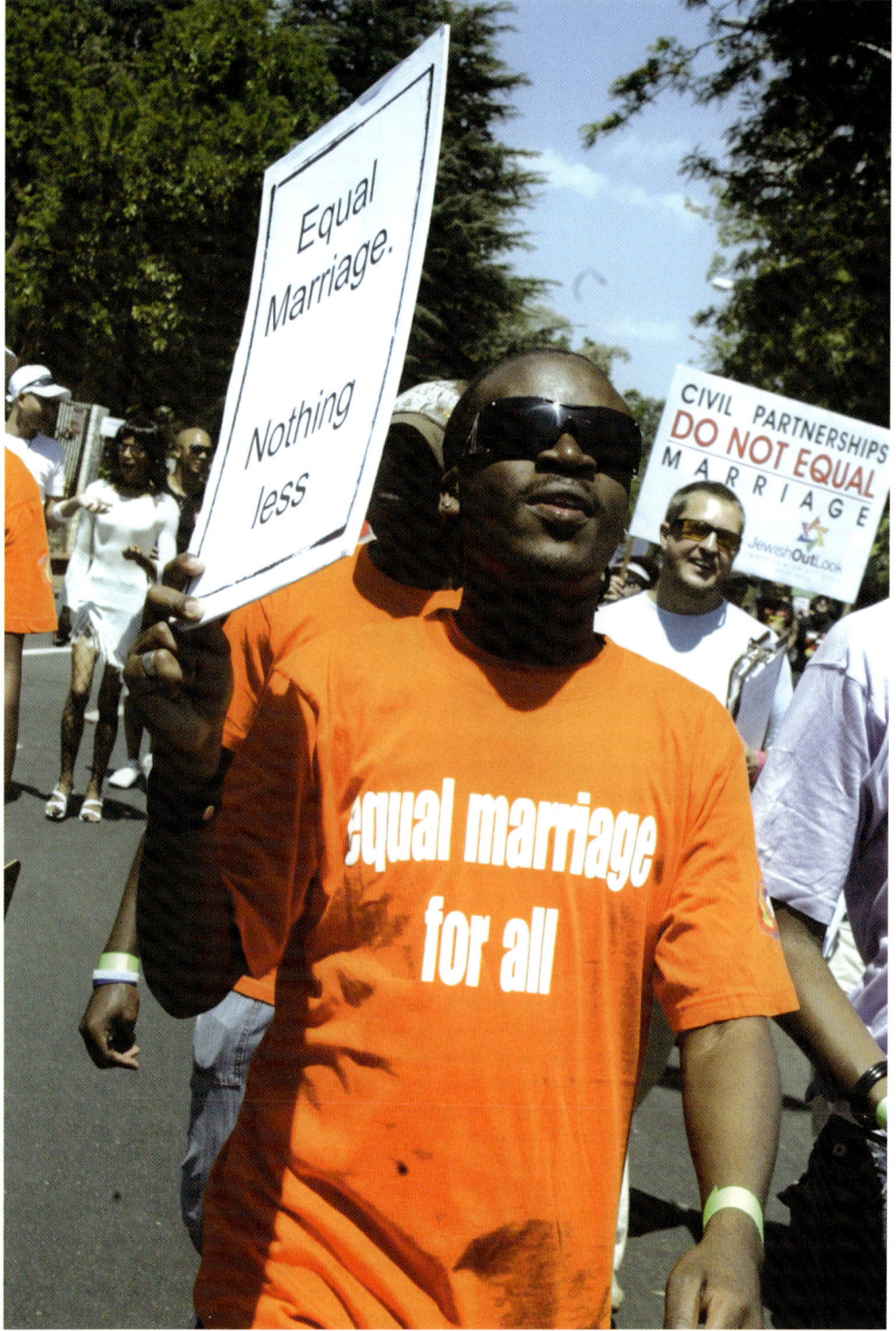

Nothing less: An OUT supporter makes LGBTI activists' demands known at Pride 2006.

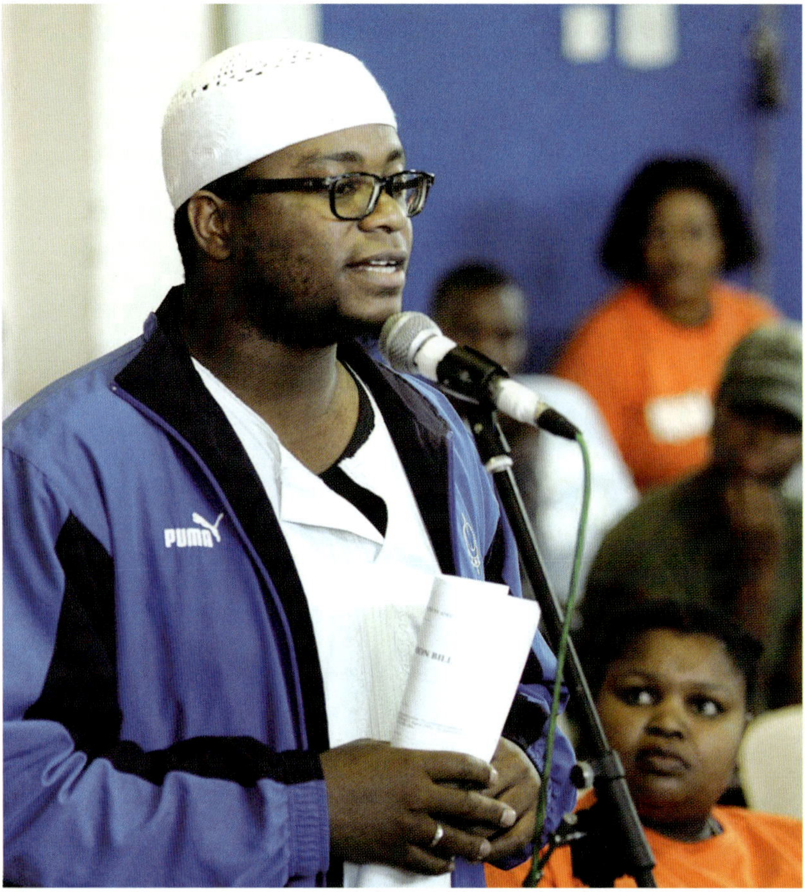

Making their voices heard: Moulan Sleinle (left) of the Council of Muslim Theologians, and Mama Grace (below) make oral submissions at the public hearings on the Civil Union Bill, held at the Jabavu community hall in Soweto on 20 September 2006.

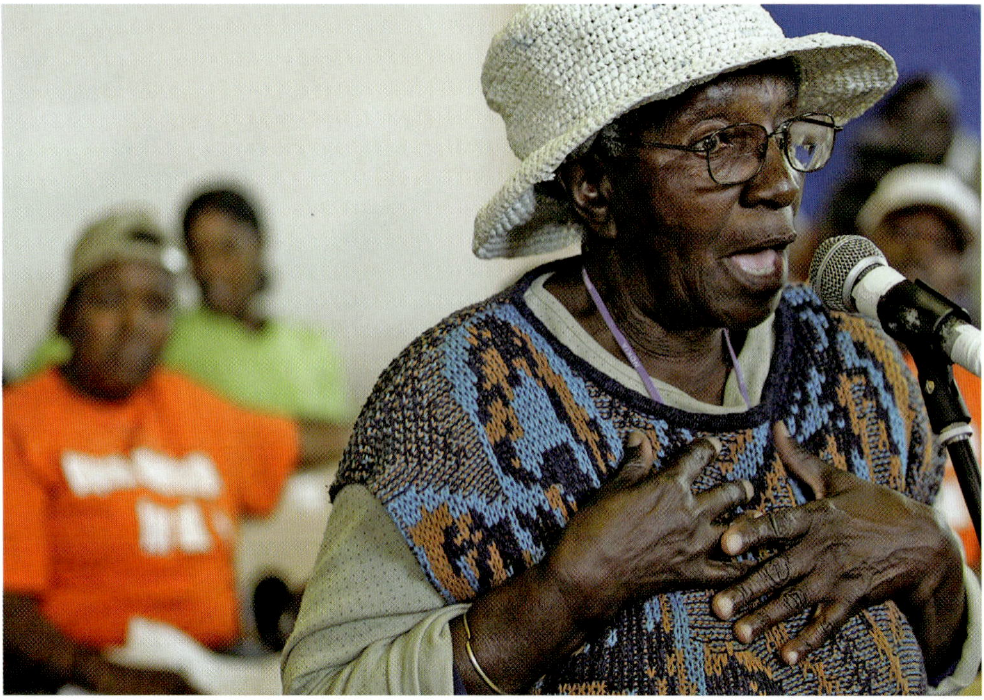

ALL PHOTOS OF SOWETO HEARINGS: DENVOR DE WEE / CITY PRESS / IMAGES24.CO.ZA

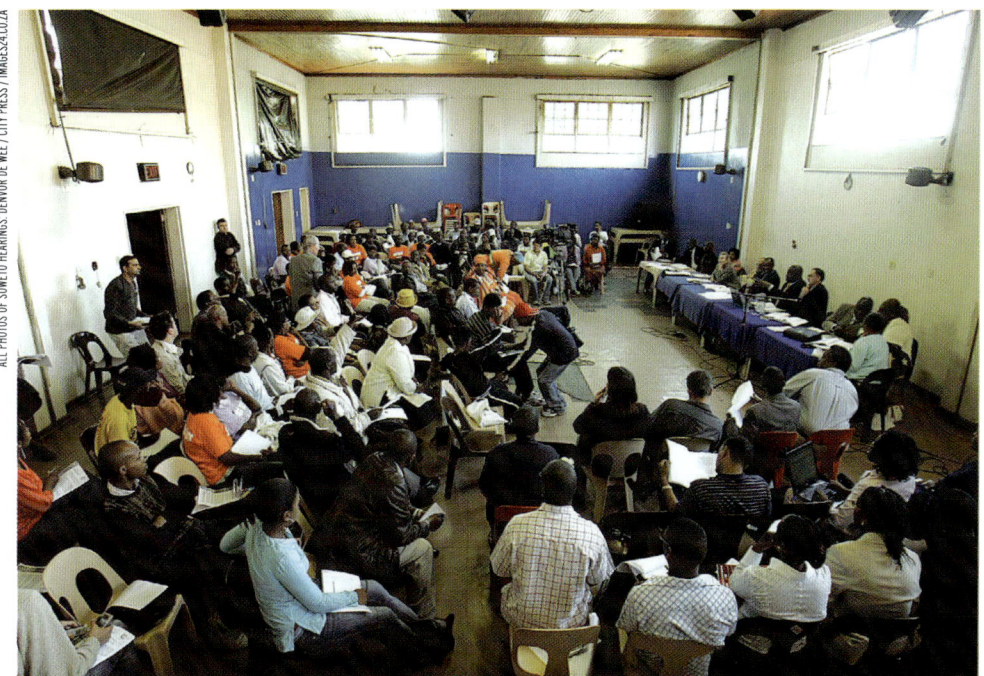

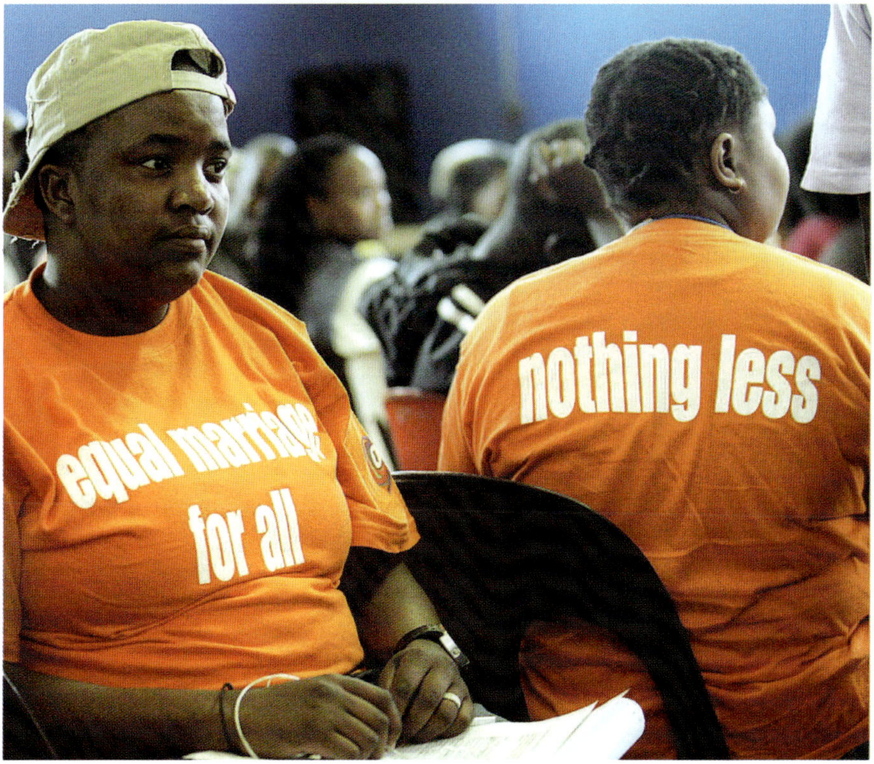

Listen carefully: Soweto debates same-sex marriage on 20 September 2006. Mmapaseka 'Steve' Letsike and Fikile Vilakazi of OUT LGBT Well-being were among the LGBTI activists who attended the hearing. (See page 87.)

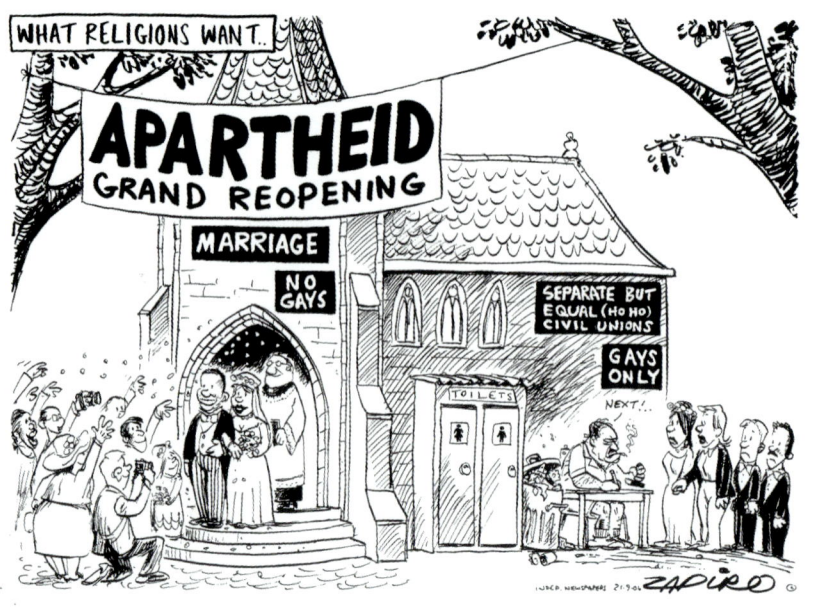

Echoes of the past: Cartoonist Zapiro's take on the calls for a 'separate but equal' system for same-sex unions. Independent Newspapers, 21 September 2006.

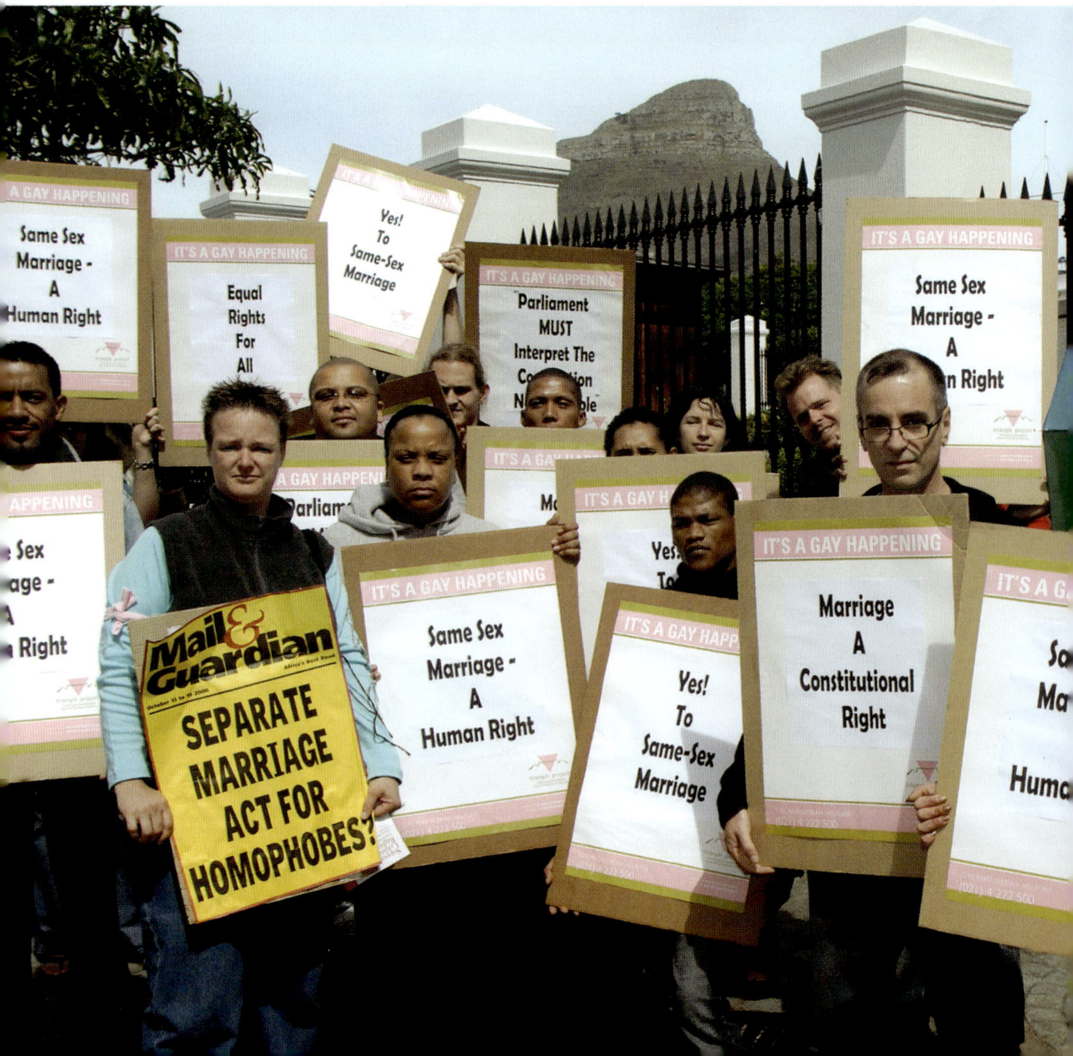

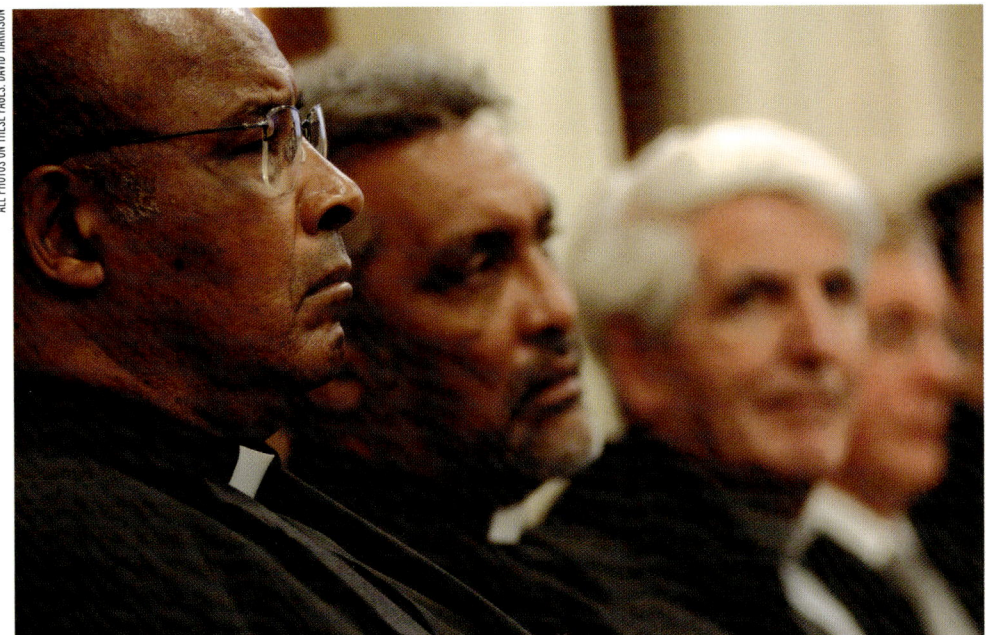

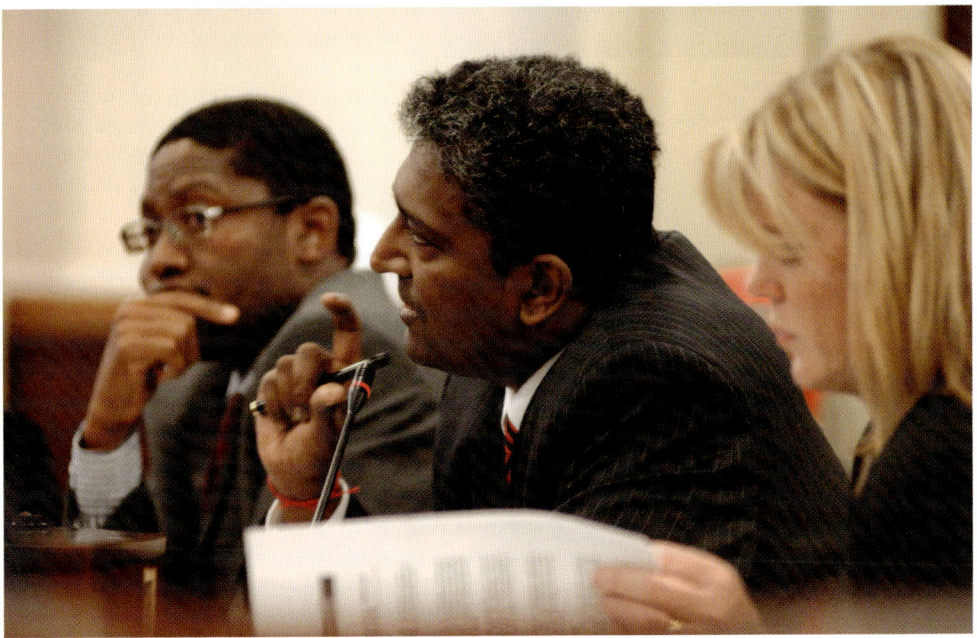

Standing up for our rights: Opposite page, below, Triangle Project and supporters picket outside Parliament during the public hearings on the Civil Union Bill, 16 October 2006, among them Tracy Smith (holding *Mail & Guardian* poster), Glenn de Swardt (far right) and Marlow Valentine (far left, holding the 'same-sex marriage – a human right' sign), from Triangle. (See page 111.)

Arguing it out: This page, above, Catholic Cardinal Wilfred Napier (far left), an outspoken voice opposed to same-sex marriage, at the hearings in Parliament. (See page 119.) Below, the South African Human Rights Commission, including Judith Cohen (far right), delivers its presentation to Parliament on the Civil Union Bill. (See page 117.)

MUNTU VILAKAZI / SUNDAY TIMES

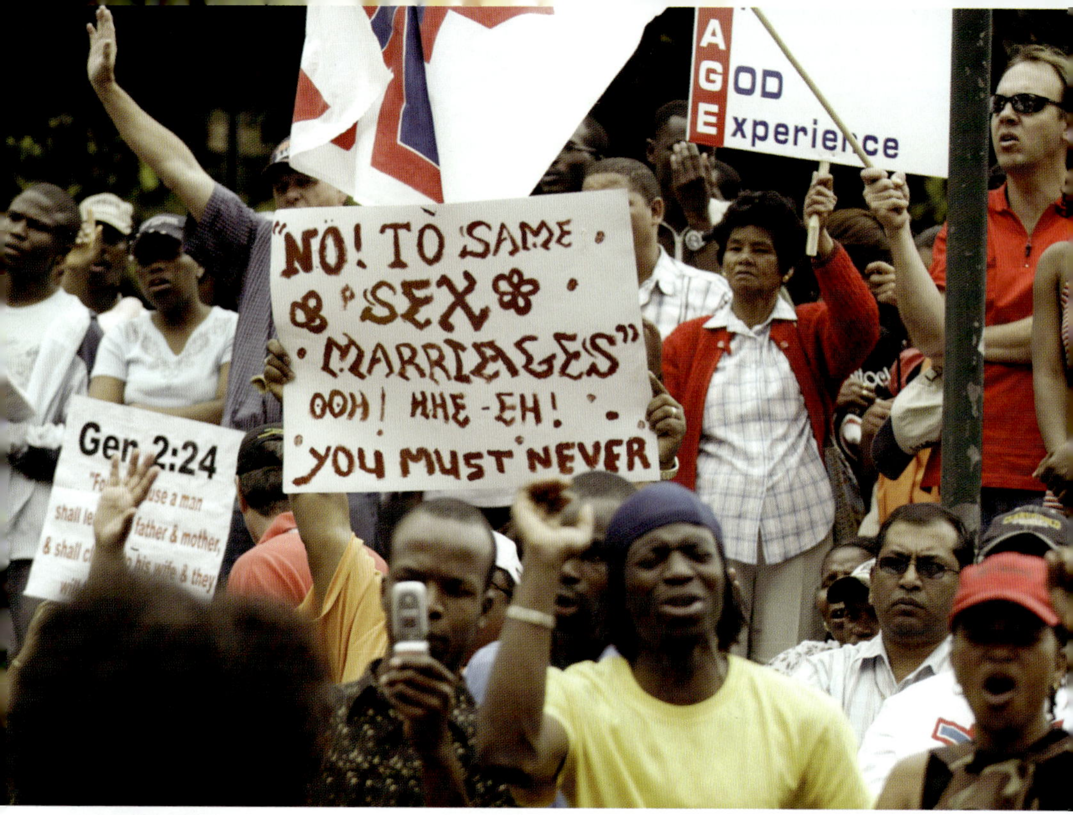

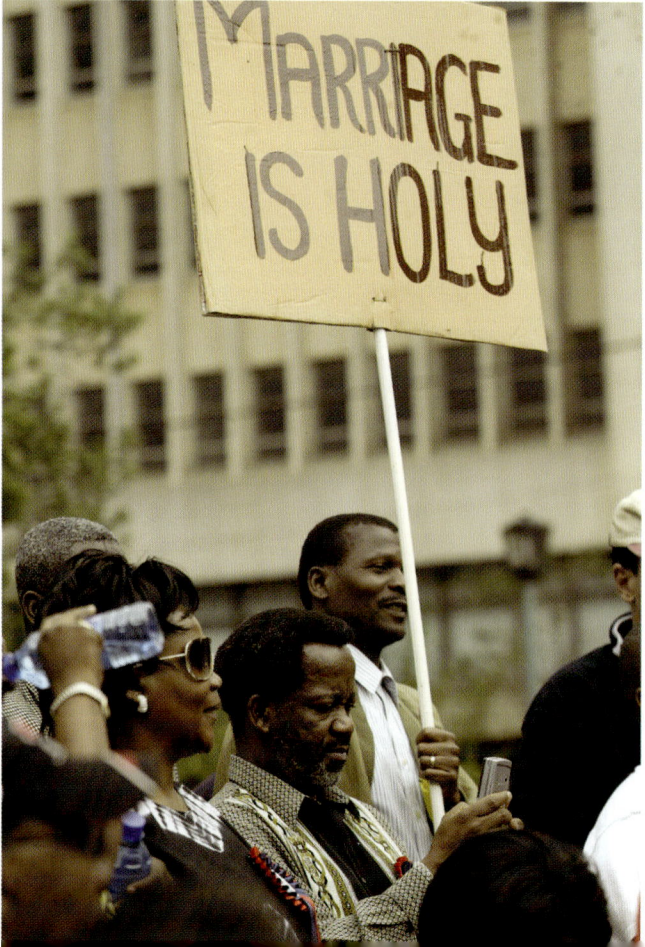

Against and for:
On 16 September 2006, The Marriage Alliance organized marches in a number of cities to protest against the Civil Union Bill. Below, the Reverend Kenneth Meshoe, leader of the African Christian Democratic Party (ACDP), at the Johannesburg march.

ALET PRETORIUS / BEELD / IMAGES24.CO.ZA

JUAN NEL

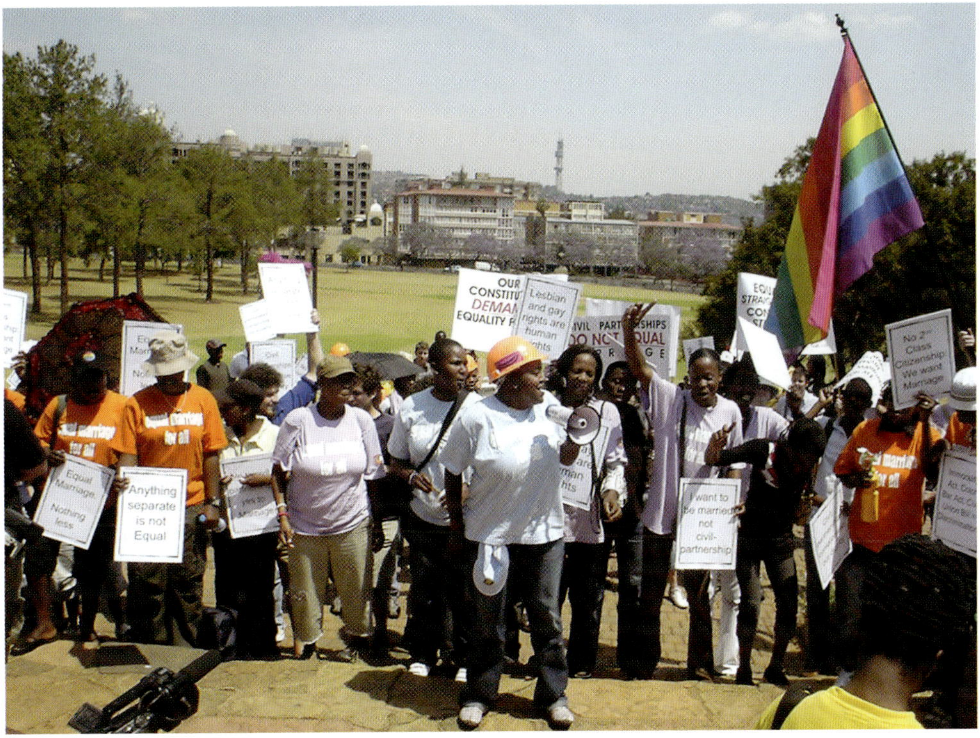

Flying the flag: On 17 October 2006, members of LGBTI organizations – including OUT, Jewish OutLook, GALA, Forum for the Empowerment of Women (FEW), *Exit*, Wits Activate, UP&OUT, Behind the Mask – marched to the Union Buildings in Tshwane to demand full and equal marriage rights for same-sex couples . The marchers handed a memorandum to the Department of Home Affairs. Top, Phumla Masuku (far left) of FEW keeps the flag flying outside the Union Buildings.

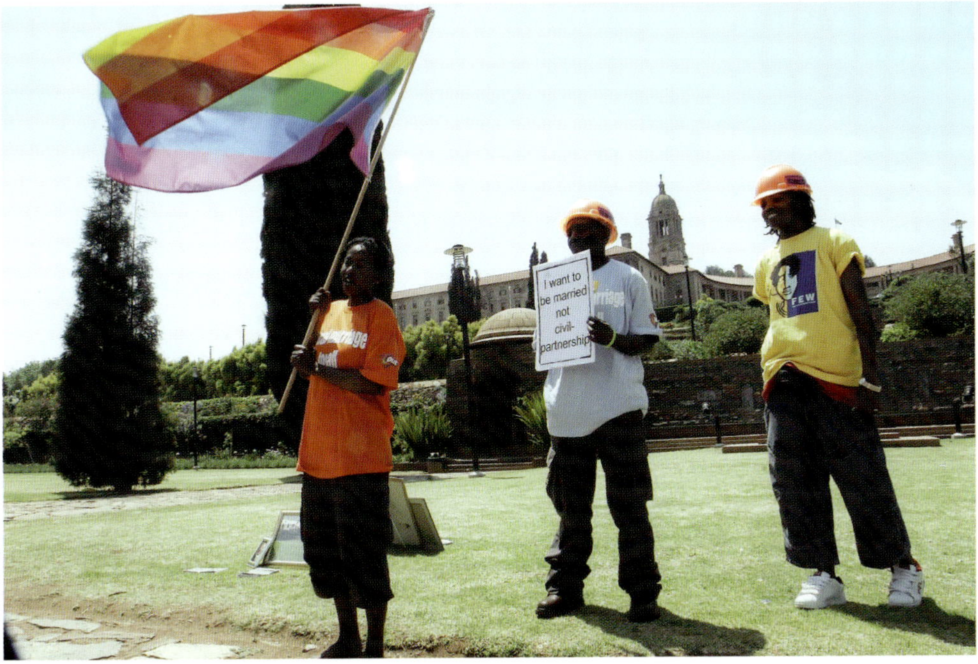

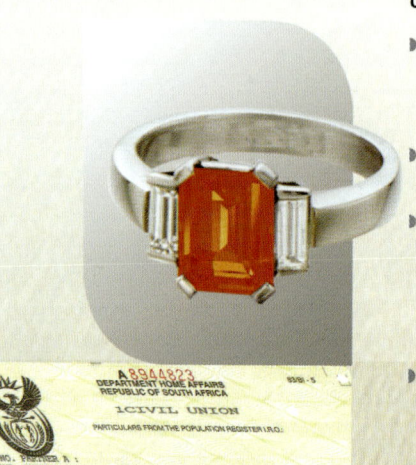

Now it's official: Poster released by the Department of Home Affairs following the promulgation of the Civil Union Act on 30 November 2006.

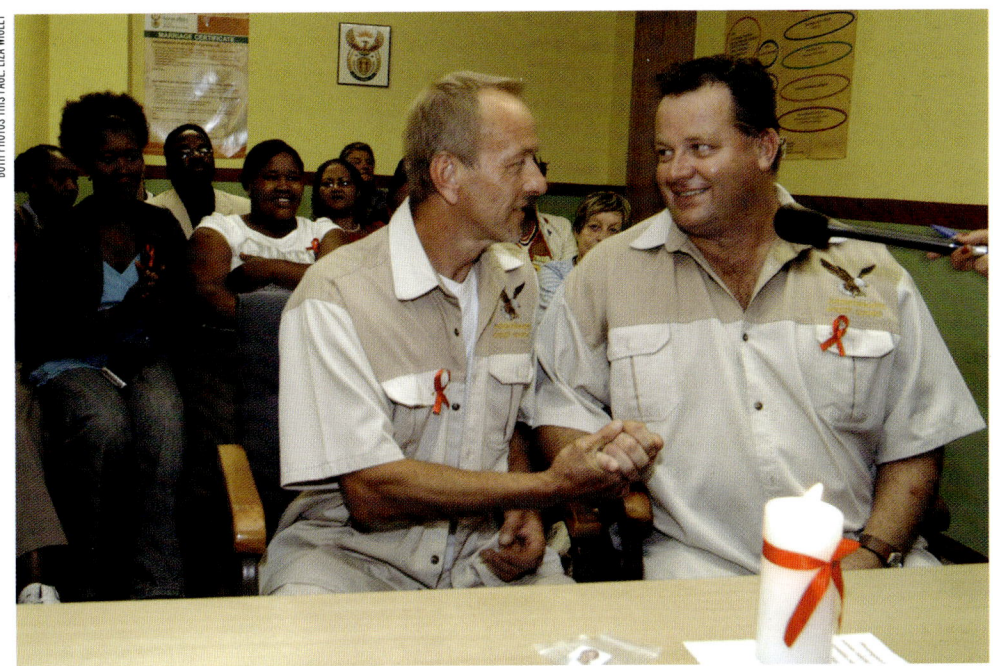

First in line: On 1 December 2006, a day after the Civil Union Act came into effect, Tony Halls (left) and Vernon Gibbs became the first same-sex couple to be legally married in South Africa. They were married at the Home Affairs office at George in the Western Cape. Vernon told British paper *The Guardian*, 'We are so pleased we did it on December 1, World Aids Day. We dedicate our marriage to all HIV/AIDS sufferers and gay people who have experienced discrimination.'

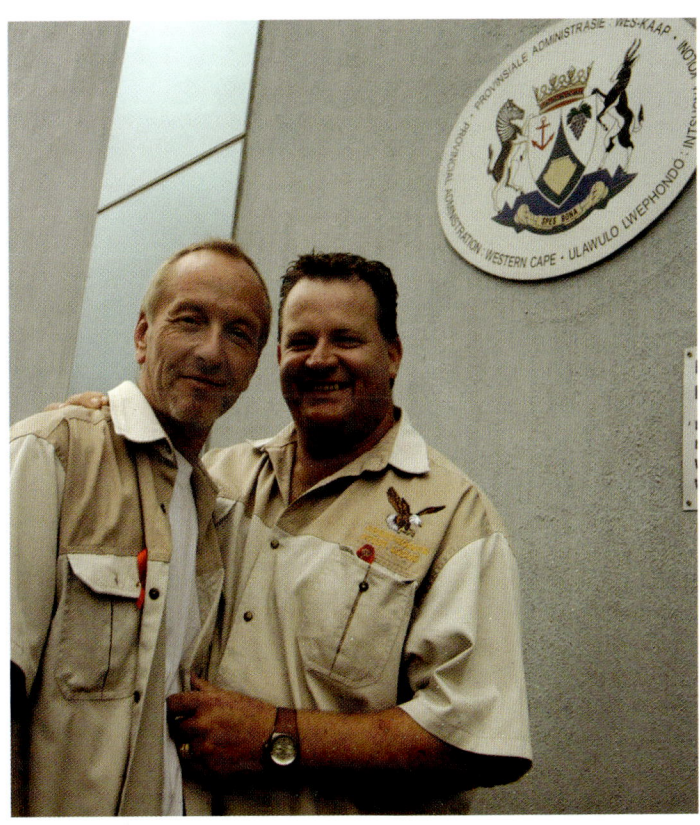

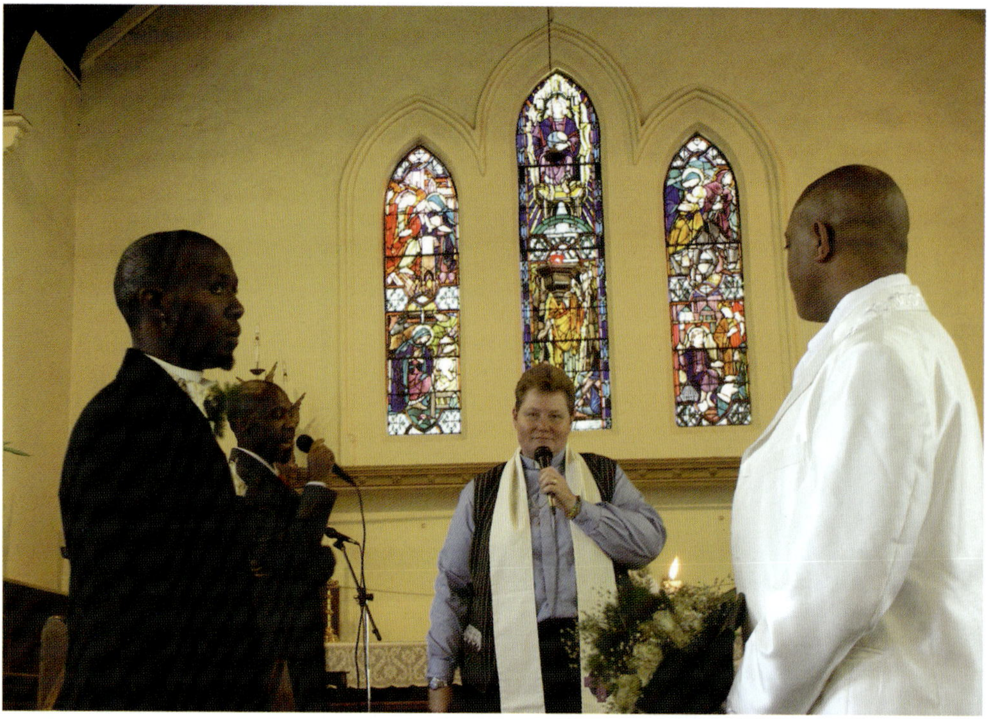

ZANELE MUHOLI

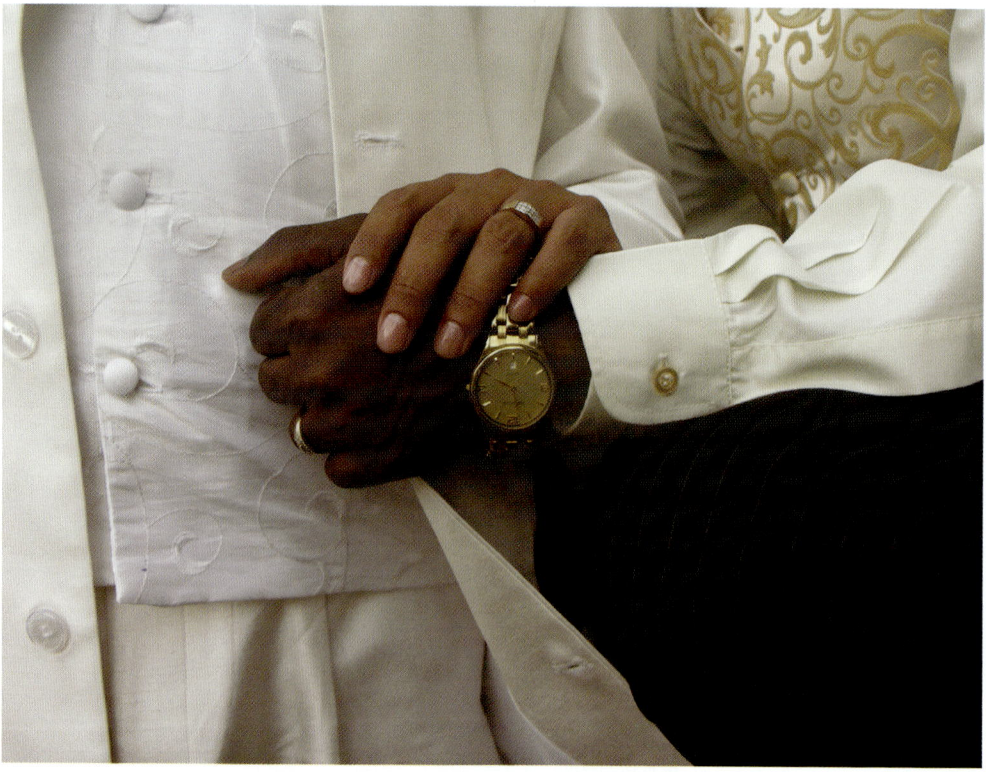

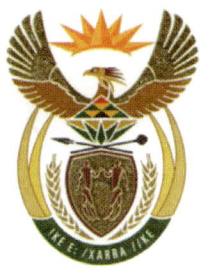

MINISTRY: HOME AFFAIRS
REPUBLIC OF SOUTH AFRICA

Private Bag X741, Pretoria, 0001, Tel: (012) 326 8081, Fax: (012) 312 6491
Private Bag X9102, Cape Town, 8000, Tel: (021) 461 5818, Fax: (021) 461 2359

The Senior Pastor
Glorious Light MCC
771 13th Avenue
Wonderboom South
PRETORIA
0084

Dear Pastor Preesman,

DESIGNATION IN TERMS OF SECTION 5 OF THE CIVIL UNION ACT, 2006 (ACT 17 of 2006)

I refer to your letter of 29 November 2006, together with the supporting documents.

I have designated Glorious Light, a member of the Metropolitan Community Churches, as a religious denomination or organisation that may solemnise marriages in terms of section 5(2) of the Civil Union Act.

I have also designated Pastor Janine Preesman as a marriage officer in terms of the Civil Union Act with effect from 1 December 2006.

Yours sincerely,

[signature]

MS N N MAPISA-NQAKULA, MP
MINISTER OF HOME AFFAIRS
DATE: 30 NOVEMBER, 2006

I thee wed: Opposite page, Sifiso and Skumbuzo Tigare were married at the Hope and Unity Metropolitan Community Church (HUMCC) in Mayfair, Johannesburg, on 2 December 2006, becoming the first same-sex couple to be legally married in a religious ceremony in South Africa. Pastors Janine Preesman (top, centre), Nokuthula Dhladhla and Paul Mokgethi presided. (See pages 228, 232.) This page, Pastor Preesman's certificate allowing her to perform marriages under the Civil Union Act. She was the first minister so designated.

White wedding: This page and opposite, Nozipho Ngcobo and Thulile Gasa were the first same-sex couple in Pietermaritzburg to have their wedding featured in the local newspapers. They were married in a legal ceremony and later in a religious one in September 2007. (See page 321.)

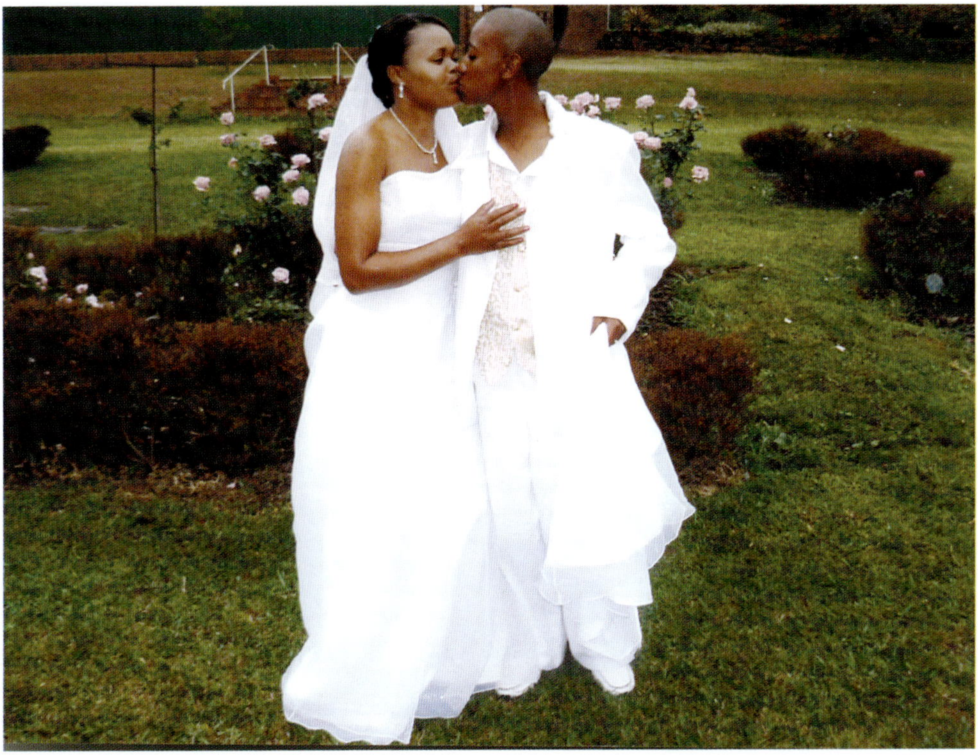

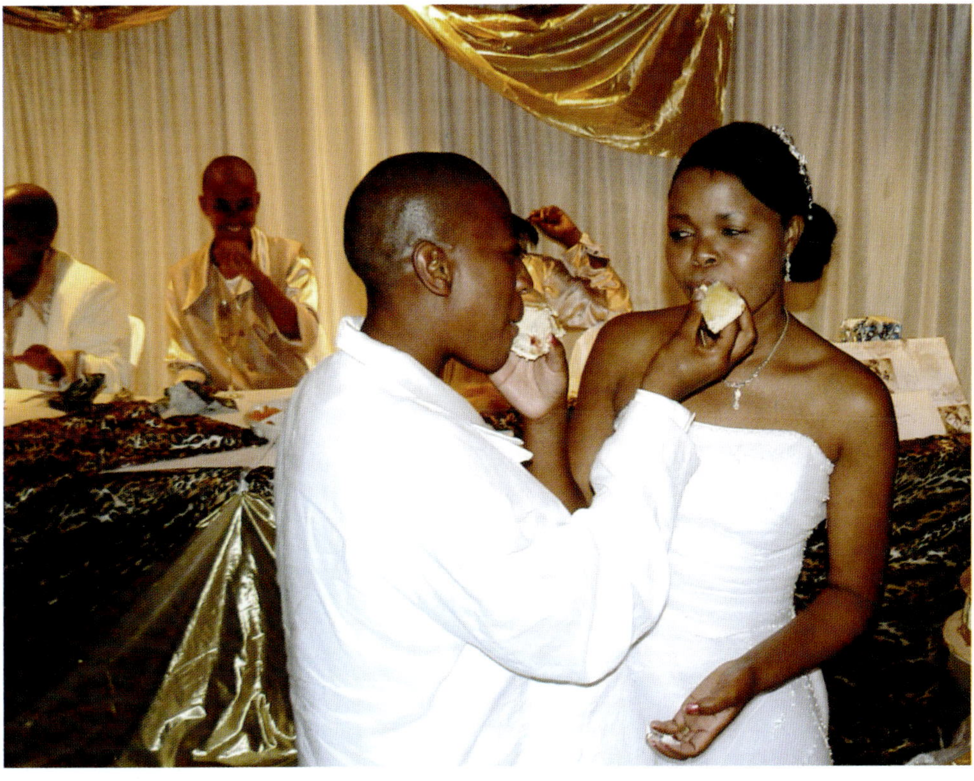

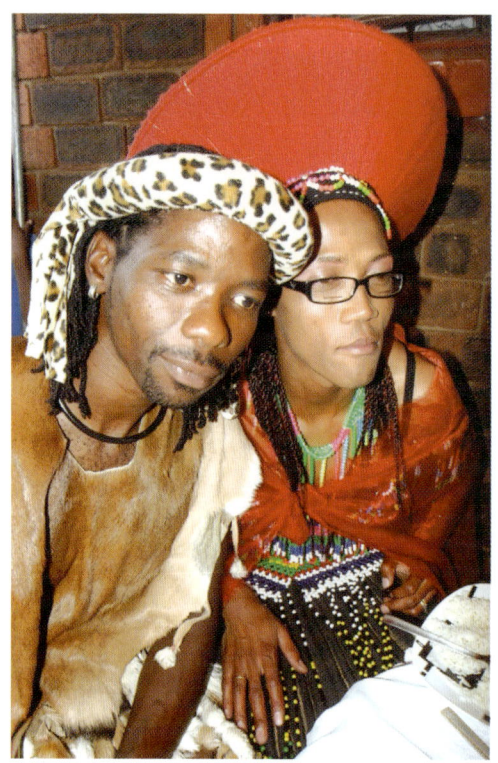

Traditional style: After having been together for 11 years, Wiseman Mndaweni (left, in both pictures) and Jackie van Rooyen of Katlehong married on 3 February 2007 at the Home Affairs office in Alberton, Ekurhuleni. They also had a traditional Zulu wedding in Katlehong (below). Said Wiseman, 'One of my uncles was fair in saying that he was a traditional man, and that he does not know this thing. But he said he will do it [the lobola negotiations] for the sake of his sister's son.'

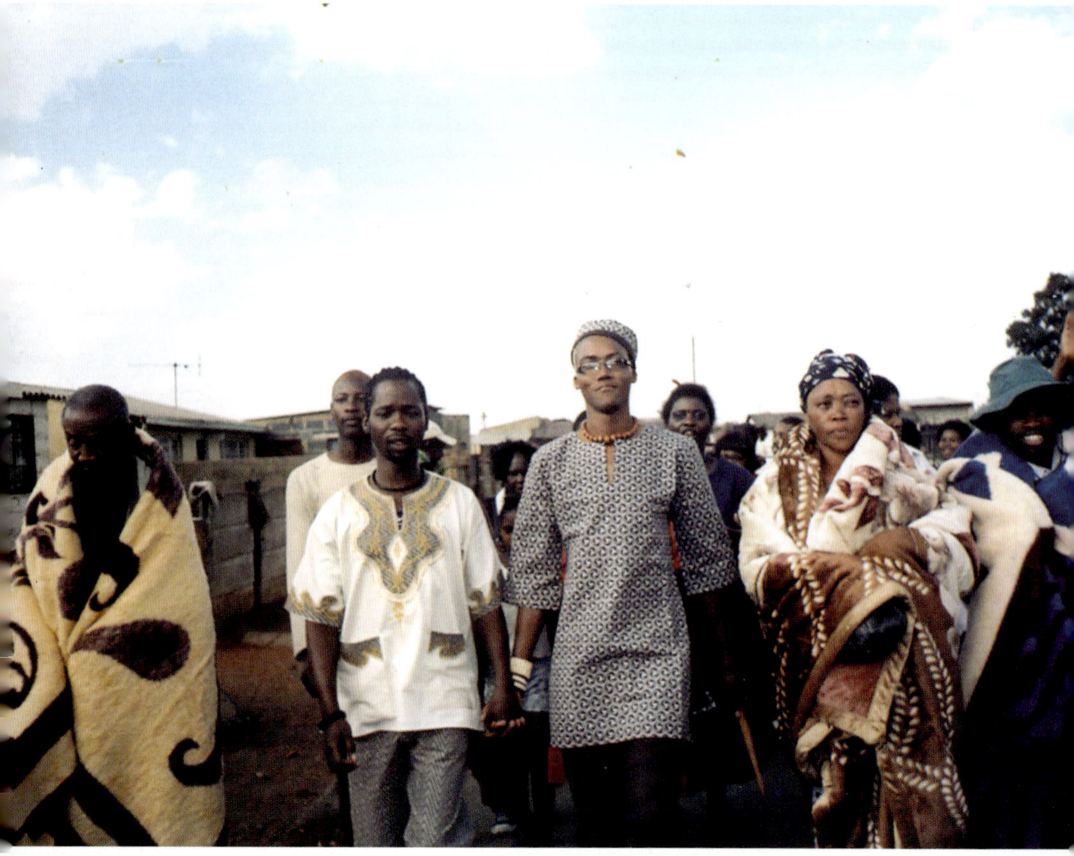

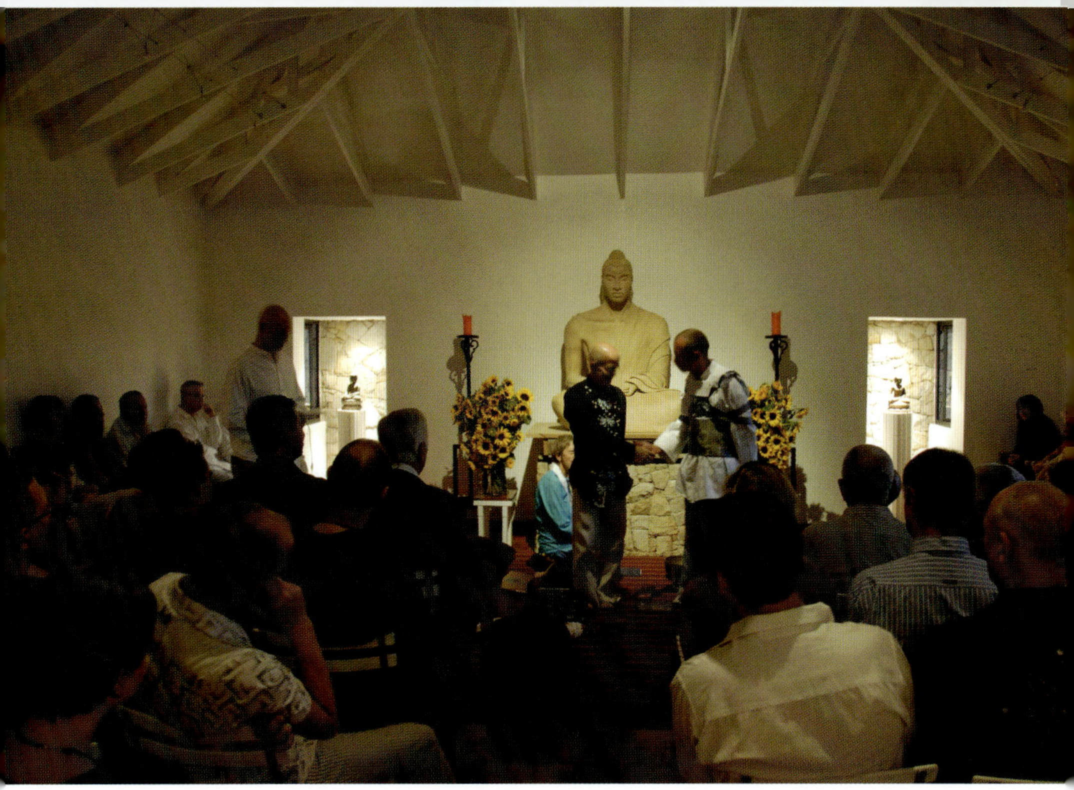

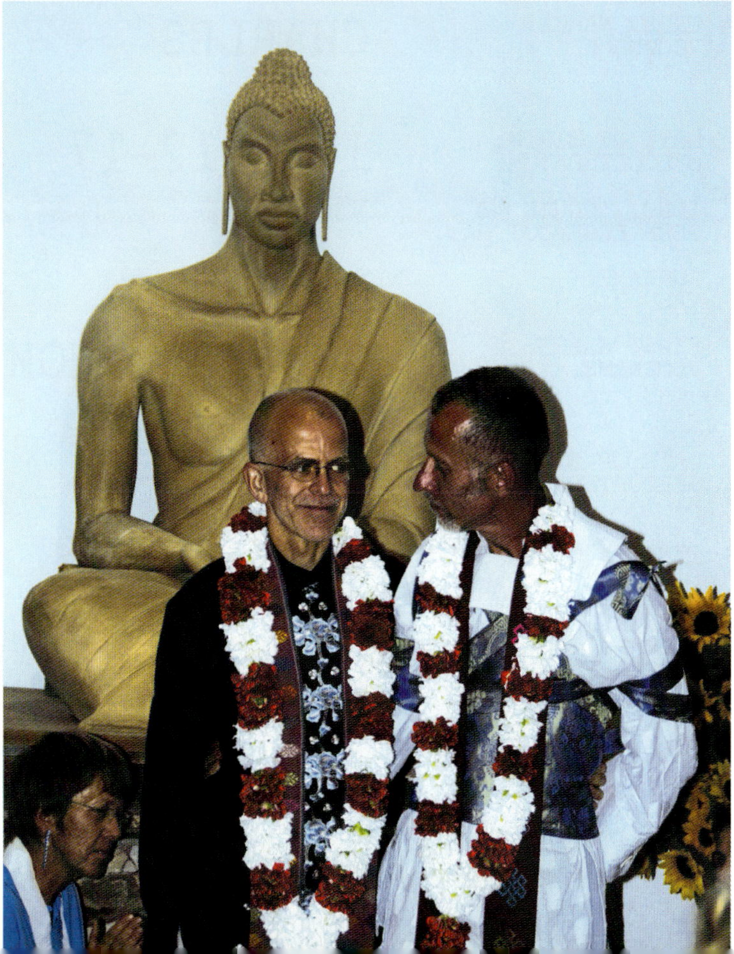

As the spirit moves: Vajradhara (left, in both pictures) and Wayne Sampson were married on 24 March 2007 at the Buddhist centre they run in Johannesburg. (See page 341.)

B 2566338
DEPARTMENT HOME AFFAIRS
REPUBLIC OF SOUTH AFRICA

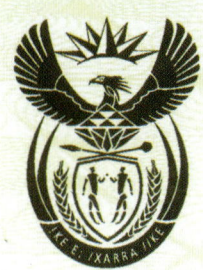

PARTICULARS FROM THE POPULATION REGISTER I.R.O.:

CIVIL UNION

IDNO. SPOUSE A :
IDNR. EGGENOOT A :

SURNAME: / VAN : JANUARIE

FIRST NAMES: / VOORNAME : CHARLES

DATE OF BIRTH: / GEBOORTEDATUM: 1967-12-17

IDNO. SPOUSE B :
IDNR. EGGENOOT B :

SURNAME: / VAN : NDIMANDE

FIRST NAMES: / VOORNAME : CROSSBEE HOMPI

DATE OF BIRTH: / GEBOORTEDATUM: 1970-09-16

TYPE OF CIVIL UNION : MARRIAGE

DATE OF MARRIAGE : 2007-03-28

PLACE OF MARRIAGE : BRAKPAN

DATE ISSUED : / DATUM UITGEREIK: 2007-04-02   ISSUED BY : / UITGEREIK DEUR: YD0211

ZANELE MUHOLI

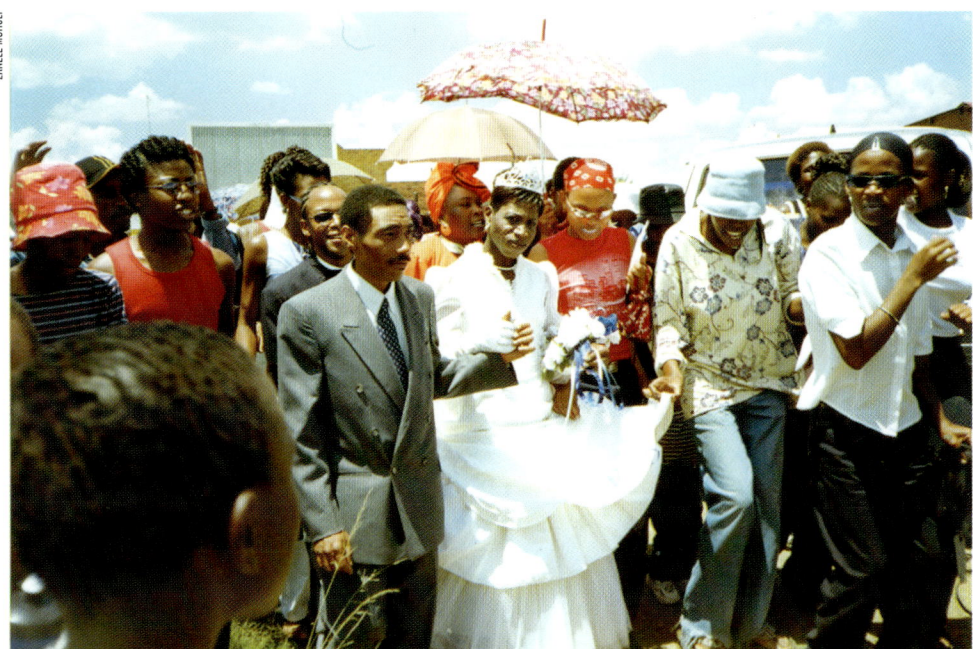

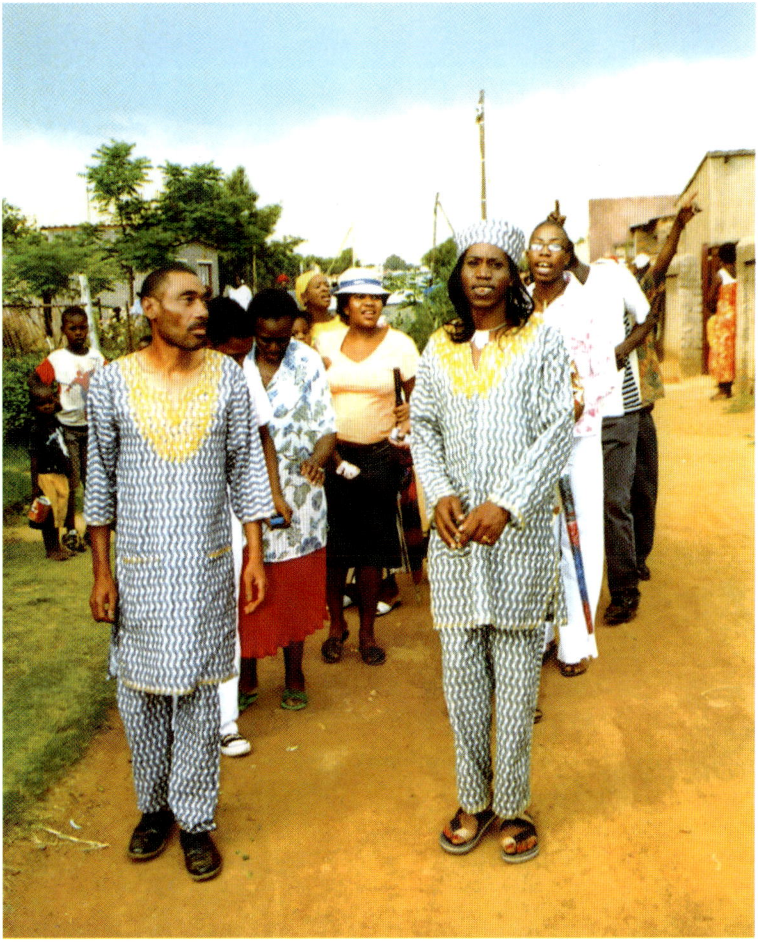

Wed twice over: Charles (left, in both pictures) and Hompi Januarie of KwaThema had a public wedding ceremony in 2002 (above). After the passing of the Civil Union Act, they got married for a second time (below), so that their relationship could be legally recognized. (See page 317.) Opposite page: The Januaries' marriage certificate.

AMANDA VAN WYK

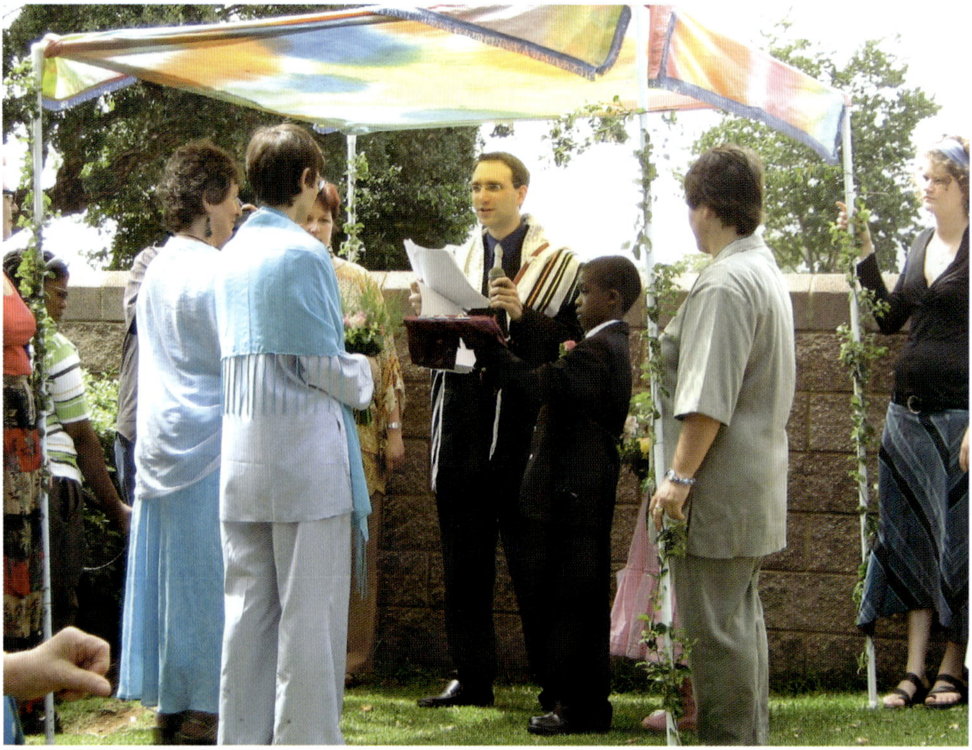

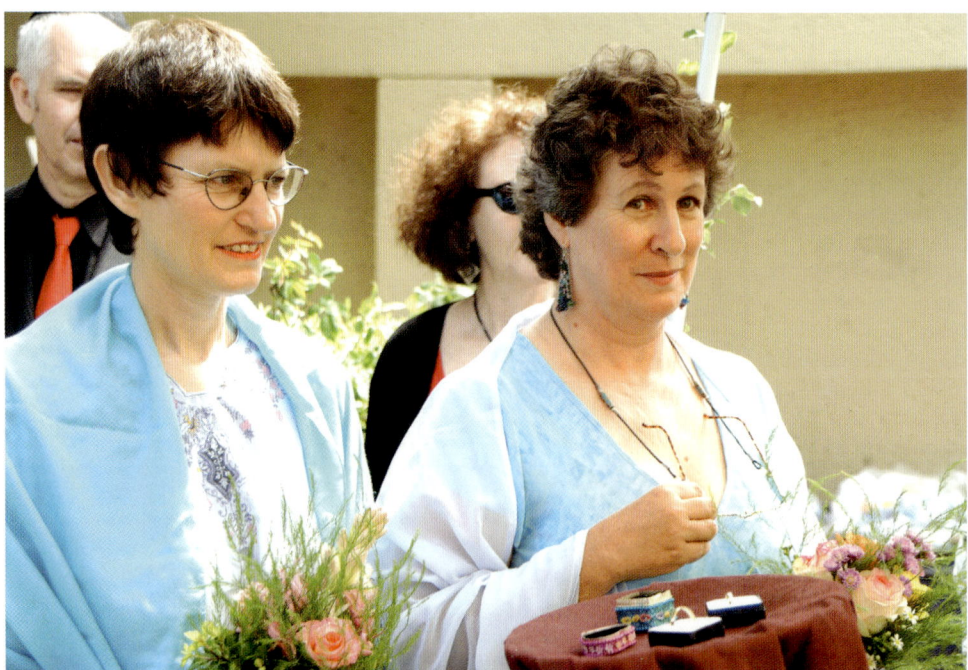

Mazeltov: Margaret Auerbach (below, left) and Liebe Kellen became the first same-sex couple to be legally married in a Jewish religious ceremony in South Africa. (See page 345.) The religious part of the ceremony was conducted by David Bilchitz (above, centre).

WEDDING BELLES

Flats lesbians go down the aisle with passion

THIS Cape Flats lesbian couple have finally tied the knot after 14 years of living together.

And they made sure they would never forget the special occasion for the rest of their lives.

Now many of their lesbian friends are considering following their lead and getting married as well.

Sadia Kruger, 48, looked dashing in a fish tail suit with silver waistcoat and cravat.

And bride Zukayna Leonard, 31, went the more traditional way and wore a white wedding dress complete with veil and tiara.

But she allowed her bridesmaids to choose their fabric

By LAUREN KANSLEY
Pics by SHAWN UYS

most exciting thing she's ever done.

Sadia says: "*The day the Home Affairs minister signed the papers to say gay marriages were legal I knew I would propose.*

Love

HAPPINESS: The couple

"We started talking and that's how everything started. But I was a taxi queen."

Zukayna says her family have been very supportive.

"I have been this way since I was 13 years old.

"All of my family are very happy for me," she says.

Sadia says she has been preparing Zukayna to be her wife since they moved in together.

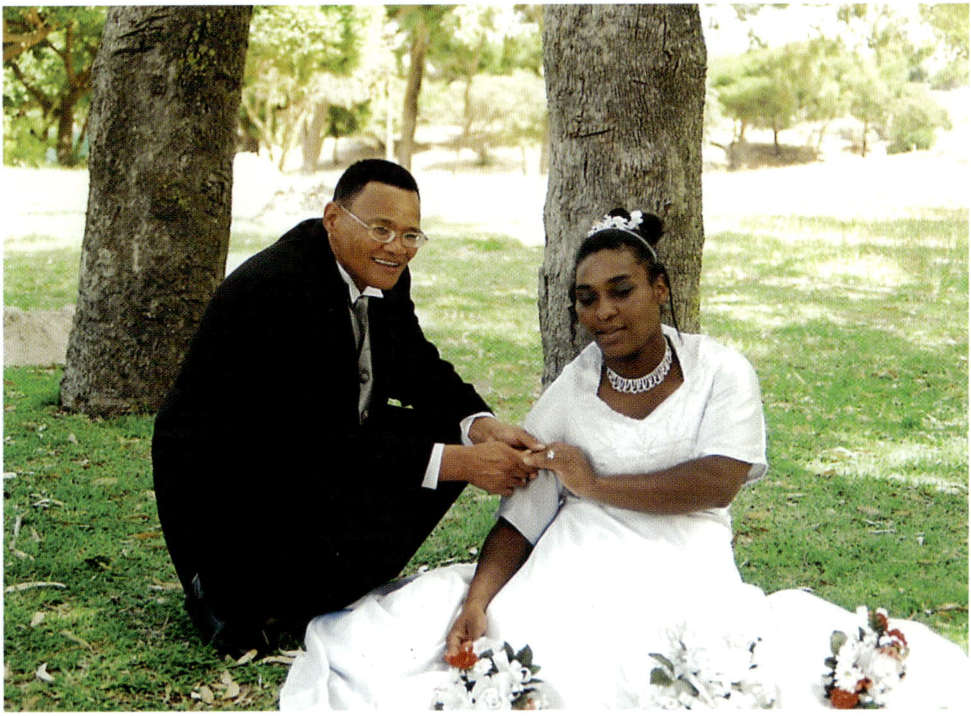

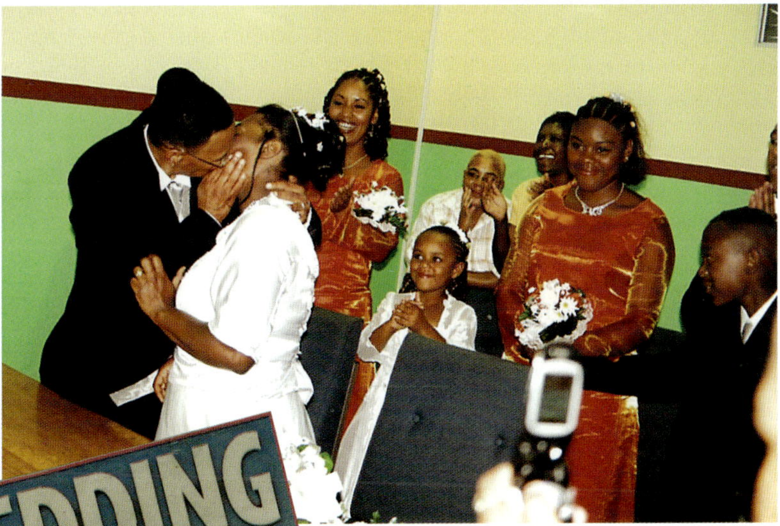

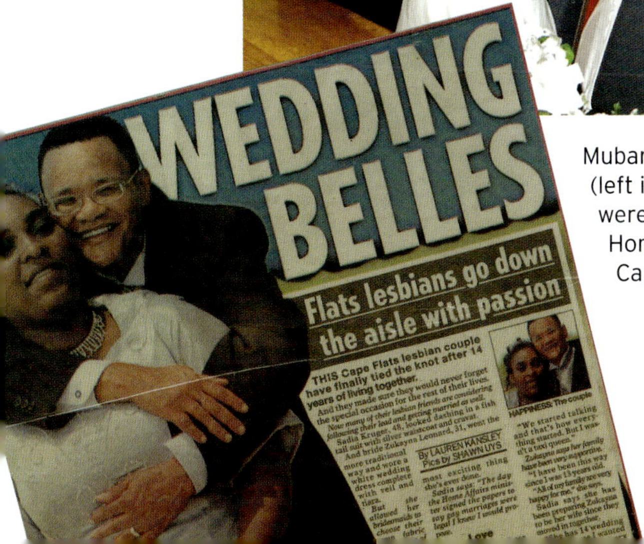

Mubarak: Muslim couple Sadia Kruger (left in top picture) and Zukayna Leonard were married on 3 February 2007 at the Home Affairs office at Mitchell's Plain, Cape Town. (See page 338.)

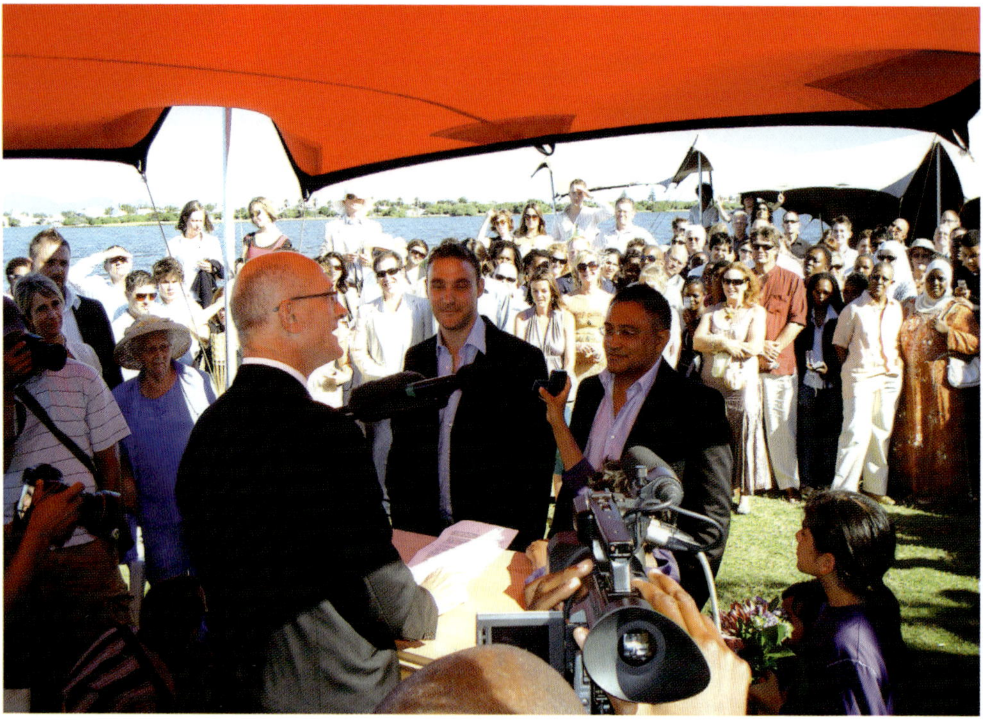

Hitched in style: LGBTI activist (former director of the National Coalition for Gay and Lesbian Equality) and renowned HIV/AIDS campaigner Zackie Achmat (right, above) ties the knot with Dalli Weyers on 5 January 2008 in Lakeside, Cape Town. Supreme Court of Appeal Justice Edwin Cameron (below, right) officiated.

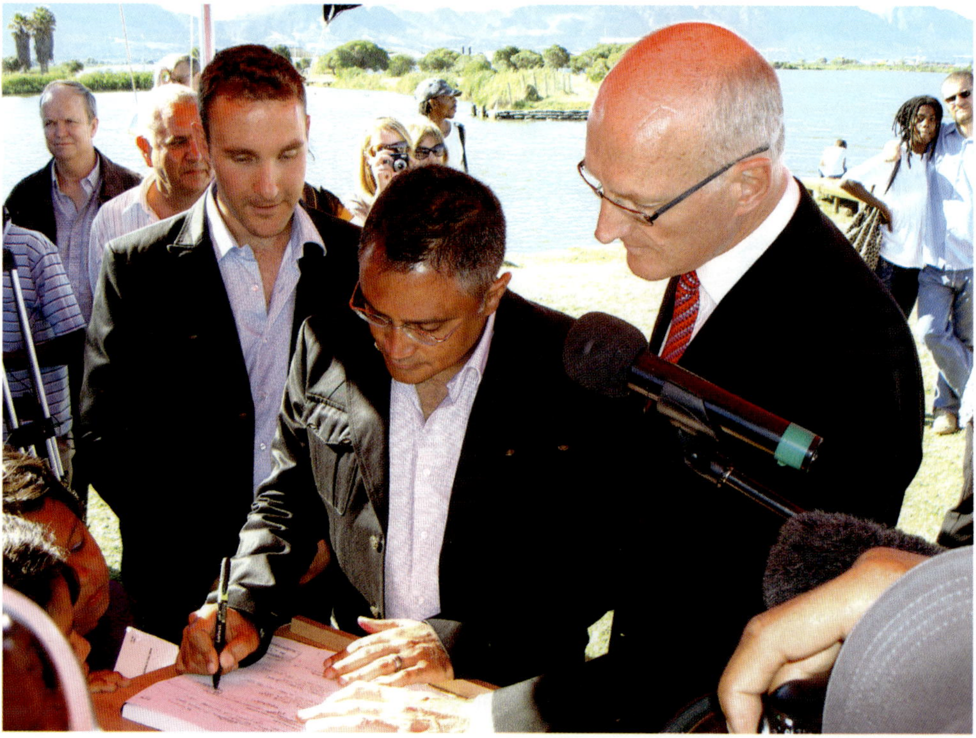

1996 to remove colonial influences and prejudices from local family law. When asked whether the new legislation would allow for marriages between women, which were known and practiced in pre-colonial times, a senior member of the committee drafting the legislation vehemently denied it.[28] It may well be that African legislatures will themselves draw upon the dichotomy between culture/religion and human rights deliberately to erase same-sex marriages from 'official' accounts of customary law in an attempt to preserve the fiction of a 'pure' or 'real' African culture, uncontaminated by same-sex practices.

Finally, the vision underpinning the Civil Union Act – of gay or lesbian identity as exclusive, immutable and irrevocable – does not reflect the identities or practices of African people who have sex with others of the same sex.[29] Lesbian and gay scholars have long identified the 'modern' 'Western' notion of lesbian and gay identity as problematic. One of the problems is that it excludes some people who have same-sex relationships, but who do not comply with the criteria for 'authentic' lesbian or gay identity.[30] This critique forms the basis of my argument that, at a symbolic and a practical level, the Act excludes African people who have sex with others of the same sex. A different problem is the reliance, at the heart of lesbian and gay identity, upon the very same dichotomous categories that currently structure and justify conservative and anti-gay beliefs.

In our society sex, gender and sexual orientation form a seemingly consistent whole where sex is assigned at birth, appropriate gender behaviour should follow and, when the time is ripe, sexual desire should be directed to a person of the other sex. This is presented as the natural order of life and our whole social system is organized accordingly.[31]

The Civil Union Act relies upon this very same sexual economy of male/female, masculine/feminine and 'hetero'/'homo'-sexuality, even as it grants legitimacy and respectability to some lesbian and gay couples. However, the practices of African people in same-sex relationships, which are far more radically disruptive of this system, are not acknowledged. Instead of destabilizing sex, gender and sexual orientation, the Act represents just more of the same old gender and more of the same old sexual orientation. Ruthann Robson wrote, in relation to lesbian women, that '[i]f we are no longer "riveted" to the extant categories, there is the possibility that we can create new categories that reflect lesbian diversity'.[32] Taking account of diverse African same-sex practices could have allowed us to move beyond the categories which currently define sex and sexuality and to start thinking about a system of family law in which the needs of family members, rather than conservative sexual mores, determine the legal rules. Unfortunately, that opportunity has been lost in the haste to adopt the Civil Union Act.

Notes

1 Joe Oloko-Onyango and Sylvia Tamale, '"The Personal Is Political" or Why Women's Rights Are Indeed Human Rights: An African Perspective on International Feminism', *Human Rights Quarterly* 17 (1995), 691-731; Oyeronke Oyewumí, 'The White Woman's Burden: African Women in Western Feminist Discourse', in Oyewumí (ed.), *African Women and Feminism: Reflecting on the Politics of Sisterhood* (Africa World Press, 2003); Martin Chanock, '"Culture" and Human Rights: Orientalising, Occidentalising and Authenticity', in Mahmood Mamdani (ed.), *Beyond Rights and Culture Talk* (David Philip, 2000)
2 Lawrence Schäfer, 'Marriage and Marriage-like Relationships: Constructing a New Hierarchy of Life Partnerships', *South African Law Journal* 123 (2006), 626-647
3 Elsje Bonthuys and Marius Pieterse, 'Still Unclear: The Validity of Certain Customary Marriages', *Journal of Contemporary Roman-Dutch Law* 63 (2000), 616-625; Likhapha Mbatha, Najma Moosa and Elsje Bonthuys, 'Culture and Religion', in Elsje Bonthuys and Cathi Albertyn (eds.), *Gender, Law and Justice* (Juta & Co, 2007)
4 Nicola Barker, 'Sex and the Civil Partnership Act: The Future of (Non)Conjugality', *Feminist Legal Studies* 14 (2006), 241; Claire Young and Susan B Boyd, 'Losing the Feminist Voice? Debates on the Legal Recognition of Same-Sex Partnerships in Canada', *Feminist Legal Studies* 14 (2006), 213-240; Nan Seuffert, 'Sexual Citizenship and the Civil Union Act', *Victoria Wellington University Law Review* 37 (2006), 283-306; Carl F Stychin, 'Not (Quite) a Horse and Carriage: The Civil Partnership Act 2004', *Feminist Legal Studies* 14 (2006), 79-86
5 Elsje Bonthuys, 'Gender, Race, Culture and Religion: Outside Legal Subjectivity', *South African Journal on Human Rights* 18:1 (2002), 41-58
6 Madelene Isaacks with Ruth Morgan, '"I Don't Force My Feelings for Other Women, My Feelings Have to Force Me": Same-Sexuality amongst Ovambo Women in Namibia', in Ruth Morgan and Saskia Wieringa (eds.), *Tommy Boys, Lesbian Men and Ancestral Wives: Female Same-Sex Practices in Africa* (Jacana, 2005)
7 Ruth Morgan and Saskia Wieringa, 'Present-Day Same-Sex Practices in Africa: Conclusions from the African Women's Life Story Project', in Morgan and Wieringa (eds.), op. cit.
8 Barbara Oomen, 'Traditional Woman-to-Woman Marriages and the Recognition of Customary Marriages Act', *Journal of Contemporary Roman-Dutch Law* 63 (2000), 274-282; Tom W Bennett, *Customary Law in South Africa* (Juta & Co, 2004)
9 Nancy Baraka with Ruth Morgan, '"I Want to Marry the Woman of My Choice without Fear of Being Stoned": Female Marriages and Bisexual Women in Kenya', in Morgan and Wieringa (eds.), op. cit.
10 Saskia Wieringa, 'Woman Marriages and Other Same-Sex Practices: Historical Reflections on African Women's Same-Sex Relations', in Morgan and Wieringa (eds.), op. cit.
11 Nkunzi Nkabinde with Ruth Morgan, '"This Has Happened since Ancient Times ... It's Something You Are Born with": Ancestral Wives amongst Same-Sex Sangomas in South Africa', in Morgan and Wieringa (eds.), op. cit.
12 Marc Epprecht, '"Good God Almighty, What is This!' Homosexual "Crime" in Early Colonial Zimbabwe', in Stephen O Murray and Will Roscoe (eds.), *Boy-Wives and Female Husbands: Studies of African Homosexualities* (St Martin's Press/Palgrave, 1998)
13 Isak Niehaus, 'Renegotiating Masculinity in the South African Lowveld: Narratives of Male-Male Sex in Labour Compounds and Prisons', *African Studies* 61 (2002), 77-97; T Dunbar Moodie, 'Black Migrant Mine Labourers and the Vicissitudes of Male Desire', in Robert Morrell (ed.), *Changing Men in Southern Africa* (Zed Books, 2001); Donald L Donham, 'Freeing South Africa: The Modernization of Male-Male Sexuality in Soweto', *Cultural Anthropology* 13 (1998), 3-21

14 Ronald Louw, 'Mkhumbane and the New Traditions of (un)African Same-Sex Weddings', in Morrell (ed.), op. cit.
15 Stychin, op. cit.
16 Pierre de Vos, 'Same-Sex Sexual Desire and the Re-Imagining of the South African Family', *South African Journal on Human Rights* 20 (2004), 179-206
17 Elizabeth Khaxas with Saskia Wieringa, '"I Am a Pet Goat, I Will Not Be Slaughtered": Female Masculinity and Femme Strength amongst the Damara in Namibia', in Morgan and Wieringa (eds.), op. cit.
18 Donham, op. cit.
19 Hugh McLean and Linda Ngcobo, '"*Abangibhamayo Bathi Ngimnandi* (Those Who Fuck Me Say I'm Tasty)": Gay Sexuality in Reef Townships', in Edwin Cameron and Mark Gevisser (eds.), *Defiant Desire: Gay and Lesbian Lives in South Africa* (Ravan, 1994)
20 Niehaus, op. cit.
21 McLean and Ngcobo, op. cit.; Khaxas and Wieringa, op. cit.
22 Isaacks with Morgan, op. cit.; Busi Kheswa and Saskia Wieringa, '"My Attitude Is Manly ... A Girl Needs to Walk on the Aisle": Butch-Femme Subculture in Johannesburg", in Morgan and Wieringa (eds.), op. cit.
23 Khaxas and Wieringa; Isaacks and Morgan; Kheswa and Wieringa, op. cit. (note 6)
24 Morgan and Wieringa (eds.), op. cit.
25 Kendall, '"When a Woman Loves a Woman" in Lesotho: Love, Sex and the (Western) Construction of Homophobia', in Murray and Roscoe (eds.), op. cit.
26 Wieringa, op. cit.
27 Signe Arnfred, introduction, in Anfred (ed.), *Re-Thinking Sexualities in Africa* (Nordafrikainstitutet, 2004)
28 Morgan and Wieringa (eds.), op. cit., 18 (introduction)
29 Angelo Pantazis and Elsje Bonthuys, 'Gender and Sexual Orientation', in *Gender, Law, and Justice* (Juta & Co, 2007)
30 Angelo Pantazis, 'The Problematic Nature of Gay Identity', in *South African Journal on Human Rights* 12 (1996), 291-307
31 Pantazis and Bonthuys, op. cit., 139
32 Ruthann Robson, *Sappho Goes to Law School* (Columbia University Press, 1998), 169

This essay also draws upon the following works:
Edwin Cameron, 'Constitutional Protection of Sexual Orientation and African Conceptions of Humanity', *South African Law Journal* 118 (2001), 642-650
Angela Quintal, 'Wrong to Legalise Same-Sex Marriage – Chiefs', *Cape Times,* 25 October 2006
Leila Samodien, 'Churches Bar Gay Marriages', *Cape Argus,* 17 May 2007

Marriage and murder

Tim Trengove-Jones

On 7 July 2007 Sizakele Sigasa and Salome Masooa were killed in Meadowlands, Soweto, allegedly because they were lesbians.[1] The Joint Working Group (JWG) – a network of organizations intimately connected with lobbying for the Civil Union Act – issued a statement expressing understandable outrage.[2] Beneath this outrage was bewilderment born of the perceived incongruence between the Constitutional ideals of the new South Africa and the brute fact of these murders: '[P]eople who inflict harm upon and kill lesbians and gays do not belong in South Africa,' opined the statement.

The anger is heartfelt. The bewilderment is axiomatic of much that comes with living in a time of transition. But the anger here is at once right and wrong. Crucially, its statement ignores a different kind of anger. The Meadowlands murders tell us, bleakly, a crucial truth about our belonging here. In our national coming out, one traced in our equality jurisprudence, lesbians and gays have come – with bewildering inevitability – to embody the highest aspirations of the nation. In being aligned with that ideal, we are at once exemplary and shocking. This paradox, at the heart of our personal and national identity, sets us up for murder.

The semiotic space that is our contemporary culture jangles with competing signs. The murders of Sigasa and Masooa are one such complex set of contradictory signs. To inhabit an 'alternative sexuality' in South Africa is to be a raw receptor for the clash of cultures currently underway. To understand ourselves, to be less angry and possibly less bewildered, we need to attempt a rigorous reading of our problematic present.

An account of the road to the Civil Union Act will make this clear.

Bildung and paradox

Our unfolding equality jurisprudence, especially as it attaches to gays and lesbians, starting with 'Polmed'[3] in January 1998 and culminating in *Fourie* in the Constitutional Court in December 2005, constitutes a single *oeuvre*, with each case forming different chapters in a single narrative. (See pages 55-57.) This narrative provides a site for many of the key cultural struggles that define what former Chief Justice Arthur Chaskalson has called 'a time of great social change'.[4] The jurisprudence itself provides a reassuring tale of incremental social, legal and political amelioration, but challenging this is a discourse of panic occasioned by a fear of derealization and dissipation. These two narratives contended in what was very clearly a culture war. That the reasoned jurisprudential narrative triumphed alerts us to the first of many paradoxes in our time: what was confirmed as a new orthodoxy provoked widespread hostility precisely because it was widely regarded as damningly heterodox.

It is in the Constitution itself that the seeds of this clash between the orthodox and the heterodox are lodged. Within that founding document of the new South Africa, nothing was more new – locally and internationally – than the explicit mention of sexual orientation in the equality clause. Here resides the unlikely twinning of the fates of an often reviled minority ('gays and lesbians') and that of the nation generally. This twinning houses an inevitable cultural and political struggle that finds its culmination in the Civil Union Act. Paradoxically, an ideal might set us up for murder.

Taking the Constitution as a prelude to the *oeuvre* that is our equality jurisprudence allows this narrative to acquire the status of national biography. Viewed as a single text, it assumes, instructively, the shape of the *Bildungsroman*. The protagonist is a composite called 'gays and lesbians'. As is the case in the traditional *Bildungsroman*, the protagonist is initially unwanted, oppressed and discriminated against. We have 'known protracted and bitter oppression', and been 'made to feel like outsiders' as Justice Albie Sachs put it in *Fourie*.[5] The *Bildungsroman* characteristically presses towards marriage. It starts with the protagonist outside those weighty institutions of family and marriage, and artfully engineers her ultimate incorporation into the very institutions that, initially, sought to (negatively) define her identity.

Our equality jurisprudence replicates this paradigm exactly. In 'Polmed' the seeds of marriage are immanent: 'The stability and permanence of [the] relationships [of same-sex couples] is no different from the many married couples I know,' Justice Pierre Roux announced, going on to declare that 'if our law does not accord protection to same-sex unions, then it is time it did so'.[6] Here the 'good' authority figure (the judge) recognizes the innate worthiness of the protagonists and urges their incorporation within dominant structures. So, a mere eight years later (very swift in terms of *Bildung*) the traditional happy ending is announced in *Fourie*, and made possible in the Civil Union Act. The plot from 'Polmed' to *Fourie* is a typical developmental trajectory, where marriage marks a happy ending and is the signifier of social, personal, and cultural integration. In this outcome, a society which for most of the plot is radically divided congratulates itself on its ultimate viability: as Sachs puts it in *Fourie*, the nation will now 'embrace all its members with dignity and respect'.[7] It is an old story and, put like this, it elides, as one reading of the old story always does, the challenges to this 'happy ending'. In our own translation of this form, the hostilities articulated by religious and Africanist lobbies ensured that a level of realism prevailed.

I spoke of the many paradoxes of our time. It was Oscar Wilde – in many ways our progenitor – who said that 'the way of paradoxes is the way of truth'.[8] He also contended that 'when the Verities become acrobats, we can judge them'. To grasp some of the truth of the current cultural climate we need to be alert to paradoxes. The founding document of the new South Africa is the Constitution. According to Justice Edwin Cameron, who is himself the founding figure in the theorizing and strategizing of gay rights in this country, the pre-eminence accorded to constitutionalism in the new South Africa rests upon a crucial paradox. Under apartheid the law had been used as an instrument of oppression. But, in the new order, this (il)legal supremacy might be made to mean that the 'law itself could be used to curb the excesses of domination and oppression'.[9]

In his *Fourie* judgment in the Supreme Court of Appeal (SCA) Cameron repeated this history. A key paradox 'lies at the core of our national project – that we came from oppression by law, but resolved to seek our future, free from oppression, in regulation by law'.[10] Some of our current bewilderment might be clarified if we grasped more fully that our time of transition is founded on paradox. Through our equality jurisprudence, the old Verities – most notably those of religion and African nationalism – were made to become acrobats and, as the vituperative nature of their protestations indicated, they feared for their footing.

If the Constitution is the founding document of the new South Africa, then Cameron's inaugural lecture, delivered at the University of the Witwatersrand on 27 October 1992, is the seminal document for understanding the course of our equality jurisprudence. Its terms and ideas provided key interpretative parameters in the sodomy case,[11] reappeared in the judge's own ruling in *Fourie* in the SCA on 30 November 2004, and culminated in the passage into law of the Civil Union Act in December 2006.

Cameron's inaugural initiates that paradoxical amplification of minority interest into majority concern that becomes a leitmotif in our equality jurisprudence. This amplification inheres in his title – 'Sexual Orientation and the Constitution: A Test Case for Human Rights' – and is refined in his central thesis: 'the question whether sexual orientation should be included in our Constitution as a specially protected condition is a crucial test of our good faith and integrity ... in making our Constitution'.[12] This is the foundational moment where the treatment of gays and lesbians is elevated into a litmus test of what Cameron elsewhere calls our 'fragile venture into constitutionalism'.[13] A minority, we are to loom large in assessments of the success of our democratic revolution. The link between the treatment of gays and lesbians and the success of a post-apartheid South Africa lies in a history of shared oppression. Gays have lived, often, in 'misery and fear [and] ... violence ("queer bashing") and peripheral discrimination' (paragraph 456). We have been legally and politically disempowered, so experiencing from the inside our own version of the wider oppression characterizing apartheid South Africa. Being a minority, however, we are 'uniquely vulnerable' (456) to sustained oppression and discrimination. Paradoxically, sexual orientation should be explicitly included in the Constitution because it should be a matter of indifference morally and constitutionally. The inclusion of an equality clause 'becomes a moral focus in our Constitution-making' (471):

> In the past we South Africans signalled to each other through our differences – the distinctions of race, sex, colour, creed and religion that separated us. The debate about non-discrimination on the basis of sexual orientation offers an invitation to us to deal not in this coinage but in something different [472].

Far from its being legitimate to regard us as a threat to established order, our equal treatment would now (have to) be the litmus test with which to measure the success of 'our search for transformation' (472) and of 'our commitment to creating a common future for ourselves' (472). This is a brilliant tactical manoeuvre. But there are crucial elisions at work in aligning legal equality for gay and lesbian people with the national democratic revolution, and these foreground why we have become so (im)pertinent. In barely six years, Cameron's view of gay rights as a test case for human rights had become orthodoxy. In *Sodomy* Sachs would repeat Cameron's insistences: 'It is no exaggeration to say that the success of the whole constitutional endeavour in South Africa will depend in large measure on how successfully sameness and difference are reconciled, an issue central to the present matter' (paragraph 131). Again we see the paradox of those who suffer 'institutionally imposed exclusion from the mainstream' (129), as Sachs put it, becoming 'central'.

In the *Fourie* judgment in the Constitutional Court, Sachs repeated this view. Not gay rights, but national identity was at issue: '[W]hat is at stake is not simply removing an injustice experienced by a particular section of the community. At issue is a need to affirm the very character of our society as one based on tolerance and mutual respect' (60). Further, 'the hallmark of an open and democratic society is its capacity to accommodate and manage difference of intensely-held world views and lifestyles in a reasonable and fair manner' (95). Our (im)pertinence has solidified into this paradox: the 'deviant' now promises/threatens to become the establishment.

This re-cognition and management of difference seeks to displace the doctrinal absolutism and political autocracy that had punished – what Cameron called 'queer-bashing' – the gay body. Where there had been the dismemberment of the gay mind and body in physical and psychological assaults, the re-cognition of difference now means that the options open to the gay body become the definitive gauge of the wellness of the body politic. Unsurprisingly, this is what provoked the enormous outcry at the passing of the Civil Union Act: what was allegedly our shared vision of transformation, loaded with paradoxes as it was, strained some of our minds and authorities close to breaking point.

Shared values?

The amplification of the treatment of a minority into a test case for the well-being of the nation was allied to another key expansion. Post-apartheid is not just a time term: it is also a value one. The Constitution as founding document is described by Cameron as espousing 'shared commitments spring[ing] from shared values, and shared values from shared interests'.[14] After the divisive conception of difference under apartheid, our Constitutional values offer a powerfully ameliorative vision of ourselves. Our equality jurisprudence embodies this mitigation.

But the necessary optimism about shared values and commitments could issue in an over-stated distinction between apartheid and post-apartheid worlds. Perhaps nowhere has this amplification been more marked than in our equality jurisprudence. In *Fourie*, Sachs exemplifies this zeal: 'our Constitution represents a radical rupture with a past based on intolerance and exclusion' (paragraph 59). 'Our society,' he claims, 'is completely different.' As such, difference itself is now regarded differently, he contends: 'the world in which [gays] live ... has evolved from repudiating expressions of [gay] desire to accepting the reality of [gay] presence' (78).

This amplification is misleadingly roseate and introduces an element of fantasy into our national narrative. Optimistically meliorative visions energize. Fantasy endangers. The twinned amplifications at work meant that arguments about same-sex rights were made to bear more weight than they could comfortably carry. Whether supporting or opposing gay rights, amplification issued in bewilderment or anger on both sides of the question. The juridical orthodoxy of achieved difference was out of step with tardy attitudinal transformation. The litmus-test positioning meant those who still saw us as repugnant felt alarmed, even betrayed. What our jurisprudence asserted as current orthodoxy offended many who did not recognize themselves, their time or place, in what was offered as the incarnation of their shared values and interests.

The amplification of our cultural positioning predetermined the amplified hostility provoked by the Civil Union Bill. Defence Minister Mosiuoa Lekota, friend and comrade to Simon Nkoli, could insist that many gay and lesbian people had been part of the anti-apartheid struggle. But this attempt at legitimation merely provoked a rictus of disapproval, with Lekota accused of suggesting the struggle was 'for sodomy and not for freedom'.[15] In miniature, these responses persuade me that the founding paradoxes of the new South Africa continue in post-apartheid South Africa. On a conceptual level, the linkage between gay liberation and black liberation is compelling. In practice it proves less so. The alliance between anti-apartheid and anti-homophobic struggles is in some ways a flattering (mis)conception. Instances of a troubling experience of distance between the anti-apartheid struggle and gayness have been recorded.[16] The 'piggybacking' of gay rights on the anti-apartheid struggle meant that with the Civil Union Act something latent within that struggle became, finally, for many uncomfortably patent.

Given the Constitution's equality clause, the findings of unconstitutionality in all the cases from 'Polmed' to *Fourie* were inevitable. Because the courts have borne the brunt of this transformational energy, the reservoir of apartheid-engendered scepticism about the law resurfaced worryingly, since the new orthodoxy articulated in these judgments ran ahead of still largely untransformed personal and religious ideologies. In *Fourie* Sachs asserted that in 'vindicating the rights enshrined in the Bill of Rights ... the legislature is in the frontline' (138). But the fact is that it is the courts that have had to be in the frontline largely because of the seemingly tardy transformational commitment of the legislature itself in matters of gay rights, something tactfully gestured at in both *Fourie* judgments.[17] Because it fell to the courts to articulate what is, officially, the new orthodoxy within our non-racist and non-sexist society, apartheid-engendered scepticism about the law resurfaced in the pronounced hostility towards the courts and the Constitution itself. This scepticism represents a hazardous tendency in our national project.

Because the rulings of unconstitutionality were inevitable, the significance of these judgments really lies elsewhere. Read as a single text, the judgments are both *Bildungsroman* and textbook. Given the foot-dragging of the legislature, given the largely untransformed nature of individuals and institutions, given the renewed scepticism that the rulings *per se* provoked, we must turn to these judgments to see our national aspirations defined, argued for, and defended. Read as an *oeuvre* the jurisprudence becomes a narrative of explication and exemplification: it strives to serve as a model for the reformation of our priorly re-imagined national and cultural life. The judgments' reiterations form an incremental dynamic that is, of course, fundamental to what is called legal precedent. This repetition compulsion is a key to the process of re-education required for nation-building. It is not just that 'the law ... would now form the basis for our national aspirations', as Cameron puts it in *Fourie* (paragraph 8), but that jurisprudence, through esteeming precedent and thereby becoming one of the oldest intertextual practices we have, becomes itself a model and engine for transformative processes.

As litmus test, the controversy elicited by the Civil Union Bill suggests that the allegedly shared values inscribed in the Constitution have not yet been naturalized. Because the legitimating narrative offered from 'Polmed' onwards has not taken root yet, the Bill couldn't provide unambiguously happy confirmation of the health of our national democratic revolution. The very fact that gay liberation sought to piggyback on a national liberation struggle meant that when, finally, our liberation narrative got to the issue of same-sex marriage – a genuinely cross-racial, cross-cultural, and cross-class issue – the alliance between (gay) sexual liberation and national liberation was subjected to severe deconstructive pressures. The moral and the popular wills remain incongruent. While temporally we are in post-apartheid South Africa, ideologically it is not in all of us.

Limitation and expressiveness

The Constitution is the closest thing we have to a sacred text in what is officially now a secular state. It offers not only a new paradigm for political relationships but a new moral norm. In the sodomy case, Sachs made this clear, stating that the Bill of Rights is 'a document founded on deep political morality'; that 'a State that recognizes difference does not mean a State without morality'; and that 'what is central to the character and functioning of the State ... is that the dictates of the morality which it enforces, and the limits to which it may go, are to be found in the text and spirit of the Constitution itself' (136). In *Fourie* in the SCA, Cameron noted that the Constitution established an 'imperative normative setting' (5), and, extending this in *Fourie* in the Constitutional Court, Sachs claimed that the 'law serves as a great teacher [and] establishes public norms that become assimilated into daily life' (138). Inevitably, this new moral law came into conflict with the older normative moralities it seeks to replace.

In his *Fourie* judgment, Cameron quoted Sachs quoting Cameron's inaugural lecture: 'As Sachs J has observed in a different setting, "because neither power nor specific resource allocation are at issue, sexual orientation becomes a moral focus in our constitutional order"' (19). Religious institutions knew that a decisive shift in power was occurring and that their status as final arbiters of moral teaching and authority was under threat. 'The far-reaching doctrines ... of inclusive moral citizenship' (13) that the country's new high priests were disseminating reached very far indeed: they reached to Mecca and to Canterbury, to Jerusalem and to Rome.

Sachs was clear about this challenge to traditionally religious moral law in *Fourie*:

> It is one thing for the Court to acknowledge the important role that religion plays in our public life. It is quite another to use religious doctrine as a source for interpreting the Constitution. It would be out of order to employ the religious sentiments of some as a guide to the constitutional rights of others [92].

Crucially, Sachs declares the separation of church and state and scuppers claims by religious authorities to dictate state policy. He also confirms a link between our national project and what traditionalists regard as deviance.

The Constitution is a foundational covenant, and covenants, being instruments of authority, at once enable and curtail. This being so, Sachs's claim in the sodomy case that 'respect for human rights requires the affirmation of self not the denial of self' (132) is a little misleading. Under the Civil Union Act, same-sex marriages are enabled. But this is not simply an expression of new freedom. It also extends the limits exacted by culture and so asserts its affinities with the establishment. Sachs argued that, if we were unable to marry we were 'made to feel like outsiders who do not fully belong in the universe of equals' (61). At best this is mere whimsy. I do not feel an insider because I now have the choice to marry. Sachs's claim stems from his continuing to view marriage as the pinnacle in the hierarchy of relationship modes. Consider another rhapsodic Sachsian moment. Unable to marry, we 'are not entitled to celebrate [our] commitment to each other in a joyous public event' and our 'unions remain unmarked by the showering of presents and the commemoration of anniversaries so celebrated in our culture' (72). Sachs's enthusiasm for the 'new' is buoyed by a delightful fiction underwritten by the traditional. His sentimentalism *tries* to defuse controversy by construing a radical challenge to the old order in affectionate terms that hope to keep its translation firmly within the imaginary of the traditional.

Separation of powers

If in *Fourie* Sachs redefined the boundaries between church and state, he was less scrupulous in defining those between the judiciary and the legislature. In his *Fourie* ruling in the SCA, Cameron recognized the supremacy of the Constitution and claimed that it 'assigns an imperative role to the court' whereby, 'subject to limitation, it is obliged to develop the common law appropriately' (40). In the Constitutional Court, however, Sachs fell back on a majoritarian discourse that had been explicitly rejected by the Court itself.

In *S v Makwanyane*, Justice Chaskalson stated that were the 'protection of rights left to Parliament … this would be a return to parliamentary sovereignty and a retreat from the new legal order' (88).[18] If the limits of religion are redefined in post-apartheid South Africa, so are those of the judiciary and legislature. Yet, despite the Constitutional Court precedent in *Makwanyane* and his own sentiments in *Fourie*, Sachs effected a partial return to a damaging form of parliamentary sovereignty and flirted with a retreat from the obligations vested in the new legal order. He claimed that 'in the search for effective ways to provide an appropriate remedy that enjoys the widest public support' (113) it would be best that 'Parliament be given an opportunity to deal appropriately with the matter' (139). We see here a moment of apostasy. Sachs's decision to suspend the Court's order for 12 months while Parliament developed a legislative response showed a certain disrespect for the status and mission of the law. In a negative sense this time, the fate of the body of gay citizens became, once more, a gauge of the fate of the body politic.

Justice Sachs has been a long-time companion of gay rights, going back to the message of support he sent to the first Pride parade in 1990 and his comments in the sodomy case. In *Fourie* he committed himself firmly to a fundamental principle in our secular democratic constitutionalism by refusing religions the final say in what was or was not allowed in the new order. Yet, in suspending his order and referring the matter to Parliament, his ruling in *Fourie* offers us a final paradox: he succumbs to a new form of deviancy of his own.

Perhaps the seeds of his *Fourie* apostasy were latent. In the sodomy case he did allude to the 'danger of over-intrusive judicial intervention in matters of broad social policy' (123). From that caveat it was perhaps only a short step to his proclaiming in *Fourie* that 'I believe that Parliament is well-suited to finding the best ways of ensuring that same-sex couples are brought in from the legal cold' (138). All but one of the Constitutional Court judges followed Sachs into this heresy. In her dissenting judgment, Justice Kate O'Regan reminded us of the orthodoxy in the new order: 'The power and duty to protect constitutional rights is conferred upon the courts and courts should not shrink from that duty.' She also insisted on the source of ultimate legitimacy in the new order: 'the legitimacy of an order made by the Court does not flow from the status of the institution itself, but from the fact that it gives effect to the provisions of our Constitution'. And, finally, O'Regan reiterated the Constitution's hostility to majoritarianism: 'Time and again there will be those in our broader community who do not wish to see constitutional rights protected, but that can never be a reason for a court not to protect those rights' (171).

O'Regan's points are salutary. The superficial discourse of radical rupture with the past was exposed in the parliamentary hearings that followed: they showed that many in the new South Africa have not agreed to the replacement of traditional, older forms of law and norm with the new norms of the Constitution.

History is now

Fourie, the Civil Union Act and the controversies they excited are hugely significant indices of our present. They allow us to note more precisely how our own social transformation occurs, and to gauge the appropriateness of some of the descriptive and evaluative terms – 'the miracle of the new South Africa', 'the rainbow nation', 'post-apartheid' – routinely used to describe our present. In suggesting something of the limitations of these terms, we are encouraged to look more deeply at our own place and role in our national democratic revolution. Justice Cameron has constituted a seminal, informing presence in what I have written. It is fitting that he reappear at the close. In June 2001 he generously noted that as gay citizens in South Africa we 'approach [our] constitutional and legal entitlements with civility and also with humility'.[19] This is generous in being a prescription couched as a description. Humility requires that we do not meet resistance to our presence with the often routine and all-too-easy cry of 'homophobia'.[20] We – as much as our fellow citizens – must accept the limits of the new conception of difference that we are helping to define. In the sodomy case Sachs clarified this as follows: 'What becomes normal in an open society is, then, not an imposed and standardized form of behaviour that refuses to acknowledge difference, but the acceptance of the principle of difference itself, which accepts the variability of human behaviour' (134).

That the limits articulated in this conception of difference are as challenging for many of us as they are for our fellow citizens is made clear when, in the same judgment, Sachs noted that 'those persons who for religious or other belief disagree with or condemn homosexual conduct are free to hold and articulate such beliefs' (137). Our antagonists took full advantage of this freedom during discussions on the Bill. Seven months after the Act was passed, reactions to the Meadowlands murders showed a steady persistence of old attitudes towards homosexuality: 'We'd have to change the facts of *ubuntu*' for lesbianism to be accepted; the best response to lesbianism is 'to rape the lesbianism out of them'; 'it is time that our Constitution be revisited'.[21] There is no convincing evidence that the year's suspension of the Constitutional Court's order or the process of parliamentary hearings on the Civil Union Bill altered broadly held views on the unAfrican, unnatural, socially compromising nature of same-sex relations. We know the delay allowed for a crescendo of hostility to mount. The 'violence' perceived in our disrupting previous forms of social and legal restriction provokes, with seeming inevitability, an echoic violence. Our demonization elicits demonic responses.

Opposition to our rights is only feebly categorized as 'homophobia'. Rather, the months of vituperation exemplified the difference between having an argument and making one.[22] As religious groupings confronted the limits of their own power in what George Steiner calls the 'after-Word',[23] we were asked to engage with the limits of our own tolerance and endurance. To remember, too, that those holding religious views that disapprove of us and of our marrying are not, as Justice Laurie Ackermann put it in the sodomy case, 'crude bigots only' (38). Humility requires that, even as we engage with our own 'right to be different', we are nuanced enough to acknowledge that right in others, and not meet signs of prejudice with prejudices of our own. We should note that our *Bildungsroman* points to a 'deep re-ordering or dis-ordering of long-established frontiers'.[24]

It is clear that many of our fellow citizens are disconcerted by this. The Meadowlands murders remind us of the hazards of openness in what is officially a 'free and open society.' I doubt whether within our own sub-culture we have as yet always arrived at a mature engagement with difference. To do so will qualify us for another paradox: in appropriate humility, alert to our own special history, we will also, as Cameron put it, 'exercise our constitutional equality with pride'.[25] If we do this then, perhaps, the Verities will not only dance, but dance in step. If we do not do this, we will remain mired in anger and bewilderment. And if we are uninterrogatively ignorant of the processes at work in our history, we might well continue to be murdered.

Notes

1 'Outrage at Lesbian Murders', www.mambaonline.com/article.asp?artid=1136 (last accessed 9 January 2008)
2 'Community Orgs Meet on Lesbian Murders', www.mambaonline.com/article.asp?artid=1153 (last accessed 9 January 2008)

3 *Langemaat v Minister of Safety and Security and Others* (hereinafter referred to as 'Polmed')
4 *S v Makwanyane and Another* 1995 (3) SA 391
5 *Minister of Home Affairs and Another v Fourie and Another* 2005 (3) BCLR 355 (CC); 2006 (1) SA 524 (CC), hereafter *'Fourie';* paragraphs 136; 61
6 *Langemaat v Minister of Safety and Security and Others* 1998 (3) SA 312, 316
7 *Fourie*, paragraph 61
8 Oscar Wilde, *The Picture of Dorian Gray* (Penguin, 1985), 64
9 Edwin Cameron, 'Our Legal System – Precious and Precarious', *South African Law Journal* 117 (2000), 371-372
10 *Fourie and Another v Minister of Home Affairs and Another* 2005 (3) SA 429 (SCA); 2005 (3) BCLR 241 (SCA), hereafter *'Fourie (SCA)'*, paragraph 8
11 *National Coalition for Gay and Lesbian Equality and Another v Minister of Justice and Others*, CCT 11/98, paragraphs 20, 128. Known as 'the decriminalization case' or 'the sodomy case'; see page 56.
12 Edwin Cameron, 'Sexual Orientation and the Constitution: A Test Case for Human Rights', *South African Law Journal* 110 (1993), 450-472; 451-452
13 Cameron, 'Our Legal System', op. cit., 375
14 Ibid., 373
15 The quoted words are those of the United Christian Democratic Party's Edmund Pule. See Angela Quintal, 'Civil Union Bill Approved in Historic Vote', http://www.iol.co.za/index.php?set_id=1&click_id=124&art_id=vn20061115043713495C702320 (last accessed 9 January 2008)
16 See, for instance, Gerald Kraak, 'Homosexuality and the South African Left: The Ambiguities of Exile', in Neville Hoad, Karen Martin and Graeme Reid (eds.), *Sex and Politics in South Africa* (Double Storey, 2005), 118-134. Ruth Mompati's apology for comments made about homosexuality is in the foreword to the same text (7). The notorious instance of the banner proclaiming that 'Homosex is not in black culture', displayed outside the house of struggle icon Winnie Mandela during the Stompie murder trial in 1991, is a further example of the uneasy relationship between the struggles for sexual and political liberation.
17 See *Fourie* (SCA), paragraph 47; *Fourie* (CC), paragraph 116; O'Regan J dissenting, *Fourie* (CC), paragraph 171
18 Once more it is crucial to note that in every instance, from 'Polmed' on, the state, for a variety of different reasons, opposed the moves to extend equal rights to gay and lesbian citizens. This placed the courts firmly in the firing line and, in my view, added greatly to those hostile claims accusing the courts and the Constitution itself of being on the side of depravity.
19 Edwin Cameron, 'Constitutional Protection of Sexual Orientation and African Conceptions of Humanity', *South African Law Journal* 118 (2001), 648
20 Just one recent example. Choreographer Somizi Mhlongo appeared in the Randburg magistrate's court on 30 November 2007, after being arrested for indecent assault. A report on Mambaonline claimed that 'Media reports on the weekend smacked of homophobia, with the *Saturday Star* including the incident within an article on paedophilia and celebrities, while others chose to focus on Mhlongo's clothing and flamboyance.' 'Gay Celeb in Court', http://www.mambaonline.com/article.asp?artid=1519 (accessed 9 January 2008)
21 Comments on AM Live's 'After 8 Debate', 11 July 2007
22 See Deborah Tannen, *The Argument Culture* (Virago, 1999), 6: 'Public discourse requires *making* an argument for a point of view, not *having* an argument – as in having a fight.'
23 George Steiner, *Real Presences* (Faber, 1989, 1991), 231
24 George Steiner, *In Bluebeard's Castle* (Faber, 1971), 66
25 Cameron, 'Constitutional Protection of Sexual Orientation ...', op. cit., 649

On rupture and rhyme: Perspectives on the past, present, and future of same-sex marriage

Ruthann Robson

> 'Finally, our Constitution represents a radical rupture with a past based on intolerance and exclusion ...' – Justice Albie Sachs in *Fourie*
>
> 'The past does not repeat itself, but it rhymes'
> – widely attributed to American writer Mark Twain

Prologue

Circa 1979, same-sex marriage and South Africa were equally far on my horizons. I was living in North America, in the subtropical state of Florida in the United States, and had just graduated from law school. I filled my mind with concepts such as the 'rule against perpetuities', which I had needed to master for the Bar Examination and have never used since. To the extent I thought about same-sex marriage as a personal or political option, I reviled it as bourgeois and patriarchal, perspectives that I have not entirely abandoned.

Yet I marveled at the power of same-sex marriage in conservative rhetoric. Indeed, along with the spectre of unisex toilet facilities, same-sex marriage was successfully deployed to defeat the proposed Equal Rights Amendment to the US Constitution that would have provided that 'equality of rights' shall not be denied by the government 'on account of sex'. In Florida, not only did the state legislature refuse to ratify the Equal Rights Amendment, it passed a statute prohibiting 'homosexuals' from adopting children. The adoption ban and referenda repealing local anti-discrimination laws were a direct result of the efforts of Anita Bryant. Her political activism marked the rise of the conservative religious right throughout the US, as she spearheaded an anti-gay campaign called 'Save Our Children'. Previously, she had seemed a rather innocuous figure. As the spokeswoman for Florida orange juice, the former pop singer had been smiling on television advertisements accompanied by a cartoon bird and crooning 'breakfast without orange juice is like a day without sunshine'.

Boycotting Florida orange juice was one response of the queer community to Bryant's anti-gay campaign. Although it involved a bit of personal sacrifice (orange juice seemed a cheap and healthful drink, with the added bonus of mixing well with an assortment of liquors), it was effective as a collective effort. The Florida Citrus Commission let Bryant's contract lapse because of her controversial status.

In addition to her professional problems, Anita Bryant's personal life suffered. Soon, she divorced her husband. Her status as a divorced woman substantially decreased her popularity among fundamentalist Christians and conservatives.

Boycotts were a fact of political and daily life at that time. Complying with some was effortless, including boycotting diamonds and gold from South Africa in support of anti-apartheid efforts. Unlike the suggestion of a glass of orange juice, the advertisements proclaiming 'a diamond is forever' did not tempt me. The scenarios of heterosexual romance, in which the woman was presented with an expensive gift, seemed designed to be deconstructed in a women's studies class. Students in business classes meanwhile studied De Beers' long-standing and successful promotion of the relatively plentiful diamond as a symbol of love and eternity, creating demand for diamonds as a luxury yet necessary item, with the bonus of making the resale of diamonds seem tawdry. Personally, I had no plans or sufficient funds to buy a diamond for myself and certainly was not hoping for any man to offer up an engagement ring.

As for gold, I wasn't rushing to fill a safe with bullion, despite currency scares, and even when I wore jewellery, I preferred silver or string. Any affection I had for gold was sullied by a skit on the television show *Saturday Night Live*, specifically linking the purchase of the gold coin to supporting apartheid and white supremacy. I can still remember the scene, constructed as a mock advertisement for the Krugerrand that was renamed in an inflammatory manner.

Despite these recollections, in those days I was not always watching television or thinking about possible purchases. I recall commemorating the tenth anniversary of Stonewall, the watershed resistance of queer people in New York City to law-enforcement repression, in a bar in Florida. I remember studying the 'rule against perpetuities' and learning that I had passed the examination and thus gained admission to another type of bar in Florida, that which certified attorneys. I felt ready to use the law as an instrument of social change.

On most days, I was convinced that 'liberation' was right around the corner. I would admit that there was in lull in the counterculture, but rationalize that this was merely a bit of breathing space, until the women's movement and the gay movement and the black-power movement and the anti-poverty movement and lesbian-feminism and indigenous cultures gained ascendancy. There was a global movement toward liberation and it was unstoppable!

But if anyone would have asked me, circa 1979, about the future of same-sex marriage or South Africa, my wildest guesses would not have approximated the present state of affairs. Certainly, I would never have connected the two.

The South African Constitution, *Fourie*, and the Civil Union Act
It is late 2005, and I am jetting from North America to South Africa for a conference on comparative constitutionalism in Durban. Only a few days before, the

Constitutional Court had rendered its decision declaring the limitation of marriage to opposite-sex couples unconstitutional. On the long flight, I try to revise the paper I had intended to present. My analysis of judicial power to promote sexual freedom in constitutional democracies needs to include this new development. But I am tired and soon fall asleep on my lover's shoulder. When the flight attendant serves orange juice for breakfast, I notice that she sports what looks like a diamond ring.

Upon hearing about the *Fourie* decision, many people in the US envied my travel plans. It seemed that South Africa was definitely at the apex of 'gay liberation'. For sexual minorities in other nations, including the US, the Constitution of the Republic of South Africa has become an inspiration. The prohibition of unfair discrimination by the government and private actors on a numerous grounds, including sexual orientation, remains unique. This constitutional provision provided the clear basis for the Constitutional Court to declare the criminalization of sodomy unconstitutional, which did not occur in the US until 2003, when the Court reversed a case decided 17 years earlier. The South African constitutional text also provided firm grounding for the Constitutional Court to recognize rights for sexual minorities in same-sex partner relationships, including immigration, government pensions, joint legal parent status through adoption, joint-parent status for children born through alternative insemination, and later, intestate succession. This jurisprudence has a special resonance for queer legal advocates in other constitutional democracies, but is certainly the object of global craving.

Yet there is something about marriage that still rankles with me. At the conference, full of legal progressives, heterosexuals almost unerringly assumed that my lover and I were thrilled with the prospect of our impending marriage. At times, it could feel rude to engage in a conversation that, at bottom, informed the well-meaning heterosexual that I had absolutely no desire to emulate him or her. Colleagues whom I had believed knew me better – or had read my work – gaily imagined the ceremony and the party and even the honeymoon. 'You two have lived together for years and years,' a friend said to us, laughing. 'Don't you think it's high time you got married?' The unarticulated assumption was that surely we did not want to remain in what Justice Albie Sachs in *Fourie* described as a 'state of legal blankness', in which our union would remain 'unmarked by the showering of presents and the commemoration of anniversaries so celebrated in our culture'. Sachs did acknowledge that a same-sex couple might 'abjure mimicking or subordinating themselves to heterosexual norms', but concluded that what was important was 'not the decision to be taken, but the choice that is available'. Nevertheless, surrounded by well-meaning heterosexuals, I felt distinctly that there was a correct choice and a less-correct (if not entirely wrong) choice.

My discomfort was complicated by the fact that if the Constitutional Court had decided differently, I would be distressed. In the US, heirs to Anita Bryant had been busily promoting anti-same-sex-marriage laws and even constitutional amendments to circumvent or forestall 'judicial activism' protecting queer rights. The Massachusetts Supreme Judicial Court, under the leadership of South African native Margaret Marshall, had declared same-sex marriage as constitutionally mandated. At that moment (and still), Massachusetts was the only state in the US where same-sex marriage was lawful. A handful of other states had what some named a 'separate but equal' regime of relationship recognition for same-sex couples, usually denominated as 'civil union'. The large majority of states, however, had laws preventing the courts from ruling same-sex marriage constitutionally required, or even recognizing same-sex unions from other states. These laws were often passed through direct ballot measures. This was the same strategy that Bryant had so successfully employed years earlier, and the contemporary electoral rhetoric was similarly ugly.

Meanwhile, in the cafés and on the streets of Durban and later in our travels throughout KwaZulu-Natal, my lover and I were repeatedly asked if we were 'sisters'. We speculated on various cultural customs to explain this question, which we had only been asked a few times previously, all of them in hospital. After a while, it was tempting to answer 'yes'. After all, sisterhood was powerful, as we had learned in those women's studies classes decades ago.

In addition to my personal qualms, and despite its status as an object of envy, the achievement of the *Fourie* decision is not as untroubled as it first appears to casual international observers. Notably, the Court did not remedy the unconstitutional condition, but allowed Parliament 'to cure the defect within 12 months'. Writing for the Court, Sachs reasoned that Parliament might later choose a remedy other than a simply 'reading-in of the words "or spouse"' in legislation that was sex-specific, as the Court would do, and the Court's 'temporary remedial measure would be far less likely to achieve the enjoyment of equality as promised by the Constitution than would lasting legislative action compliant with the Constitution'.

The process of Parliamentary approval, including what some have a called a 'roadshow' that provided a vehicle for 'homophobic hate speech', resulted in the Civil Union Act of 2006. Returning to South Africa in 2007, I was lucky to be able to spend a month in Johannesburg at Wits Law School and have amazing opportunities to speak to advocates, academics, activists, and judges from all over the nation about the *Fourie* decision and Civil Union Act. As to be expected, there were various views. Those expressing doubts about the institution of marriage expressed the same conundrum I did, and many others believed the Act fell short of equality. There were critiques, satisfactions, pride, and wonder. Despite these differences, almost everyone agreed that there was more work to be done on queer liberation. The subsequent murder of Sizakele Sigasa and Salome Masooa served as a chilling reminder that no judicial decision or legislative act will cure homophobia.

Backlash, including violent backlash, to advances in queer liberation is a worldwide phenomenon. Also common are troublesome compromises, such as the Constitutional Court's deferral to Parliament and Parliament's inclusion of the opt-out conscience clause, and our often ambiguous and inconsistent reactions to legal reforms. Trying to imagine the future under such circumstances is a fraught endeavour.

And yet, conceptualizing the future is a temptation that is almost impossible to resist.

The Permanent Partners Judgment of 2027
I imagine myself at a party for the 'diamond anniversary' of Stonewall, in a rather well-appointed apartment, overlooking an ocean that may be a bit warmer than it once was but still tumbles a beautiful blue. My imagination includes my lover and I – I refuse to say 'spouse' although we had to get married years ago in order to benefit from our pension accounts – drinking orange juice with a splash of champagne. My imagination tends towards the pleasant, in part because I believe it should; and in part because I believe that one has a duty to hope for the best. Yet my imagination also veers toward my fears, a less controllable response. Even as I can visualize myself in a festive mood, I can anticipate my celebratory humour being ruptured.

As detailed as a dream, in this imagined future, I read from this hypothetical decision rendered by the South Africa Constitutional Court:

CONSTITUTIONAL COURT OF SOUTH AFRICA
Case CCT 117/2027

RIGHTS OF SINGLES TASKFORCE
First Applicant
CORINNA ZAZO SMITH
Second Applicant
And others
versus

MINISTER OF HOME AFFAIRS
First Respondent

THE PRESIDENT OF
THE REPUBLIC OF SOUTH AFRICA
Second Respondent

Heard on: 10 February 2027
Decided on: 27 June 2027

JUDGMENT
Mori, J:
Introduction
[1] This case raises the vital issue of the importance of marriage in our society. The Applicants challenge the Permanent Partners Act, Act 17 of 2025, also known as the 'Rule in Favour of Perpetuities', which eliminates divorce or other dissolution of marriage except in cases in which one of the partners is confined by court order to a mental institution for at least five years or who has left the country and not returned for at least ten years. Parliament passed this Act after extensive hearings regarding the rate of divorce and the destruction of families, including but not limited to families with children. Amongst the findings of Parliament is a rise in the incidence of divorce, so that more than fifty percent of the adults in our nation are no longer in a marriage because the marriage was terminated by legal processes rather than death. Parliament also found that children are more apt to thrive when they are raised by two persons who remain married to each other.

[2] The Applicants argue a deprivation of their constitutional rights to be free from unfair discrimination on the basis of marital status, sexual orientation, and gender, and their right to dignity, as well as raising an 'ex post facto' argument. We reject each of their arguments and will treat them briefly in turn.

Marital Status
[3] The Permanent Partners Act does not discriminate unfairly on the basis of marital status. The Act apportions neither private nor public goods on the basis of a person's marital status. What the Act does provide is that once a person chooses to marry that choice is a permanent one, except in certain circumstances.

Sexual Orientation
[4] Applicant Smith, now in a marital relationship with a woman with whom she set up house and duly married, argues that the Permanent Partners Act indirectly discriminates on the basis of sexual orientation. She relies on studies that purport to show that persons with a same-sex sexual orientation have an inherently different understanding of 'permanent' than do persons with an opposite-sex sexual orientation. Without deciding on the legitimacy of such studies, we find them inapposite. Whatever the subjective understandings of particular persons, marriage is a life-long commitment.

[5] In *Minister of Home Affairs and Another v Fourie and Another* 2006 (1) SA 524 (CC), the landmark same-sex marriage case decided over twenty years ago, we began by describing what same-sex couples routinely did: 'Finding themselves strongly attracted to each other, two people went out regularly and eventually decided to set up a home together.' At the time of that opinion, the couple was not allowed to enter into the marital commitment, a constitutional deficiency that has long since been remedied. Now, the parties cannot be heard to complain that they must be released

from their commitment. Assuming that the parties entered into the marital commitment willingly, the legislature certainly has the power to enforce that commitment. Moreover, in *Fourie*, the Court specifically based its decision on the principle that same-sex couples should have the same rights and responsibilities as heterosexual married couples should their relationship threaten to rupture (paragraph 73).

Gender
[6] Generally, marriage 'stabilizes relationships by protecting the vulnerable partner and introducing equity and stability into the relationship', as we stated in *Fourie* (paragraph 69). However, although increasingly infrequent, violence against women remains a scourge in our society of equality, Parliament's choice to exclude an ability to terminate an otherwise valid marriage on these grounds presumably occurred after reasoned and deliberate consideration. We reject any link between the availability of divorce as necessary for women to avoid violence or that the instances of violence against women are attributable to the availability of divorce for women. On that assumption, we cannot usurp the power of Parliament and 'edit' the statute. We note that organizations exist representing women suffering from violence at the hands of their lawful spouses and trust that such organizations will pursue their arguments in Parliament.

Dignity
[7] Our constitutional concept of dignity imposes on our people the responsibility to comport themselves with dignity. As Sachs and O'Regan JJ stated in the landmark judgment of *S v Jordan* 2002 (6) SA 642 (CC), it was not the criminal prohibition against prostitution that diminished the dignity of prostitutes, but the 'very character of the work they undertake devalues the respect that the Constitution regards as inherent in the human body' (paragraph 77). Similarly, just as the prostitute chooses her regrettable lifestyle and must accept the consequences attendant thereto, so must the married person. With any luck, these consequences are of a much happier quality. However, even if they are not, the choice must be honoured and enforced.

'Ex Post Facto'
[8] The Applicants also raise an argument that the change in marriage laws constitutes an impressible 'ex post facto' law, operating impermissibly retroactively in regard to persons who were married at the time Parliament passed the Permanent Partners Act of 2027. Our Constitution provides in Section 35, regarding 'arrested, detained, and accused persons', in Subsection 3, that every 'accused person' has certain rights, which include, in Subsection I, 'not to be convicted for an act or omission that was not an offence under either national or international law at the time it was committed or omitted'. As is obvious from the explicit language of the Constitutional text, this right accrues in the criminal context. Marriage, obviously, is not such a context. Instead, marriage is a civil contract, and as our native countrywoman Margaret Marshall asserted, in her landmark

decision declaring same-sex marriage constitutionally mandated for the people of the state of Massachusetts, where she had become the Chief Justice of the state's Supreme Judicial Court, there are three parties to any marriage: two willing spouses and the state - *Goodridge v Department of Public Health* 798 NE 2d 941, 954 (Mass. 2003). Parliament has altered the terms of the contract, as the parties were always aware that it could, and they cannot be heard to complain.

International Law
[9] Pursuant to Section 39 of our Constitution, requiring us, when interpreting the Bill of Rights, to consider international law, we again note that there is presently no extant body of law that qualifies as 'international law'. However, we also note that South Africa is not alone in passing legislation and in upholding such legislation against constitutional challenge, promoting the permanence of marriage. Amongst constitutional democracies, Australia, the United States, and the Consolidated Republic of South America, have passed and upheld similar laws. In Aortearoa (formerly known as New Zealand), East Timor, Iran, Iceland, and Israel, amongst others, the respective Parliaments have passed similar provisions deemed consistent with their national interests. The situations in the European Union and Asian Confederacy are understandably more complex given current conditions, but cannot be said to be inconsistent with our present opinion.

Conclusion and Order
[10] The Court finding that arguments of the Applicants challenging the Permanent Partners Act of 2027 are without merit, and the Court certifying that this Judgment complies with the 1 000-word limit for all judicial opinions, excluding this paragraph and the caption, as recommended by the Chief Justice, the appeal is dismissed.

Epilogue
I do not mean to suggest that the hypothetical Permanent Partners Act of 2027 and the hypothetical judgment upholding it are inevitable, predictable, or even likely outcomes, either globally or as a consequence of present South African Constitutional Court doctrine, the Civil Union Act, or social conditions. Nevertheless, this dystopian portrait is not unimaginable. The celebratory rhetoric marriage in *Fourie* might be extended to its perhaps illogical conclusion. Further, the reasoning in *S v Jordan* (the sex-workers case) about 'choice' might be extended to make the choice of marriage irrevocable. In the US, so-called 'covenant marriage', prohibiting no-fault divorce, has been adopted as an option in a few states.

Looking back on 1979 from the perspective of 2007, one can spot the scattered seeds of same-sex marriage and the South African democratic revolution. The energy directed at stamping out both possibilities by repressive forces is perhaps one indication of the fertility of these seeds. And perhaps one can even discern how these seeds would combine and mutate to flower into the *Fourie* judgment. Yet I do not think I was alone in my inability to include such eventualities in my most adventuresome speculations.

Trying to gaze into 2027 is an equally fraught endeavour. However, I assume that the *Fourie* judgment and the Civil Union Act shelter many of the seeds of our queer future, in South Africa and globally. A pessimistic but rather simplistic prediction is that the gains that have been made will be rescinded. An optimistic forecast is that the realization of sexual liberation will only grow, with 'civil unions' being only one form of partnership and 'partnership' being only one type of sexual expression.

The reality will most likely be a tangle of rupture and rhyme with our present and past.

A short guide to the Civil Union Act

What is the main purpose of the Civil Union Act?
The Civil Union Act allows both opposite-sex and same-sex couples who are 18 years and older to form a marriage or a civil partnership, both of which can be referred to under the general category of being a 'civil union'. The Act provides the procedures through which such unions are solemnized and regulates the legal consequences that flow from registering such a relationship.

What is the legal difference between forming a marriage and forming a civil partnership in terms of the Civil Union Act?
There is *no* legal difference between forming a marriage and a civil partnership in terms of the Civil Union Act. Both forms of relationship have the same legal consequences as a marriage does under the Marriage Act (with one or two exceptions discussed in the question below).

What are the legal consequences of a marriage or a civil partnership in terms of the Civil Union Act?
All the consequences that flow from a marriage in our law flow from a marriage or civil partnership under the Civil Union Act. The only differences for same-sex couples will be in respect of the very limited number of laws which still distinguish between a husband and a wife (for instance, a wife may currently in our law choose whether to adopt the surname of her husband, to retain her existing surname or to create a double-barrelled name; the husband does not have a similar right): in terms of the Civil Union Act, these laws need to be adapted to cater for a gender-neutral context (for instance, in a same-sex relationship, both parties may be given the choice to decide on the surname they wish to assume).

Most importantly, this means that couples who marry or form a civil partnership must consider the marital property regime they wish to effect between them: without an ante-nuptial contract, the default position is that the marriage will be in community of property (all assets and liabilities of both parties will form part of a joint estate). If an ante-nuptial contract is chosen, then it is possible to include or exclude the accrual system. Excluding the accrual system means that the assets and liabilities of each partner remain theirs alone and they have separate estates. Including the accrual system, means that the assets and liabilities that the partners accrue during the course of their marriage are shared but their estates are still regarded as separate. Legal advice should be taken as to the advantages and disadvantages of the various property regimes. Importantly, an ante-nuptial contract, if decided upon, must be signed prior to the marriage or civil partnership.

If there is no legal difference between a marriage and a civil partnership, what is the difference between these two forms of relationship?
The difference between a marriage and a civil partnership is not entirely clear at present. Since there is no difference in legal consequences, it seems that the difference lies in the individual and social meanings that are created around these two terms. The word 'marriage' has a particular resonance and significance that many people wish to associate with their relationships; others may wish their relationships to be free of such meanings and thus would prefer to form a civil partnership. The choice allows individuals to decide how they wish their relationships to be characterized as well as the term they wish to use to refer to their relationship, that is: as a marriage or as a civil partnership.

What is the difference between a civil union and a marriage or civil partnership?
A civil union is just the general category that refers to two forms of relationships: a marriage or a civil partnership. Thus the links between these terms can be characterized as follows:

CIVIL UNION = A MARRIAGE **OR** A CIVIL PARTNERSHIP

Who can solemnize a marriage or a civil partnership?
Only a marriage officer recognized by the state may solemnize a marriage or civil partnership. Such a marriage officer may be either:
- A 'civil marriage officer' is an official of the state such as a magistrate or an official in the Department of Home Affairs who has been given the authority to be a marriage officer by the Minister of Home Affairs.
- A 'religious marriage officer' is a person holding a position of authority (a religious or lay leader) in any religious denomination or organization recognized in terms of the Act.

How does one become a religious marriage officer?
Religious marriage officers who are presently designated under the Marriage Act cannot automatically solemnize civil unions. There are two steps necessary to become a religious marriage officer under the Civil Union Act:
- The religious denomination or organization one belongs to must apply in writing to the Director General of the Department of Home Affairs to be designated as a religious organization that may solemnize marriage in terms of the Civil Union Act and such designation must be granted. A constitution or founding statement of such organization is often required.

- The individual who wishes to become a marriage officer must apply in writing to the Minister for designation as a marriage officer and such designation must be granted. A written test is often required prior to approval of individuals as marriage officers.

Can a marriage officer refuse to solemnize a civil union?
A religious marriage officer may refuse to perform any marriage that does not conform to the tenets and beliefs of their religion. The Civil Union Act goes further, allowing civil marriage officers (officials of the state) to refuse to perform civil unions between persons of the same sex on grounds of conscience, religion or belief.

What types of civil union are prohibited?
- You must only be involved in one marriage or civil partnership at one any time, and this applies to marriages under the Marriage Act and those under the Customary Marriages Act as well (and you may be married under only one of these acts);
- Civil Unions cannot be registered between close family members such as a father and son, brother and sister.
- No person can enter into a civil union through any other person acting on their behalf but must do so personally.

What documentation is necessary to form a civil union?
- You need proof of identity which can either be in the form of an identity book or through signing a prescribed affidavit;
- You need a certified copy of a divorce certificate or death certificate if you were previously married (or civil-partnered) under the Marriage Act, Customary Marriages Act or Civil Union Act.
- The partners must sign in writing a declaration (on an official form) indicating their willingness to enter into the civil union with each other, which must be signed in the presence of two witnesses. The marriage officer and two witnesses must sign this form.

What documentation does the marriage officer complete to ensure registration of the civil union?
- The marriage officer must issue the partners to a civil union with a registration certificate stating they have under the Act entered into a marriage or civil partnership and this constitutes *prima facie* proof that a valid civil union exists.
- Each marriage officer must keep a record of all civil unions conducted by him or her.
- The marriage officer must transmit the civil union register and records to the

official in the public service with the responsibility for the population register in that area and that official must enter information about the civil union into the population register.

Where and when do civil unions take place?
- Civil unions may take place at any time on any day of the week, though a marriage officer is not obliged to solemnize such a union at any other time than between 8am and 4pm.
- A civil union must be solemnized in a public office or private home with open doors and in the presence of the parties themselves and at least two witnesses. These provisions do not apply where for reasons of long-standing illness or serious bodily injury it is not possible to hold the ceremony in such a place.

What does a civil union ceremony involve?
For a valid civil union to be contracted, a marriage officer must perform the ceremony and the documentation discussed above be completed. The marriage officer will then ask the parties whether they want their civil union to be known as a marriage or a civil partnership. Their choice will determine the designation of the relationship in law and how it is referred to in the ceremony. The marriage officer will then put the following question to each of the parties, to which each person must reply in the affirmative:

'Do you, X, declare that as far as you know there are no lawful impediments to your proposed marriage/civil partnership to Y here present, and that you call all here present to witness that you take Y as your lawful spouse/civil partner?'

The parties then must give each other their right hands and the marriage officer must declare the marriage/civil partnership solemnized in the following words:

'I declare that X and Y here present have been lawfully joined in a marriage/civil partnership.'

Both parties to the marriage, the marriage officer and two witnesses must sign the prescribed document at the solemnization ceremony. A certificate will be issued stating that the parties have entered into a marriage/civil partnership. The certificate is proof that a valid civil union exists between the parties.

Where can you go to get married?
In order to enter into a marriage or a civil partnership, you can go to your nearest Home Affairs office and make an appointment for the solemnization to take place. You and your partner will need all the relevant documentation (see above) and you will then be required to set a date for your solemnization ceremony.

Alternatively a religious marriage officer, who has applied and been designated under the Civil Union Act, can also perform your solemnization ceremony. For the details of religious marriage officers who can do this, contact the organizations below.

For more information about the Civil Union Act contact one of the following organizations:

Durban Lesbian and Gay Community and Health Centre
The Community Centre is an organization that serves the LGBTI communities of Durban and surrounding areas.
Phone: 031 301 2145
Website: www.gaycentre.org.za

Gender DynamiX
Gender DynamiX is a human-rights organization promoting freedom of expression of gender identity, and focusing on transgender and transsexual issues.
Phone: 021 6335287
Website: www.genderdynamix.org.za

The Lesbian and Gay Equality Project (LGEP)
LGEP is an organization that works towards achieving full legal and social equality for LGBTI people in South Africa. It has offices in Johannesburg.
Phone: 011 487 3810/1
Website: www.equality.org.za

OUT LGBT Well-being (OUT)
OUT works towards LGBTI people's physical and mental health and related rights. OUT has offices in Tshwane.
Phone: 012 344 5108
Helpline: 012 344 6500
Web: www.out.org.za

Triangle Project
Triangle Project is an organization that focuses on LGBTI physical and social health and rights and on marginalized LGBTI individuals and groups. It has offices in Cape Town and offers a range of services.
Phone: 021 448 3812
Helpline: 021 422 2500
Website: www.triangle.org.za

For information about other LGBTI organizations and services contact the **Joint Working Group (JWG)**.
Tel: 011 4035566
Website: www.jwg.org.za

Note
This guide to the law was compiled by David Bilchitz. It is in effect the author's interpretation of the best construction that can be placed on particular provisions of the Act and is also designed to provide a simplified understanding of the law in this area. The meaning of a number of these provisions are themselves the subject of discussion among lawyers and may change over time through judicial interpretations of the Act. The Civil Union Act is available at www.info.gov.za/gazette/acts/2006/a17-06.pdf (last accessed 29 February 2008).

4: DEARLY BELOVED ...
Religion and same-sex marriage

'Equality of the vineyard': Challenge and celebration for faith communities

Keith Anthony Vermeulen

'Just as there is not one view on marriage, there is also no single authoritative interpretation of scripture. We view the Bible as God's living word. As such, it is capable of speaking afresh to humanity at different times and in different places and circumstances ... Government ... [at] the same time ... must defend religious freedom by ensuring that churches retain control over decisions regarding religious rites and sacraments, including the religious aspects of marriage.' – Eddie Makue, General Secretary of the South Africa Council of Churches, clarifies the role of religion and politics during a period of public outcry against the recognition of same-sex marriages during provincial hearings on the Civil Union Bill in 2006[1]

'Yet, despite all of the difficulties we face, I have faith that acknowledging the inherent dignity and respect due us can lead to greater respect for our human rights. Silence creates vulnerability. I urge you, members of the Commission on Human Rights, to break the silence. You can help us achieve our full rights and freedoms, in every society, including my beloved Sierra Leone.'
– A plea by Fanny Ann Eddy, a human-rights activist and founder of the gay and lesbian association of Sierra Leone to the United Nations Commission for Human Rights. Eddy was brutally raped and murdered in October 2004[2]

Christians and churches have, throughout history, located themselves or been placed in positions of social power and thereby became arch supporters – wittingly and unwittingly – of the socio-economic and political status quo. From time immemorial the appropriate blend of politics (described by some as 'the art of the possible' as opposed to an exact science) and religion has been a vexed question. The Constantinian era – during which the Emperor Constantine allied political power and military violence in order to arbitrate the outcomes of Christian doctrine at successive councils – exacerbated an ethos of church-state relationships that compromised Judaeo-Christian ideals for human life, dignity and care of the marginalized with the politics of global domination and expansion. While an in-depth study of politics and religion or church-state relationships is not the object of this essay, suffice it to say that Constantine diverted 300 years of church-state relationships, giving rise to the 'Two Swords' doctrine adopted by the church. Bishop Ossius of Cordoba[3] is credited with advising the Emperor Constantius that, according to the scriptures – 'Render unto Caesar the things that are Caesar's and unto God the things that are God's ...' – governance of the empire was the God-ordained responsibility of the emperor in the same way that bishops were ordained to administer the affairs of the church.

The essential point here is that Jesus's commands that his followers love and care for the social well-being of their fellow human beings – especially the poor, vulnerable, marginalized and excluded, and for one another – had become wholly subverted by one of the most powerful decision-makers and empire-builders of his time: Constantine. This vexed relationship between political power and organized religion has produced systems of 'justice' having more to do with expunging of guilt through punishment and divine retribution, and, I argue, lies at the heart of the contemporary church's refusal to acknowledge and bless same-sex marriages. In a nutshell, this justice brings very little understanding of the human, social and cultural differences that affirm dignity, respect and equality of the human being. This co-option of religion is recognizable later in the Western and European colonial and imperial conquests of the 'two-thirds world', including and especially that of the African continent. The legal enforcement of political power that presumed social transformation through punitive justice – a 'justice' that included the rape, pillage, theft of national resources and the reduction of human beings to chattel as slaves – was accompanied by organized Christian religion spreading a message of 'salvation by faith'. This 'salvation', combined with political and technological power – guns, ships, military occupation – has so captured the minds and shaped the mindsets of the world that, to this day, South African and African notions of civil morality are at odds in attempts at ridding themselves from belief in colonial power and (Christian) religion being sufficient for resolving contemporary, social conflicts.

So power – in the minds of men and women – to punish and correct what is different (and by extrapolation morally wrong) lies at the heart of a paradigm that projects religiously defined mores and values as the core of a stable society. Since gay, lesbian and bisexual people are not perceived to fit into this norm of social values – and thereby are removed from the mainstream of society to its fringes – society, dominant cultures, especially the churches, continue to promote a punitive form of justice as a norm of correction. The powerful and dominant require, however, a justification for the outlet of any curative actions and subtly promote stigma and generate 'fear images' as an apparently legitimate form of social hatred that may be expunged by social cleansing. Such stigmata range from contemporary judgments on HIV and AIDS sufferers as well as theological slogans like 'loving the sinner but hating the sin'. Some Christian leaders are known to preach that the pandemic and the sufferer's condition are a direct result of God's punishment for their disobedience and immorality. Another popular form of religious interpretation – closer to our theme – is the misinterpretation of the biblical story of Sodom and Gomorrah as wreaking God's vengeance on 'homosexuality'. In reality that story is about the misuse of sex as power when a group of males in the city seek to humiliate and subdue strangers and visitors in their midst. Be that as it may, and while organized society and religion are motivated by power – especially mind-power – to 'correct', 'cure' and 'save', contemporary leaders of the Christian faith ought to know better.

The debate on civil unions and civil marriages in the Civil Union Bill and subsequent Act was an ideal time to rediscover the power of love that revolutionized the world and which continues to grip the minds of many philosophers and people in the third millennium of its existence. I refer to the words in the Gospel of John – its writer generally known as 'the disciple whom Jesus loved' – that describe the nature of their friendship: 'No man has greater love than the one who is prepared to lay down his life for a friend'; or, 'Everyone will know that you are my followers if you love one another'; or, 'The one who says he loves God and hates his neighbour is a liar for, how is it possible to love God whom you have not seen if you do not love your neighbour whom you are able to see?' How, then, to relate the power of love to society, and how to deal with fear of the ruin of social and moral fabric? These remain the challenges posed by the Civil Union Act to South Africa and Africa's faith communities. The celebration, however, is that (for the Christian faith especially) an acceptance of same-sex love may unlock that secret to spiritual cohesion – unity – which, in turn, might just be able to advance social equity, human dignity and respect in our nation, continent and in the world.

Power, family and the institution of marriage
The challenge to African and South African religious communities in the wake of the Civil Union Act, therefore, remains how to live alongside and relate as equal human beings to gay, lesbian, bisexual and transgender people, and with their international right to same-sex orientation. This right challenges all previous South African social and legal formations that outlawed, stigmatized and ridiculed same-sex orientation and denounced any recognition of *same-sex love*. I refrain from speaking of 'homosexuality' because of the emotive and religious stigmata attached to the term. The derogatory references in Christian terms to the 'homo' and the 'homosexual', as though curative and spiritual 'conversion' would lead to their ultimate salvation, now require serious revision and thought. The rights of gay, lesbian or bisexual persons, on the other hand, gives a power to which political, social and religious formations need to adapt their thought and actions. Just as society was required to transform its attitude, behaviour and practice towards former slaves after the introduction of anti-

slavery legislation 200 years ago, the same requirements apply to our modern, medical and scientific understanding of sexual orientation.

The rights to equality of respect and dignity emerge not so much from the choice of partner or sexual practice as it does, first and foremost, from the right to being human and different. As a right – in the spirit of our Constitution – equality of sexual orientation demands respect as citizens and human beings for gay, lesbian, bisexual and transgender people. This is important for religion and civil society if we are to forge a sense of social cohesion as envisaged in the Bill of Rights. If the guesstimate that two out of every five of current heterosexual marriages are doomed to failure and, if the assumption is that family life is at the heart of the moral basis of the nation, then heterosexual marriage is failing the nation. If the family is the moral basis of the nation then the heterosexual model leaves too much to be desired. I will allude later to the corollary that models of fidelity, love and trust in same-sex relationships are not a threat to heterosexual relationships but desirable and necessary if heterosexual relationships are in some way able to restore the foundations of South Africa's national project of building social cohesion. Furthermore, then, persistent religious attempts at curative therapy for 'homosexuals' require a two-pronged caveat. At one level, the denial, rejection and attempts at 'redemption' of the same-sex-oriented is a violation of their international and – in the case of South Africa – constitutional right to respect, dignity and equity with all of humanity. At the religious level, this mindset that views gay, lesbian and bisexual people as 'sinners' who can be badgered into salvation lies both at the heart of a need for modern theological review as well as at the base of thought that generates hate crimes – the result of belief and attitude – against South Africa's and Africa's gay and lesbian communities.

The challenge to religions for the promotion of a dignified, respectful and humane world in the 21st century is to recognize that homophobia – not 'homosexuality' – is both a category of sin as well as crime against humanity. The sooner Christian and religious communities acknowledge the danger and depravity caused by homophobia – and that it constitutes a breach of law – the sooner they would realize that equity of unions, partnership and marriage for same-sex partners would be a blessing – not a threat – to their high regard for the institution of marriage. One of the moral arguments against same-sex marriages, used during the passage of the Civil Union Bill, is that they would undermine the fabric of society, its moral foundation and the traditional notion of the family. The assumed notion of a family is, however, frequently grounded in the concept of a heterosexual and nuclear family comprising a mother, a father and 2.3 children. This argument against social decline – and the premise that same-sex unions would precipitate it – is further based on the assumption that there has been an immutable Christian concept and structure of family. The reality is rather different.

The precise blend of family and marriage has changed enormously over time. For example, in the New Testament scriptures, St Paul counselled his followers not to marry since he believed the second coming of Jesus was imminent. Judgment and damnation on the return of Jesus could be avoided, however, if sexual desire were channelled through marriage. But prior to this New Testament construct, Hebraic and Roman societies accepted polygynous marriages in which paternal authority was absolute over wife and children, even to the point of death. In the 12th century, the increasing numbers of children fathered by priests who claimed church property as inheritance gave rise to the idea of marriage as a 'sacrament', along with the reinforcement of primogeniture and priestly celibacy. In more modern Western traditions, it was not until the 15th century and Henry VIII's efforts to subordinate ecclesiastical authority to the monarchy in England that the state began to assume a greater role in refereeing human relationships. In subsequent centuries, the roles of the family, religious communities and the state in recognizing and giving effect to marriages became even more hopelessly entangled.

It might be argued that in contemporary South African society marriage has emotional, social and cultural significance independent of and possibly even superseding any meaning ascribed to it by a particular religious community. The notion of *ubuntu* – a construct of the supremacy of humane relations for human society acceptable to most religions – would need to redefine religious notions of social cohesion and moral fibre as they relate to state power and legal processes on same-sex relations. In a recent Constitutional Court judgment regarding social assistance to an expatriate Mozambican community living in Limpopo, the concept of *ubuntu* – while not explicitly mentioned – became the basis of a ruling that they and their families, which had for generations lived here, would qualify for access to social security and assistance. This ruling, by virtue of their connection to South Africa – *ubuntu* – guaranteed their protection and assistance under the South African Constitution.[4]

The exclusion of gay men and lesbian women from African society as a Western problem – as claimed, for example, by the Anglican Archbishop of Nigeria, Peter Akinola[5] – would find little support in the South African Constitutional Court. I suspect that such and similar views in other parts of Africa would be found unacceptable by the United Nations Human Rights Commission. The passage of the Civil Union Act through the South African Parliament, twelve years after the advent of democracy, may have been timeous for those who are bold enough to stand up and out in society, but has come regrettably too late for those who have fallen prey to South Africa and Africa's hate crimes against gay and lesbian people.

Fear, homophobia and the challenge of love

In a bid to rescue its member churches from an embarrassing and complex web of biblical interpretation, politics and religion, as well as from psychosocial pressures that were brought to bear as they faced the passage of the Civil Union Bill through Parliament, the South African Council of Churches (SACC) General Secretary, Eddie Makue, tabled an open letter before the Portfolio Committee for Home Affairs, chaired by Patrick Chauke. The letter – a portion of which is quoted above – unravelled the strands that weave the engagement of religion and public policy as they unfold within a constitutional democracy. The state, the letter indicated, has a duty to apply and interpret the Constitution. In the case of the Civil Union Bill, this meant applying the rights of equity to same-sex unions or marriage – the complexity of which we have already indicated – something hitherto denied same-sex couples.

While the legislative problem was posed as the need for a change of formula – simply replacing the words 'man and woman' or 'husband and wife' with the word 'spouse' – the deeper issue at stake was a denial by the churches to provide the social, legal and religious affirmation – tied up in the Marriage Act of 1961 – for gay and lesbian choice to committed long-term relationships. In the related Constitutional Court ruling, Justice Albie Sachs made it abundantly clear that legislation was to provide an equal affirmation for same-sex unions in the same manner that the Marriage Act provided for civil and social affirmation of opposite-sex unions. The revised marriage legislation was to provide 'equality of the vineyard and not equality of the graveyard'.[6]

Makue pre-empts the spite and denial of affirmation that religious communities would bring to the Civil Union legislation, and indicates that it is the duty of the churches to interpret the Bible in the same sense that the state is to interpret the Constitution. Granted the diverse interpretations of same-sex-relations by churches and Christians alike, Makue intimated that any permission for the state to base a policy decision on one or other Christian interpretation of the Bible would be tantamount to the state arbitrating on biblical interpretation. That would be an unacceptable intrusion on religious thought, as much as it would infringe upon South African society's right to freedom of religious belief and practice. And if this fear was not uppermost in the minds of religious practitioners in standing against the rights of same-sex couples, then we must conclude that they were willing to entertain a position of power-play politics which would give political clout to their interpretation of morality or vice versa. Interestingly, the very same Christian groups who object to making civil space and affirmation for same-sex unions would also oppose the right of women to determine their reproductive and sexual health and would promote capital punishment, as well as the right of the West to wage war in order to determine 'order' and pursue empire-building. It is this ethical hodgepodge that is scary, especially the argument that the divine can bring order out of human-induced chaos such as war. One can only conclude that there is an absence – or at most an inconsistent understanding – of the concept of justice, peace and human dignity in these religious camps.

Let us take our reflection on homophobia, fear and love further. I believe that Makue is urging the Christian community to take a further look at the sacred texts and traditions, while Sachs looks beyond the law to the psychosocial and religious to explore 'the equality of the vineyard' for marriage as an institution of social respect, dignity and inclusion for all. From within a Christian hermeneutic, the biblical reference to Jesus's performing the first of his 'signs and wonders' at a wedding feast is significant. Jesus turns water into wine at the request of his mother and associates, intimating that love, friendship, social affirmation and joy as the foundation of an enduring love would stand the test of time. The point of the quality of love in this story is that this love goes beyond community relations with his followers. It is to last in their relationships but extend to and beyond his death.[7] As a basis for his future relationship with his followers, this faith-seeking, society-changing relationship lies at the heart of (Christian) religious partnerships and is the essence of friendship. We are not told about the relationship between the bride and the groom, and their sexual orientation is never mentioned or made the point of departure for this story. What is certain is that Jesus's own relationship with his followers – male and female – was to stand the test of enduring love and faithfulness. It was never about the power of control and domination (even Jesus's relationship with his mother is severely strained by her instructions), as so many heterosexual relationships bear testimony to these days. John tells the story of the wedding feast at Cana of Galilee, a paradigm for a 'vineyard of equality', and tells more about fidelity and trust between partners equally affirmed for their mutual dignity (it matters not that the story is about a heterosexual wedding) rather than for the domination of the male over the female or the offspring that may later ensue. The story of the wedding feast also celebrates an enduring love by Jesus's followers, one for the other, which supersedes any claim to 'heterosexual' – male – supremacy.

While I am not using the Bible to claim recognition for same-sex unions, what I am adamant about is that the model relationships that Christians are to emulate are certainly not about male 'possession' or 'possessiveness' over women and their bodies, as though women were chattel in the way that Africans were slaves and remain commodities of the West. At a stroke, an affirmation of same-sex relationships, partnerships, unions or marriages challenges us to rethink the *telos* or goal of such socialized relationships. During the public hearings on the Civil Union Bill, I was struck by the regularity of news reports on family murders by fathers, rapes by known partners, abuse of children in opposite-sex marriages and families. By contrast, many same-sex partners are constrained to silence within the church community despite admirable levels of faithfulness and trust that lie at the heart of their 'different' love. Yet, either because of fear of ridicule or a sense that it is not yet safe to come out of the closet – despite our equality laws – prudence rather than valour is the order of wisdom. Ultimately, the reality is that gay and lesbian people – as with all spiritual and religious beings – will need to claim equality through participation in the life of the church and religious community, difficult as such interaction may be.

So, two challenges emerge for the churches in considering the religious implications of adopting an affirmation of same-sex unions or marriages. The one has to do with the recognition that the gay and lesbian lobby is doing the faith communities an enormous favour in assisting us to evaluate the quality and equity of love and trust within existing relationships, be they partnerships or marriages. For the follower of Jesus, true greatness and power lie in centring our attention on the vulnerable, weak and marginalized – even the child – of society.[8] The Jesus model is not about domination or possessiveness but about faithfulness, not about perpetuating the status quo through procreation, but rather an affirmation of an enduring trust and love that bonds the agreed partnership in a covenant of love. This has very little to do with eroticism but links the partnership in trust with care, love and cooperation in fidelity, in order to promote and advance a more humane society and world. This society and world in turn are called to promote dignity, love and respect for every difference in humanity – known and unknown, comprehensible and incomprehensible. Such is the depth of religious understanding of love and trust, and we need to celebrate the manner in which the gay and lesbian lobby has challenged our staid and 'unalterable' religious traditions as witnessed through the Civil Union Act.

Why, then, reduce the *telos* of human relationships to a sexual act? Why perpetuate dominance of one gender over another and hinder our progress towards human and gender equity? The debate and dialogue within the religious community requires, however, a safe space for engaging the human right for gay, lesbian, bisexual and transgender people to be included in love, respect and dignity. I suspect that such an exercise – difficult as it may be in changing archaic mindsets – will begin the path to discovery of the pristine intentions of the Christian community together with religious and spiritual friendships – as the progenitors of our faiths intended us to live.

Conclusion

If love and trust rather than possession and domination (of women) are what same-sex unions challenge the religions in South Africa and Africa to reconsider, I believe that the churches also need to re-examine just how 'different' – if at all – the love of the same-sexed is from opposite-sex love. A great deal more hermeneutic and theological studies will be required in order to bolster the support for a progressive inclusion and interaction with gay and lesbian people and same-sex couples. Furthermore, a more in-depth understanding of gay, lesbian, bisexual and transgender people will emerge as space is available and claimed to present gay, lesbian, bisexual and transgender people as beings with desires, aspirations and foibles equal to those of any other human beings. Such interaction is necessary to challenge false beliefs and myths about gay and lesbian people, especially those beliefs that emerge from anti-gay and homophobic theologies and especially from within the diversity of Christian communities so frequently bolstered by 'right-wing religion'.

The legal and social parameters of discussion have now been clearly defined and accepted in South Africa. The religious – especially Christian – communities bear the onus of opening the boundaries of dialogue in the best religious traditions across Africa. Failure to do so will result in a judgment of complicity with political power that thwarts the right of equity for those who have an innate sense or choice for same-sex love. The celebration of same-sex unions carries with it, however, a grave danger that relates to an increase in homophobia-related incidents of deaths – symbolized by the deaths of Sizakele Sigasa and Salome Masooa in July 2007. Should this safe space for social dialogue not be created, the question is: Will the religious communities of Africa accept their share of guilt – morally and legally – for homophobia and further homophobia-related deaths? For surely death, murder and human brutality must rank as a sin and a religious concern – especially within the Christian community – way beyond any dispute on sexual orientation and same-sex love.

Notes

1 Taken from an open letter, addressed to the Chairs of the Parliamentary Portfolio Committees on Home Affairs and Justice and Constitutional Development, sent by Eddie Makue, General Secretary of the SACC. Available at www.sacc.org.za/news06/marriage.html (last accessed 18 February 2008)
2 http://www.hrw.org/english/docs/2004/10/04/sierra9440.htm (last accessed 13 December 2007). Fanny Ann Eddy was the founder of the Sierra Leone Lesbian and Gay Association and a lesbian rights activist known across Africa. Human Rights Watch reported that Eddy, 30, was found dead on the morning of 29 September 2004. While working alone in the Association's offices the previous night, she was raped repeatedly, stabbed and her neck was broken.
3 See 'Protest by Ossius of Cordova to Constantius II', in James Stevenson (ed.), *Creeds, Councils and Controversies: Documents Illustrative of the History of the Church AD 337-461* (Seabury, 1966; revised edition SPCK, 1981), 37-39
4 This point was clarified by Constitutional Court Judge Yvonne Makgoro at a conference entitled 'What Is Law without Morality?' at the University of the Western Cape. She argued for the extension of *ubuntu* justiciability in South Africa's Bill of Rights.
5 See a concise analysis of gay and lesbian relationships and rights in Africa (as at December 2006) in the article 'Still a Long, Hard Road to Gay Rights in Africa' by Alex Duval Smith at http://www.nzherald.co.nz/topic/story.cfm?c_id=177&objectid=10415047 (last accessed 13 December 2007)
6 Judgment in *Minister of Home Affairs and Another v Fourie and Another* 2005 (3) BCLR 355

(CC); 2006 (1) SA 524 (CC). In his decision to reject equality of marriage by levelling down or denying access to civil marriage, Justice Albie Sachs contends that 'such parity of exclusion rather than of inclusion would distribute resentment evenly, instead of dissipating it equally for all. The law concerned with family formation and marriage requires equal celebration, not equal marginalisation; it calls for equality of the vineyard and not equality of the graveyard' (paragraph 149).
7 Holy Bible, New International Version, John 2:1-11
8 Ibid., Mark 9:33-37; 10:1-16

A way forward through *ijtihad*: A Muslim perspective on same-sex marriage

Muhsin Hendricks

The passing of the Civil Union Act in South Africa has given Muslims an opportunity to reflect on what Islamic traditions have to say on the subject of marriage, and to interrogate its meanings in terms of same-sex couples. Of course this implies a consideration of Islam's attitude towards homosexuality in general, which has often taken the form of outright condemnation from the pulpit, or, within Muslim communities, the silence accorded a taboo. At the same time, there is a growing openness among gay and lesbian Muslims, encouraged by liberal legislation such as South Africa's Constitution. Moreover, a close look at Islamic thought reveals a conception of marriage that is more in tune with legislation such as the Civil Union Act than with the way marriage is often presented in conservative circles.

This essay will trace some of the lines of Islamic thought on marriage, and then look at Islam in South Africa specifically. In such communities, openly flamboyant homosexuality has in fact often been tolerated. I will then provide a snapshot of gay and lesbian Muslim attitudes towards organizations such as The Inner Circle (which I run and which forms a support network for queer Muslims) and their thoughts on same-sex marriage.

The Islamic tradition on marriage

Modern Muslim scholars assert that both homosexual sex and homosexual orientation are sinful and prohibited by Islamic law. The only verses in the Quran itself that refer specifically to homosexuality are those which speak of the people of Lot or Lut (Sodom and Gomorrah). Muslim scholars also quote several *hadith* – sayings attributed to the Prophet Muhammad (peace be upon him) – to directly condemn homosexuality. For example, *At-Tirmidhi*, Hadith 1376 states: 'Whoever you find committing the sin of the people of Lut, kill the one who does it and the one to whom it is done.' It can be argued that this condemnation is based on patriarchal assumptions and beliefs rather than on a clear reading of scriptural texts.

It is difficult for lesbian and gay Muslims to find answers within orthodox Islamic thinking. As such, it is important that we make use of one of the principles of Islam that has been lost over the years – *ijtihad* or 'independent reasoning' – to contribute to an alternative vision of Islam that has space for lesbian and gay people.

Historically, there is evidence that homoeroticism persisted for a long time in Muslim societies, even if it was not spoken of openly. There were renowned gay Muslim poets such as Abu Nawas (750-810). The prophetic traditions teach Muslims to hide a same-sex relationship outside wedlock, and homosexuality is treated as a shame that should not be spoken of.

All four Sunni schools of thought, and the Shi'a schools, assume that marriage is an essentially heterosexual institution, but they differ in the prerequisites for marriage and the 'pillars' that constitute a marriage. It is interesting to note how vast the difference of opinion between these schools are, which indicates that there have been many varying views on marriage among scholars from the 8th to the 11th centuries, when Islamic jurisprudence was developed into the more formal Sunni schools of Hanafi, Shafi, Maliki and Hanbali. After these schools were formed, the majority of Sunni Muslims felt that it was necessary to follow one of these schools (*taqleed*) as opposed to independent reasoning (*ijtihad*). Although there were still varying views on marriage after the imams of these schools passed away, these schools of thought still formed the basis of debate around marriage. Today, orthodox Sunni Muslims do not allow any differences of opinion other than those represented by the four schools.

The basic orthodox argument against same-sex marriage is that marriage is for procreation and hence a marriage between two men or two women is 'fruitless'. The Quran, however, clearly mentions that taking a partner (in marriage) is for love and tenderness and to place tranquility in the hearts of the partners:

> And among His wonders is this: He creates for you *mates out of your own kind* [direct translation from Arabic] so that you may find tranquility with them, and He engenders love and tenderness between you: in this, behold, there are messages indeed for people who think! [30:21]

If marriage were for procreation only, then a marriage with sexual intercourse between a sterile man and a 'barren' woman would have been forbidden. Even the Arabic word for marriage (*nikah*) is derived from the root letters (*na-ka-ha*) meaning 'to have sex'.[1] Hence, the term *nikah* can also be applied socially to same-sex couples who feel that marriage legitimizes the enjoyments and comforts of sexual interaction.

Numerous *hadith*[2] mention temporary (*mut'a*) marriage as a form of marriage accepted within Islam. Shi'a Muslims still practice this form of marriage, an agreement between two parties to marry for a stated term, which could be as short as three nights. This type of marriage was specifically granted by the Prophet Muhammad to fighters in his army, who had no means to satisfy their sexual appetites. Instead of allowing them to have sex with females captured in battle, he offered his warriors the option of marrying them by providing them gifts. After the death of the Prophet Muhammad (in 632), the Caliph Umar abolished *mut'a* marriage, an abolition staunchly upheld thereafter by Sunni Muslims. The Caliph Umar said: 'Two types of Mut'a were legal during the time of the Prophet and I forbid them both, and I punish those who commit it. They are: Mut'a of pilgrimage and Mut'a of women.'[3] It is clear from these *hadith* that marriage in this instance was not for procreation and that the Prophet Muhammad took into consideration the natural needs of human beings.

In the Hanafi jurisprudence, the offer *(ijaab)* and the acceptance *(qabul)* are the only pillars of the marriage, in their definition of a pillar *(rukn)*. Furthermore, in Hanafi jurisprudence, the offer/acceptance can begin from either party. If this pillar is in place, the marriage contract is legal, be it verbal or written. In fact, many marriages at the advent of Islam were contracted verbally and in the desert. This belief broadens the scope for the inclusion of same-sex marriages: the offer and acceptance are not defined in terms of sex or gender, and there is nothing in the conception of the pillars of marriage that indicates the two parties should be from opposite sexes. The terminology used in the marriage contract is not gender-specific. What seems to be more important in this Hanafi rule is that there should be no force or deceit in the contract, but that there should be a clear understanding of the contract between the two parties involved.

Much of what Muslims practice today in terms of marriage has been borrowed from Judaeo-Christian traditions and Hindu and Indonesian cultural heritages. A marriage in Islam is not as sacrosanct as in the Judaic and Christian faiths, and divorce is not as frowned upon as in Hindu culture. Divorce in Islam is more easily obtained. All the wedding paraphernalia – flowers, lavish banquets, pageboys and pretty dresses – is unimportant and in fact discouraged in Islam. Hence the seriousness of the matter lies within the contract that binds the two parties. In the light of this historical tradition, it may be argued that Islam makes space for the kinds of marriages envisaged by the Civil Union Act in South Africa.

Islam in South Africa

Islam arrived at the Cape in the 17th century, when the Dutch East India Company imported slaves from the Malay Archipelago. Also, political dissidents and religious leaders who opposed the presence of the Dutch in what is now Indonesia were banished to the Cape. This group first introduced Islam to South Africa. Muslims settled in the Bo-Kaap, formerly known as the Malay Quarter, in Cape Town, and in the late 1800s occupied the District Six area.[4] In such areas, homosexuality was tolerated when it took the form of men dressing like and behaving as women, especially when they took the role of entertainers. Hadji Galiema, a 76-year-old woman who lived in District Six, remembers that same-sex-identified people were fairly visible and tolerated among Muslims in the Bo-Kaap and District Six while she was growing up, from the 1940s to the 1960s: 'Moffies[5] used to dress up like women. They were funny and used to put up shows for us in the streets ... They were protected by gangs in District Six, so there was no such a thing as gay-bashing ... Moffies were part of the community. They were part of the entertainment ... They use to be the hairdressers and made beautiful wedding gowns and made the costumes for the Cape Coons.'

But when she was asked about their sexual escapades, she said: 'Now and then you hear about it, but it was never spoken of. Some people avoided moffies because they believed them to bring bad luck, but we used to enjoy their company and found them very funny.' She continued: 'Today's moffies are different, they don't dress up like women any more, so one does not know whether they are really moffies or not.'[6] Although 'moffies' were to a certain extent accepted socially among Cape Muslims in the Bo-Kaap and District Six,[7] homosexuality still remains a taboo and is considered a sin in Islam today.

The revolution of Iran in 1979, which brought a theocracy to power in that country, influenced the formation of fundamentalist groups such as Qibla in South Africa the early 1980s. Qibla aligned itself with the anti-apartheid struggle and aimed to promote the ideals of the Iranian revolution in South Africa, and to transform South Africa into an Islamic state. The environment created by Qibla was also a strong force in the formation of the Islamic Unity Convention and Pagad (People Against Gangsterism and Drugs) in the mid-1990s, which also called for the 'Islamization' of South Africa.[8] Many queer Muslims feared that such growing religiosity might make them targets of gay-bashing or restrict their freedom to socialize. It was assumed that the bomb blast on 25 August 1998 at the Planet Hollywood restaurant at the Victoria and Alfred Waterfront was executed by Pagad. On 6 November 1999, another bomb blast at Blah Bar, a gay nightspot, in Somerset Road in central Cape Town, scared gay Muslims who feared that Pagad might be targeting gays. It was believed by queer Muslims that Pagad would take an anti-gay stance and, it was joked, become 'People against Gays and Dykes'.[9]

This transformation in the Muslim community contributed to the dampening of the entertainment spirit of Cape Malays. Music, moffies, dance and New Year's Eve celebrations were now criticized as overly frivolous. New Year's Eve celebrations, for example, which had previously been an occasion for an ongoing carnival, were substituted with all night prayers – *qiyamul layl* – in many mosques. The Tabligh Jamaat, an Islamic revivalist movement that arrived at the Cape in the early 1960s, had preached that spending one's time on the path of Allah was much better than devoting oneself to the enjoyment this life has to offer. Many queer Muslims started to question their sexuality and accepted the Tablighi lifestyle as a means to negotiate the dilemma presented by a sexuality not in keeping with one's faith.

Yet the Prophet of Islam was very open towards sex and encouraged sex as opposed to abstinence. He even mentioned that sex with one's legal spouse is a form of worship. Although Islam is one religion that views sex in a positive light, sex and sexuality are still sensitive topics that do not get much public discussion. In Islam, sex is a private matter and, if it does occur outside wedlock, shame would lead to its being covered up. In the opinion of both Sunni and Shi'a Jurists, homosexuality in itself is a sin, whether private or public. Hence, for a long time, homosexuality was not openly discussed. (There are six nations with Muslim majorities that currently invoke the death penalty for same-sex intercourse: Iran, Mauritania, Saudi Arabia, Somalia, Sudan and Yemen.)

In recent times, many Muslims have had mixed feelings about homosexuality: effeminate behavior may have been accepted or tolerated, but disgust at the idea of anal sex, even with one's legal opposite-sex spouse, was widespread. There is no verse in the Quran prohibiting anal sex, but most orthodox Muslim jurists are of the opinion that it is prohibited in the sayings of the Prophet Muhammad, as narrated by Abu Hurayrah, who said, 'He who has intercourse with his wife through her anus is accursed.'[10]

Most Muslims prefer not to talk about homosexuality, although those Muslims associated with liberal Islamic organizations show some acceptance based on human rights and their understanding of Islam as a religion of compassion and inclusion. Very few Muslim scholars have been prepared to debate the issue, as Munadia Karan, a radio personality at The Voice of the Cape, observed: it was difficult, she said, to find scholars to debate the issue and she was often disappointed by last-minute cancellations by those who had indicated a willingness to speak on the subject.[11] Some Muslim scholars prefer gay and lesbian people to fight their own battles while, from the pulpit, others vehemently oppose homosexuality and anything related to it. One such scholar, the secretary general of the Muslim Judicial Council (MJC), Sheikh Achmat Sedick, has said that 'Prophet Muhammad condemned them to the fires of hell in the hereafter and said that God has cursed them on this earth. That wrath may come in various forms, including Aids and other venereal diseases.'[12]

A group providing a supportive network for gay and lesbian Muslims saw a fluctuation in its membership between 1998 and 2004, largely influenced by the tensions around homosexuality within the Muslim community at the time. This group is The Inner Circle, previously known as The Al-Fitrah Foundation (founded in 1998), which was an organization formed by gay men and giving social and spiritual support to queer Muslims. During this period, in the late 1990s and early 2000s, the work of Al-Fitrah became publicly known and this forced some queer Muslims into hiding; they feared being 'outed' through association with Al-Fitrah.

In recent years, queer Muslims seem to have become more comfortable with their sexuality as they open up and discuss the possibilities of reconciling their sexuality with Islam. This can be attributed to the post-apartheid anti-discriminatory laws, which offered protection to gay and lesbian people, as well as to the efforts of The Inner Circle. Except for a few Muslims who vented their anger on local Islamic radio stations, no criticism was levelled at the organization or its staff. Instead, the organization has received the support of Islamic organizations such as the Islamic Social Welfare Association (ISWA) and individuals within organizations such as Positive Muslims and the Muslim Youth Movement.

It is clear what The Inner Circle offers to gay and lesbian Muslims, and it saw an increase in membership at the beginning of 2005, largely because the fears of the queer Muslim community that the organization might be attacked proved to be unfounded. A member of The Inner Circle, who does not wish to be named, says: 'It was at this time that, through an affiliated source, I came upon an organization that dealt with the issues I found myself plagued by, calling itself The Inner Circle. I approached them seeking further education and enlightenment on my road less travelled. They never judged me. They understood entirely the need in me to know God without having to relinquish how I choose to love someone.'

Most of the debate around homosexuality took place at intervals between 2004 and 2007. Muslim media such as The Voice of the Cape and Channel Islam International conducted a number of programmes to discuss homosexuality and same-sex marriage.[13] Live on-air discussions on the issue allowed Muslims to air their views publicly. Often these discussions, coupled with the parliamentary hearings on the Civil Union Bill in October 2006, were used to try to influence Parliament to reject the Bill as 'irreligious' and 'immoral'. Most reactions to same-sex marriage were emotive, angry responses underpinned by a conservative view of the faith. Muslims who reacted sympathetically were mostly progressive in their thinking, or had been exposed to homosexuality through openly gay family or friends.

Because homosexuality is seen as a sin in Islam, conservative Muslims were outraged by the apparent lack of moral sense shown by the state in its support for gay and lesbian rights. The Muslim clergy felt that the government was completely ignoring the rights of a majority of religious people in South Africa while giving rights to an 'evil' minority. Orthodox Muslim scholar Mufti AK Hoosain said on Channel Islam International: 'All the scholars agree that homosexuals must be killed. They only differ in the manner in which they should be killed.'[14]

Mufti Bayat, a spokesman for the Jamiatul Ulama (Council of Muslim Theologians), KwaZulu-Natal, said: 'Same-sex marriages are a violation of the limits prescribed by the Almighty, a reversal of the natural order, a moral disorder and a crime against humanity. No person is born homosexual, just like no one is born a thief, a liar or murderer. People acquire these evil habits because of widespread shameless social interaction ... Homosexuality leads to the destruction of family life and is symptomatic of a decadent society.'[15]

On 9 October 2006, The Inner Circle made a submission to Parliament supporting same-sex marriages. (See pages 121-122.) Its submission stated that there is no historical evidence that the founder of Islam, Prophet Muhammad, ever persecuted same-sex-identified individuals, or gave any orders for such individuals to be persecuted on the basis of sexual orientation. The isolated incidences or banishment of some *Mukhannathun* (a group of effeminate men closely associated with the arts and who formed a part of the Medinan society during the time of the Prophet Muhammad[16]) were not based on sexual orientation, but rather irreligious behaviour on the part of the individuals in question.

A representative of the Muslim Judicial Council, Moulana Abdul Fattaag Carr, who was clearly oblivious of the instances of homoeroticism in the history of the Middle East,[17] also made a submission. In it, he stated: 'The Muslim Judicial Council is of the opinion that the spread of homosexuality and lesbianism will invite the anger of Allah, erode the family structure and expose young, innocent children to an unnatural lifestyle.'[18] After the passing of the Civil Union Act, Moulana Carr at least moderated his views and acknowledged that personal choices were to be accepted (while still maintaining his orthodox view that same-sex marriage is 'sinful'). He said that 'while the MJC understands that everyone has the right to their own choices, Muslim law recognizes marriages as being uniquely between a male and female.'[19]

The Civil Union Act and attitudes today

In short interviews conducted by The Inner Circle with queer Muslims in Cape Town, it emerged that many felt that the Act brought blessings to the queer Muslim community. 'Coming from an oppressed minority, it's a relief to know that we can share the same benefits as the "straight" community,' said one interviewee. The majority confirmed that they would use the opportunity to get married when they are ready, while only a few responded in the negative: 'Once I've been convinced from a religious point of view that being gay is OK, I will,' said another person interviewed.

Some, such as Sadia Kruger and Zukayna Kruger, two members of The Inner Circle, took advantage of this new piece of legislation. They took the bold step of marrying publicly in Tafelsig as soon as the Act was passed. (See pages 338-340.) 'We have been involved for 14 years and I have been buying her a wedding ring every year, hoping to make her my wife,' Sadia Kruger told a Cape newspaper.[20] When asked what the response was from the community, Sadia Kruger said: 'They all know me as Boeya [a term of respect, used in addressing one's father or an older male, in the Cape Malay community] and have lots of respect for me. Even religious Muslim friends came to my wedding and blessed us.' She added: 'Your acceptance by the community depends on how comfortable you are with yourself.'[21]

In general, however, there seems to be a sense of detachment on the subject of homosexuality on the part of the majority of Muslims in South Africa. There is a tendency to rely on the clergy to deal with the issue. Islamic organizations such as ISWA and Positive Muslims continue to provide services to the queer community, irrespective of the orthodox Islamic view on homosexuality, but Islamic organizations supporting gay and lesbian rights do not verbalize such support too openly for fear of being branded as unIslamic, which would affect their status and ability to work within the Muslim community. It was a difficult task, for instance, to get Islamic organizations to attend a workshop on Islam and sexual diversity. In 2003, however, The Inner Circle presented this workshop on Islam and sexual diversity and assisted organizations such as ISWA and Positive Muslims to understand homosexuality and the struggles of queer Muslims. Through the support of such mainstream Islamic organizations queer Muslims were given hope that they will one day be accepted within the Muslim community as equal partners in faith.

Muslims in South Africa are responsive to issues affecting the community, as can be observed by the many recent protest marches. Muslims took offence and protested against cartoons of the Prophet Muhammad; Muslims protested against the drug lords, and against the demolition of old mosques and Muslim cemeteries. If there was not a greater Muslim protest against the Civil Union Bill, it was perhaps because sexuality is still very much a taboo issue in the Muslim community. Many queer Muslims feel that, despite the passing of the Civil Union Act, there has been no perceptible shift in mindset in the Muslim community. If the community at large continues to sweep the matter under the carpet, it could make the process of awareness and education around sexual diversity a tedious and lengthy one. Gay and lesbian Muslims are still full of fear: fear of being mocked, ostracized, disowned, punished by God and condemned to hell. Such fears drive some queer Muslims to alcohol, drugs and promiscuity. The clergy may preach against such syndromes, while refusing to acknowledge the homophobia that engenders them.

Muslims are seldom taught that Allah is also the Allah of love. We were taught to fear God (*taqwa-allah*). But the Quran reflects the fact that Allah is the loving (*al-latif*), as well. The word '*jihad*' means a struggle, rather than the common misunderstanding of the word as 'holy war'. A *jihad-un-naff* is a struggle with the self. The lives of gay and lesbian Muslims in South Africa are a struggle to reconcile their identities as both gay or lesbian and Muslim, and to still be part of a Muslim community. This will take a *jihad* of love, and perhaps a lifetime.

Notes

1 Ectaco Online English to Arabic Dictionary, http://online.ectaco.co.uk/ (last accessed 17 October 2007)
2 http://www.juniata.edu/faculty/tuten/islamic/archive/glossary.html#H (last accessed 17 October 2007)
3 Fakhr al- Din al-Razi, *Tafsir al-Kabir*, Book III, 201
4 'A Brief History of Muslims in South Africa', November 2005, http://www.islamonline.net/english/views/2005/11/ images/south%20africa.swf/ (last accessed 20 September 2007)
5 A South African term for gay men, especially those who are effeminate in behaviour or wear women's clothing; usually derogatory, but many gay South Africans use the term of themselves in a non-pejorative way.
6 The Inner Circle's mini-survey on the Civil Union Bill, August 2007
7 Christopher Saunders, Howard Phillips, Elizabeth van Heyningen and Vivian Bickford-Smith (eds.), *Studies in the History of Cape Town* (University of Cape Town, 1984), *passim*
8 Abdulkader Tayob, 'The Function of Islam in the South African Political Process: Defining a Community in a Nation', in Abdulkader Tayob and Wolfram Weisse (eds.), *Religion and Politics in South Africa: From Apartheid to Democracy* (Waxmann, 1999)
9 Jacklyn Cock, 'Engendering Gay and Lesbian Rights: The Equality Clause in the South African Constitution', in Neville Hoad, Karen Martin and Graeme Reid (eds.), *Sex and Politics in South Africa* (Double Storey, 2005)
10 *Sunan Abu Dawood*, Book XI, Hadith 2157
11 E-mail correspondence with Muhsin Hendricks, 19 June 2007
12 Yunus Kemp, 'Gay Muslims Come Out in South Africa', *Cape Argus*, 12 November 2001
13 The Voice of the Cape (VOC), 'Debate at Ten', 2003; Channel Islam International, with Mufti AK Hoosain, October 2004; VOC, The Civil Union Bill, October 2006; VOC, debate on homosexuality, June 2007
14 Channel Islam International, radio debate on Islam and homosexuality between Imam Muhsin Hendricks and Mufti AK Hoosain, October 2004; see also Sandi DuBowski and Parvez Sharma (producers), *Jihad for Love* (documentary, 2007)
15 Aakash Bramdeo, 'No Law or Church Invented Marriage', *Sunday Times*, 4 December 2005
16 Everett K Rowson, 'The Effeminates of Early Medina', *Journal of the American Oriental Society* 111 (1991), 671-93
17 Stephen O Murray and Will Roscoe, *Islamic Homosexualities: Culture, History and Literature* (New York University Press, 1997)
18 http://www.mjc.org.za/pressreleases.aspx (last accessed 20 September 2007)
19 Leila Samodien, 'Dutch Reformed Church Rejects Gay Marriage', *Cape Argus*, 8 June 2007
20 Myolisi Gophe, 'Wedding Gives Tafelsig a Gay Day', *Cape Argus*, 4 February 2007
21 Quotes from interviews conducted by The Inner Circle

'It had such meaning'
Interview with Janine Preesman

Janine Preesman officiated at the first legally recognized religious marriage conducted under the Civil Union Act. She is a pastor at Glorious Light (a member of the Metropolitan Community Churches). Janine was the first religious marriage officer in South Africa to be designated under the Civil Union Act. Since the Act's inception she has conducted 68 civil unions, of which nine were designated as civil partnerships and 59 as marriages.

What were some of the challenges the same-sex marriage campaign faced?
I think some of the biggest challenges, and of course I speak from my own context, came from the faith communities. There were some sections of the faith community that were very open and who also participated in getting this thing going and getting this through, who made a submission to Parliament and said 'We are for this.' That was wonderful. But, generally speaking, in the faith community there is still a 'no'.

I think that the activists were successful – we have an Act that says that same-sex people have the same standing in terms of their relationships. For me, it is a pity that it couldn't have been just the Marriage Act that was amended. The fact that we have two Acts might still be discriminatory, although the standing is the same. I have made my decision to solemnize marriages under the Act because straight people can also get married under the Act. I am a marriage officer under the Marriage Act, but I have decided that I am only going to marry couples under the Civil Union Act. I will not go for something that is discriminatory.

For me, the sadness about the Civil Union Act is the section or clause where people can exclude themselves as marriage officers from marrying same-sex couples on the grounds of conscience. That should not have been there. It is a civil right and these people should perform the civil right. That is something that we need to tackle and get changed.

How did you come to be a marriage officer under the new Act?
You have two levels of marriage officers. One is what they call *ex officio*, which is like a magistrate and people working for Home Affairs – they get appointed as marriage officers. Then you have religious officers, and various faith groups then apply. You are not appointed as a marriage officer in your person – you are appointed in your position as a minister or religious officer in a particular

religious organization or denomination. Your religious organization or denomination needs to first apply to be designated under the Civil Union Act. There are specific documents to be submitted to Home Affairs. Your church board would apply on your behalf and say, 'This is our person.' It doesn't have to be a priest. Then you will get sent a lot of documents and the Act to study. You write an exam and when you pass the exam you are designated as a religious marriage officer. That is what I did for the Marriage Act. So when the Civil Union Act came through, for a couple of us they waived the writing of the exams because we were designated under the Marriage Act and there was a lot of confusion at that time. It is really ridiculous that now all ministers of religion already designated under the Marriage Act and who want to marry under the Civil Union Act will have to apply and write an exam, because the procedures in the Acts are the same.

Tell us about the first religious marriage under Civil Union Act, which you conducted on 2 December 2006.
There was this couple who wanted to marry on 2 December. I got my documentation together again and submitted it to the Minister's office. My cell phone rang and I answered it and there was this woman on other side who said to me, 'Hello, this is the legal advisor of the Minister of Home Affairs,' and my response was: 'Yeah, right, and why would the legal advisor be phoning me?' She said to me, 'I am sitting here with your letter of designation as marriage officer – how do I get it to you?' The minister had just signed it, and I thought 'Wow!' We sorted out the paperwork and at half past eight the next morning she gave me my letter. And she said to me, 'You are at the moment the only one, because the Minister is gone for two weeks.' So that's how it happened. I was just lucky. It was an amazing experience doing that first ceremony.

Can you tell us about that experience?
The Anglican church in Mayfair was absolutely packed. There were so many people. It was quite nerve-racking because the couple was two hours late. It was really funny because everybody came to the church and then we waited. Finally they came and the *Sunday Times* were there, but they were not allowed in the church because the couple didn't want any media coverage of them personally. I did the ceremony together with Paul Mokgethi and with Nokuthula Dhladhla. They did some of the religious stuff and I did the legal stuff. And it was so amazing when I got to the point of declaring them legally married. I think the words that I used were: 'Now, for the very first time ever in a religious ceremony and in a church in *South Africa*, I now declare you legally married.'

There was this fraction of a moment where there was dead silence in the church, and then the congregation exploded. People were clapping and they were shouting and they were whistling and they were laughing, and everybody was standing and dancing and hugging each other. It was just so amazing. It took a couple of minutes before we could get back to the ceremony. There were lots of people crying, and I think I was one of them. It had such power that this was now legal. It still has that effect on me and everyone that I marry. These people are making history. I really hope that it will take a very long time before we become blasé about this.

I did a ceremony for a couple who were together for 33 years and they were both on pension. They broke down and cried when I pronounced them married. They wanted to change surnames, and the one partner said, 'I have waited for so long to take your surname.' It had such meaning. Then I see the youngsters in the church – they don't feel the absolute weight of this. This is amazing for them, and this is nice and so on, but they don't have that history of what it means not to be able to get married. Most of the weddings that I have done are long-term relationships. I think the average would be about fifteen to sixteen years of people being together – that is long time.

Why are there not more same-sex couples being married?

I think there are various reasons. If I wanted to I could line up marriages every day, but people are finding it difficult if they go through Home Affairs, because they are not very helpful. I still don't have registers – we are still using photocopies from the *Government Gazette*. These kinds of things are specifically happening to try and make it difficult to make it work. Besides the difficulty with Home Affairs, there are not enough marriage officers. Also, I think the folks who are getting married are thinking about it. There are also lots of people in our [gay and lesbian] communities who do not believe in marriage, who say 'We don't want to be part of this, it is a patriarchal institution,' and that is fine. There are other ways to get legal protection. I am happy that it is not a situation where people meet today and marry tomorrow because we are gay. People are thinking about it, which is important.

Why do you think marriage is important to the same-sex couples who do get married?

I think it is the value that is added in the eyes of society – the dignity that is all of a sudden situated in these relationships. It is no longer two men playing house or two women playing house. It is linked to legal stuff, and all of a sudden the society and the world are saying, 'Hey, hang on, this is a real family.' It is something that shows, on some level for the couple, a meaning in terms of 'we are journeying together and we are committed to live together'. I think that is part of it.

What do you think the future holds for gay and lesbian Christians in South Africa?

It is difficult to say. I think it is positive and negative. I think there are a lot of negative things coming through at the moment. We see the killings and a lot of that stuff is fuelled by religion and by Christianity. Things that are happening within churches are at some level scary. In that sense, I think there is still going to be a struggle. On another level there are some straight folks within mainline denominations who are doing amazing work, who are really fighting this and bringing change.

There is still lot of work that needs to be done and I think in the future there is going to be even more in certain sections of Christianity. It is a difficult road to foresee, but for some people in certain churches it is a lot easier. In other places, and sometimes even within the same denomination, there is even more hatred and homophobia coming through at the moment. It is going to be an interesting time.

'A bright future for lesbian and gay Christians'
Interview with the Reverend Nokuthula Dhladhla

Nokuthula Dhladhla was born in Soweto and comes from a charismatic Christian background. When she told her church about her relationship with another woman she was victimized and ostracized by the pastor and other church members ('we had to sit at the back'). Nokuthula has been the pastor leading the Hope and Unity Metropolitan Community Church (an LGBTI-affirming denomination) for ten years. In December 2007 she co-conducted, along with the Reverend Janine Preesman and Paul Mokgethi, the first legally sanctioned religious marriage in South Africa.

How did you become involved with the Hope and Unity Metropolitan Community Church (HUMCC)?
Somebody told me about the church in late 1997. The Reverend Tsietsi Thandekiso was the pastor at that time, and he helped me to understand that God does not look at us in terms of our sexuality, but as people, and that we are created by God. I started making peace with my sexuality. Soon afterwards Thandekiso died. Some people in the church were feeling discouraged and hopeless, now that there was no-one to lead the church or do the sermons. I was elected to be the pastor in 1998, and have been so until now.

How does the HUMCC understand lesbian and gay relationships?
In my upbringing I was told that sex before marriage is a sin. There was no way then that, as lesbian and gay people, we would be able to get married. The only thing that we could do at HUMCC was to introduce principles and morals. People say that gay relationships do not last. But as church people we have to be an example. I said to some of the couples at the church that if we want to commit to each other we also have to make a commitment to God. Having the church bless our relationships shows the commitment that we have for each other.

Did you bless same-sex unions as pastor of the HUMCC before same-sex marriage became legal?
We called them commitment ceremonies, although some people called them marriages, and we would give the couple a certificate of the blessing of the union.

The first commitment ceremony I did was in 1998. A couple who belonged to the church came to me and said, 'We want you to bless our union in a church.' I saw that it was important to them to commit to each other and to have this witnessed by the people attending the ceremony. It made that couple happy to feel that their relationship was recognized both by people and by God, but at the same time I wondered why we had to do it like that. I felt that by now lesbian and gay people should be accepted and recognized as South Africans. I said to myself, 'Eish! These kids did something very good, but then at the end of the day who will recognise them? Why can't we marry them properly?'

What was your experience of the campaign to legalize same-sex marriage in South Africa?
I first heard about the attempts to get same-sex marriage legalized in 2004, when I attended some of the workshops held by the Lesbian and Gay Equality Project. My worry was that gay people tend not to support each other in what we do. You call people for a workshop, say, and people do not really want to participate. But if I say 'Let's party,' everybody will be there! I was very glad that a group of people had taken the initiative to mobilize and work for all of us. It made me feel proud.

What does the fact that same-sex couples can now get married mean to your congregation at HUMCC and to you as pastor of the church?
We have couples meetings once a month where we talk about different issues. We spoke about the Civil Union Act in the meetings, and people really felt happy that we can now get married and that our partnerships are recognized. This recognition has made people be more responsible in everything. We had relationships before, but people had doubted our relationships. Now our relationships will be recognized and we will be at the same level as other people. Now there is no excuse any more for all those people who have been saying, 'What's the point of having a relationship if I know for a fact that my relationship won't be recognized?'

Do you see yourself personally taking advantage of the Civil Union Act in the future?
I am engaged to this wonderful woman and we are exploring getting married. There is only one little problem that we have. My family is fine with my sexuality now, and they have accepted my partner to the extent of asking us, 'When are you getting married?' But her family is still struggling to accept our relationship. We have decided to wait so that we can work on her family and make them aware that we love each other. It is not going to be fair for my family to be there on our wedding day and not hers. We want one big family. But then

we might also wait forever, because families are like that! We need our families' support and love when we come across problems. So, for us, it is very important that both families be at our wedding. When we say that we're building a family together, it includes my partner's family.

What impact has the public discussion around same-sex marriage had on Christianity in South Africa?

The discussion has opened doors for people to talk about sexuality. For so many years Christians have not wanted to talk about sensitive issues. I remember going to do a church workshop on HIV where a young person stood up and said, 'It's so strange that my church should be the one teaching us about HIV. The only thing that the church does is to stand in front and scream, "Sex before marriage is sin!"' The discussion around same-sex marriage was often very negative, but at the end of the day it got leaders talking about these issues. It does not make sense that Christians come together on Sunday and worship, and forget that there are gay people in our churches who need our attention. I was excited that for the first time we had this kind of a dialogue.

Do you feel that organized religion in South Africa can be reconciled to lesbian and gay people?

I think there is a bright future for lesbian and gay Christians in South Africa. Instead of concentrating on the negative things that some churches are saying about them – that you are going to hell – gay Christians are concentrating on their faith and on the God who has called them. It has given them a firm standing point to say, 'I am here and God has created me, and there is nothing you can do about it.' We should be grateful that after years of struggling with these issues, we are finally recognized.

'Justice for all is a core religious value'
Religious and spiritual responses to the Civil Union Act

The editors of this book put a series of questions on same-sex marriage and the Civil Union Act to selected members from different faith groups. The aim was to present a range of the more progressive thinking that is taking place within faith structures on the topic. These responses were then collated into the discussion that follows. We approached numerous Muslim organizations and structures but were unable to find someone who felt comfortable going on the record.

The participants are:
- Rabbi Greg Alexander is a child of the Progressive Jewish Movement in South Africa. Presently the rabbi of Temple Israel (Cape Town) and a member of the South African Association of Progressive Rabbis.
- Dr André Bartlett is a minister of the Dutch Reformed Church (NGK) and the co-chairperson of the NGK study commission on the church and homosexuality as well as Centre Space, a study group on homosexuality and Christian faith.
- Dr Jillian Carman is an Anglican and a member of St Francis church in Parkview. She serves on the parish council and is secretary of Centre Space, a study group on homosexuality and Christian faith.
- Heila Downey is a Zen Buddhist and is the Guiding Teacher for The Dharma Centre, Cape Town.
- Laurie Gaum is a trained Dutch Reformed Church (NGK) minister, who was suspended by the church for being in a gay relationship and recently reinstated as a minister after a successful appeal to NGK's General Synod. He is currently linked to the Centre for Christian Spirituality.
- Damon Leff is a Pagan witch and the magus of his own coven, Clan Ysgithyrwyn; he is the convenor and elected executive member of the South African Pagan Rights Alliance (Sapra) and is national co-ordinator for Pagan Federation International in South Africa and the Pagan Freedom Day Movement and regional co-ordinator of the South African Pagan Council for the southern Cape.
- Shahindran Moonieya is a Hindu of the Shri Vidya Tantric philosophical school. He teaches Tantra and Chakra. His training in the traditional school was largely shaped by the philosophy of the Shri Ramakrishna Ashram, whose founder, Shri Ramakrishna, was the high priest in the Temple of Kali in Calcutta.
- Sangoma (traditional healer) Nkunzi Nkabinde works as a tour guide at Constitution Hill, Johannesburg.

What does the passing of the Civil Union Act, and the fact that same-sex couples can now be married by the state, mean to you as a religious or spiritual person?

Laurie (Christian): I am elated. It is a great move in the direction of the eradication of discrimination against the LGBTI community. It concurs with the best Christian values, which underwrite the equality of all people. I believe it will help a lot towards the normalization of society and will strengthen same-sex relationships.

Jillian (Christian): A victory for human rights and inclusive, loving faith – *but* it is deeply disturbing that a separate act had to be promulgated to accommodate same-sex unions (which ideally should have been included in an adapted Marriage Act), that so many faith communities reject the recognition of same-sex unions, and that unjust and unloving discrimination against homosexuality continues within many faith communities.

Heila (Zen Buddhist): The promulgation of this act will enable us to marry same-sex couples legally and this is something we have long needed and wanted to do – honouring all!

Damon (Pagan): As a homosexual it means that I and my life partner can, if we choose, be married. As a Pagan this Act means a lot more than that. Until the passage of the Civil Union Act the state would not appoint Pagan religious marriage officers. Under the provisions of the Civil Union Act any religious denomination or organization may be designated as a religious organization that may solemnize marriages in terms of this Act. The South African Pagan Rights Alliance submitted its first request to be so designated even before the passage of the Act. South African Pagans have literally had to wait for centuries to be afforded the same rights and privileges previously afforded only to Christians, Jews, Muslims and Hindus. Having succeeded with our application, Pagan religious marriage officers can now fulfill a vital and needed religious function within and for our religious communities. Without the Civil Union Act none of this would ever have been possible.

André (Christian): I see the Civil Union Act in a very positive light. It is part of an ongoing process of restoring people's dignity. That is a basic concern that I have as a Christian. Part of the problem with the way gay and lesbian people have been treated over centuries by society and the church is that their human dignity has been diminished.

Greg (Jewish): As a Progressive Jew and rabbi I believe that distinguishing the status of same-sex marriages from those of heterosexual couples is not a religious act but an act of prejudice. It has nothing to do with the Torah and everything to do with social and political bias. The Reform Jewish movement has fought for egalitarianism in Judaism since its inception in the late 18th century, and yet it was only in the late 20th century that women were ordained as rabbis and even later that openly gay and lesbian rabbis were accepted. It is not to say that the movement was not 'ready' or brave enough – they made many unpopular decisions that set them in dramatic opposition to the more Orthodox movements – but that the issue of same-sex marriage was never raised as a question to be addressed. Once feminists in the 1960s asked why there weren't any women rabbis, women rabbis began to be ordained (after a lengthy struggle): Once the wider society made it possible for gay and lesbian couples to be accepted, the issue became an issue to be discussed religiously. It is only about 2 000 years overdue, but we will try to make up time.

Nkunzi (Sangoma): It is a good sign. There are a lot of gay and lesbian sangomas that have wanted to get publicly married for a long time. Now they can!

Shahindran (Hindu): As a Hindu, the normalization of society is achieved through many forms; one of these forms is the act of marriage or the union of two souls by mutual consent. It is the duty of a Hindu to respect the love and the relationships that people have, and no Hindu has the right to question this love. Two souls that meet each other and find that the only expression of their love and desire for each is through the act of love and marriage must fulfill this destiny regardless of the gender of the body they find themselves in. The demand laid on all Hindus is the act of compassion and the absence of judgment. To deny any couple the act of marriage or civil union is to defy these very basic laws of compassion and love.

What do you think the impact of the public debate on same-sex marriage was on your religious or spiritual community?

Greg (Jewish): The Civil Union Act posed a direct question to our movement. Now that a Jewish same-sex couple could marry civilly, would our rabbis be allowed to marry them religiously? This was a movement that represented the most liberal grouping of Jews in this country and still by 2006 had never in its history taken any kind of stance (except condemnation or silence) on homosexuality. The South African Association of Progressive Rabbis (SAAPR) decided to conduct a study process throughout the national movement giving rabbis and laypeople an opportunity to look at traditional and contemporary sources on the topic and debate and discuss an appropriate response. Once we began to hold study forums we were overwhelmed with the positive response from the congregations, to the point where they wanted to know why we were talking about 'commitment ceremonies' and not 'marriages'. The decision was taken to recommend to our national movement to permit its rabbis to perform same-sex marriages. This was debated and passed at the following South African Union for Progressive Judaism (SAUPJ) executive meeting in May 2007. I am proud to say that our local movement acted decisively.

Nkunzi (Sangoma): There was a lot of debate among sangomas about this. Many straight sangomas do not understand what it really means to be gay or lesbian. There were lots of questions like 'How can a woman married to a woman have kids?' There are lots of ways to answer that question, like adoption. Many sangomas were also saying that a woman marrying a woman is 'unAfrican' and not Christian. This debate is still going on. But, for myself, I'm done debating. I'm happy with who I am.

André (Christian): The church has a history of negatively judging homosexuality. This means that gay people kept a low profile in their churches in order to survive there. This process has helped people in the church to move towards a more liberated personal position. Discussions started popping up. People felt freer to come out of the closet. But it was not a groundswell. The issue of transformation in South Africa from white, Afrikaner domination to a new non-racial system held sway in the church. It was with the issue of same-sex unions that reality dawned in the church that this was what was agreed upon in the Constitution and suddenly people asked, 'How can this be?' The parliamentary desk of the Dutch Reformed Church prepared a submission on the Civil Union Bill. It was quite controversial. The argument put forward in the submission was quite subtle, and it focused on the issue of constitutionality. It made a distinction between the position of the church and the responsibility of the state. It had to stick to the conservative position of the Church that marriage is a union between a man and a woman. But the submission acknowledged that the state had a duty to make provision for same-sex couples to marry, because we live in a pluralistic society where the laws of the state must take into account people with different points of view and keep to the Constitution.

Heila (Zen Buddhist): It had an impact only in the sense that it highlighted our own frustrations resulting from the limited and narrow views so often expressed.

Shahindran (Hindu): Hinduism is not an organized religion but a way of life. It is a synchronization of a large tapestry of philosophies and belief systems bound together by the Vedas, the Shastras, the Puranas and the Tantric texts. Debate and discussion among the varied philosophical schools of Hinduism is encouraged. As extreme as the differences often are in the practice and interpretation of Hindu philosophy, there are many common threads that run through all the various schools of thought. The debate about same-sex marriage in the Hindu community is an ongoing one. Because there is no central authority in the Hindu world, such as a papacy or a judicial council, Hindus vary in their views. Many Hindus are unaware of the normality and in fact sacred position held by gay people in our history – remnants of this are still evident in societies such as the Hijra and the Kinnar in India. Enlightened Hindus who are aware of the sacred writings and their impact in Hindu attitudes on sexuality (consider Tantric sexuality as well as the Kama Sutra in ancient Hindu society) have no issue with homosexuality or same-sex marriages, but those who have been socialized and shaped by Western, Victorian and Judaeo-Christian thought are opposed to it.

Laurie (Christian): To some extent it did cause a hardening among hardliners, but on the other hand it did confront a lot of people with the reality of same-sex relationships, causing them to have to familiarize themselves with different arguments.

Jillian (Christian): I think there has been a positive impact, in that homosexuality has come out of the closet, so to speak, and discussion has been encouraged. Having homosexual people in our congregation, who have discussed their experiences, has tremendously facilitated open and positive discussion.

Damon (Pagan): The Pagan religious community followed the public debate quite closely. I don't think we were surprised by the venom or the sheer quantity of it that emanated primarily from Christians. As Witches we're quite used to being the targets of Christian discrimination. As a homosexual the public criticism against same-sex marriage turned my stomach. But despite the rhetoric and religious conservatism I found the entire public-participation process breathtaking. Yes, people chose to use their right to freedom of speech to propagate hate speech against non-heterosexuals, but it was liberating to be able to take part in such a transparent process.

Has your religious community changed in recent years in how it thinks about sexual orientation and same-sex marriage?

Jillian (Christian): My parish has always been open to addressing issues which some might find uncomfortable to discuss. However, the arrival of our present priest about ten years ago has greatly increased sensitivity, acceptance and awareness about sexual orientation. His approach is entirely inclusive, accepting and loving, whereas the previous incumbent (although displaying similar qualities) believed physical expressions of love between homosexuals were 'unChristian'.

Damon (Pagan): Paganism promotes a very tolerant and pragmatic approach to sex, sexuality and sexual orientation. Pagan philosophies on transmigration of the soul admit the possibility that one could incarnate as either male or female at any potential incarnation. Transmigration may also imply that the question of any particular sexual orientation or skin colour is relevant only for a single lifetime and ultimately not a true reflection of the hidden potential and purpose of the soul.

Shahindran (Hindu): My place of worship is any Hindu temple, and as a Hindu I do not 'belong' to a temple. The council of a temple serves the up-keep of the temple and the maintenance of correct application of the sacred rituals and the holy festivals. If I wish to marry in a temple, I will approach the priest to officiate the ritual; if he/she refuses, then I will perform the ritual myself or get any Hindu who is willing to and is able to, to perform that ritual. Hindu marriages are not usually held in temples, but usually in any space that is conducive for this, such as a hall, and a structure (a *pandal*, like a Jewish *chupah*) where the ritual is held. The ritual can take any form, with a few common rites recognizable to all forms or styles. The view of individuals within a temple society on same-sex marriage is irrelevant. No Hindu will be excluded on these grounds by any other Hindu, as no central dogma of exclusion exists in the Hindu faith or way of life.

Laurie (Christian): Our community is reflecting very deeply on the issue. Having studied it for a number of years, and with some movement towards change, a better understanding is emerging and we are at least being more sensitive on the issue.

How do your spiritual leaders view same-sex marriage? Can gay and lesbian people assume leadership positions in your religious community?

Nkunzi (Sangoma): Some straight sangomas show that they accept and understand gay and lesbian people. But many don't accept gay and lesbian sangomas. What makes me angry is when people pretend to accept you but don't really do so. Some of the older sangomas don't want younger ones to open up about their sexual orientation in public. But if they are open about their heterosexual life, why can't I be open about mine? Some gay and lesbian sangomas hide their sexuality when they're among elder sangomas because they're afraid of what they will say. I say, 'Who cares? It's my life.'

Laurie (Christian): Talk of marriage definitely still is hair-raising to most! Openly homosexual people are tolerated but, mostly, not officially included or accepted in leadership positions.

Heila (Zen Buddhist): We have never had any restrictions or limitations in terms of gender, sexual orientation, race or creed, and continue to promote and practise an 'open-door' policy.

Jillian (Christian): The Anglican Church does not allow same-sex marriages or blessings of same-sex unions. That is the official position. But there is much dissent, and open discussion appears to be encouraged. There are openly gay priests who have their own parishes and receive support, and homosexual people are involved in leadership positions in our parish. One of our most proactive and involved parishioners left previous parishes because he sensed homophobia – I'm delighted that he feels entirely comfortable at our parish.

Greg (Jewish): There have been members, leaders and rabbis who have been less than happy with the very clear and public decision our movement has taken. They have in all cases been respectful of the democratic process that led to the decision and have not been in any way as obstructive as some feared they would be. In our national movement we have openly gay and lesbian lay readers who lead prayer services and at least one gay rabbi. In the event that a rabbi is not 'comfortable' to perform a same-sex marriage, they are required to give the couple in question the details of one of the majority of our SAAPR rabbis who are happy to perform them.

Shahindran (Hindu): There are many gays and lesbians who serve in Hindu society. I am one such person. Again, there is no room for exclusion, and sexual orientation cannot be questioned. There is no hierarchy of priesthood in Hindu society. Any person who is trained in the traditional rites can assume the role of a priest. The gender and sexual orientation of such priests is not important because the rules that govern conduct and moral behaviour are, universal whether you are gay or straight. Morality is informed by other factors. Promiscuity will be frowned on by the traditional culture of Hindu society, and monogamy encouraged.

Damon (Pagan): Many men and women in leadership positions within individual Pagan communities, groups, associations and organizations are lesbian or gay.

What do you feel about the fact that, even if she or he wants to do so, a religious marriage officer may not marry same-sex couples unless her or his denomination applies for designation to perform marriages under the Civil Union Act?

André (Christian): While it is second-best, I think it is the wisest option at the moment. It creates a necessary sanity in the debate. In the long term it creates the problem that religious marriage officers who do feel free to officiate at same-sex weddings are not in a position to act on their conscience. I would like a situation where the individual can decide according to conscience.

Jillian (Christian): This is a deeply problematic and ethical issue. I realize, listening to some priests who form part of our study group on homosexuality and Christian faith (Centre Space), that they are facing a similar sort of struggle that they experienced under apartheid rule, but this time they are not united as a church against an outside force. The antagonists are in their midst, so to speak. At Centre Space, we are looking at ways of becoming a licensing entity so priests can be licensed outside of their denominations (but this presents huge ethical dilemmas), and also at ways of supporting priests who are facing censure because of their beliefs.

Laurie (Christian): I think religious marriage officers should be allowed freedom of conscience to be able to perform marriages irrespective of the stand of their denomination.

Shahindran (Hindu): Marriage is a civil contract and I am of the view that any person who is registered as a marriage officer by the state must be bound by the letter of the Constitution and the law and should be obligated to perform such a civil union. The religious rite is just added fluff to this civil contract. Hindu priests, including myself, have been known to marry anyone who asks, regardless of race or creed. One must separate the civil act from the religious act. The legal conscience is informed by the law and as such is driven by a legal obligation. The religious conscience can only be shaped by religious leaders within a religious society – primary examples are the Dalai Lama and Bishop Desmond Tutu. A Hindu priest acts in his or her own right and may follow his or her conscience, informed either by the enlightened views of our ancestors and sacred writings or the narrow views of Western bigotry.

Heila (Zen Buddhist): They should be encouraged to deeply examine their individual commitment to dignity, honour and respect for all, as well as their direction and functioning within an organization or church opposing same-sex marriages.

What challenge does same-sex marriage present for religions in South Africa, generally, and for your community specifically?

Greg (Jewish): Everyone in the Judeo-Christian world is obsessed with Leviticus. In the Progressive Jewish world we don't hear cries of 'abomination' when women are called to read from the Torah, or because we abolished the status of *mamzer* (bastard children) or *agunah* (women unable to remarry because their husbands have refused them a divorce.) These changes are now accepted, and this will be the case in time with same-sex marriages. For the Orthodox movements or those who need to read texts literally, let them take a long hard look at Leviticus and ask if there really are other ways to read those texts, and whether it is absolutely clear that they condemn what most people assume they do. I believe there certainly are other ways to read the texts. Nothing is mentioned about lesbian relationships, and there is certainly no mention of two men committing to a lifelong monogamous relationship. At a stretch one might argue that the two verses condemn anal intercourse, but that is already reading in what one wants to read. Rather, these verses seem to condemn abusive, unequal sexual acts and need to be understood in that way. It is only when people begin to see that their attitude towards same-sex marriage has nothing to do with Leviticus and all to do with their fear of the new, the misunderstood, that they will truly be able to move on. I believe that in the Progressive Jewish community we are starting to make this happen, and where we go now the Orthodox world will go grudgingly in 25 years time. I, for one, am not waiting around.

Damon (Pagan): Generally our society has had to come to terms with an entirely new paradigm, one in which human rights supersede religious and cultural prejudices. Whether or not this shift will transform the root philosophies that tend to propagate such prejudices remains to be seen. I guess centuries of propaganda will take centuries to unravel and change. Pagan communities will continue to promote understanding and acceptance of diversity in all its forms. Mere tolerance isn't enough. We have to be committed to real change for the greater good.

Heila (Zen Buddhist): For our community the only challenge is to get fully registered in terms of the Civil Union Act. In terms of religions opposing same-sex marriages, the struggle to free themselves of homophobia might be likened to freeing our society of apartheid – a process requiring trust, wisdom and patience – enabled by time.

Shahindran (Hindu): The challenge exists to ensure that Hindus do not view same-sex unions from the perspective of our conservative sisters and brothers in the Judaeo-Christian and Islamic worlds, but from the enlightened history of India's past, within the context that Hindus are the world's oldest unbroken civilization. As such, our history does not have any record or action that is homophobic. The contrary is usually the case.

Laurie (Christian): The challenge to act justly, to recognize what justice in this case looks like, to become the inclusive communities they are supposed to be, simply to be true to the values of the gospel! The Dutch Reformed Church has the opportunity to show that they have learned hard lessons about justice in their history of biblically legitimizing apartheid.

Jillian (Christian): The bald challenge is: How can discrimination against people on the grounds of their sexual orientation be considered differently from racial discrimination under the apartheid regime? Do church leaders support the Bill of Rights? On what ethical grounds can they not support it? This is a social-justice issue, and goes to the core of the Christian belief system. Christianity was a radical movement at the time of Christ, with ministry and love bestowed on those who were socially excluded. It turned on its head the hierarchy of the religious establishment. People, not religious officers, should be the focus of this religion. The hierarchy of the Anglican Church needs to address very seriously the question: Is it more concerned about placating its religious officers or about ministering to its congregations?

André (Christian): The basic premise of all religions is adding value to life and to help people in the pursuit of happiness. For Christianity the challenge is to come to terms with a basic respect for human dignity. We need to help each other find meaningful relationships and work against all forms of discrimination. The challenge is to come to terms with who we are saying we are, and to find a morality that asks, 'What kind of moral positions would help people to lead meaningful lives and conduct non-destructive relationships and non-destructive behavior?' That is a true Christian approach. Someone else would say that there are certain eternal, absolute rules that you have to stick to. I don't think Christ thought like that. He said, 'Man is not made for sabbath, sabbath was made for man.' People are not made to conform to moral standards. Moral standards are there to help people lead meaningful lives. That is a challenge to the church to find a moral standard that is inclusive to the needs of marginalized people.

Nkunzi (Sangoma): One of the challenges is the myth that same-sex marriages do not last. To remove that myth, gay and lesbian people need to show society that same-sex relationships last, and be faithful to their partners. If you make a commitment, stick to it!

Do you think that lesbian and gay rights and organized religion can be reconciled?
André (Christian): I do not see gay and lesbian people as being in conflict with basic Christian values. The problem is that it is *perceived* as split. One of the best ways of overcoming this is to keep creating space for open dialogue and meaningful debate. Another way is to expose the run-of-the-mill straight person to real gay people and so break down stereotypes and normalize the issue. The rights that gay and lesbian people are working for are basic human rights, and if Christianity is true to itself it should be looking out for the basic rights for all people.
Damon (Pagan): Why not? A few hundred years ago Christians and Jews promoted slavery but both religions now recognize slavery as inhumane. Perhaps other religious groups will one day come to terms with the fact that prejudice promotes hatred and that hatred is ultimately the very thing religion is not meant to protect or propagate. I hope so. Paganism doesn't need to explore such reconciliation because, in my opinion, Pagans know their place in a universe of infinite possibilities.
Nkunzi (Sangoma): If we try we might be able to bring them together. I am a Christian as well as a Sangoma. My powers as a Sangoma come from the ancestors, and I think the ancestors are more accepting of gay and lesbian people than Christianity is.
Jillian (Christian): Yes. Just as the ordination of women has been accepted and the Dutch Reformed Church has realized its racial views were wrong, so will today's organized religions come to realize their discriminatory views about sexual orientation are, essentially, no different from views held in the past regarding exclusion on the grounds of race and sex.
Heila (Zen Buddhist): Not likely, but the passage of time might prove otherwise.
Laurie (Christian): Yes, faith and sexual identity can surely be integrated – justice for all is a core religious value.
Shahindran (Hindu): There is a fundamental need for such reconciliation because no oppression can last or should be tolerated. The sexual experience and sexual activity in human beings are multi-dimensional. A sexual act between consenting adults of a legal age, regardless of the nature of the act or the genders of the participants, would be embraced within the Tantric Hindu worldview. Transgender or gay people are traditionally revered in Indian society. The embodiment of this philosophy is manifested in the image of Ardhanrishwara, the Supreme Lord, who is both male and female, Shiva and Parvati, in one being. The inherent bisexual nature of every human being does not imply bisexuality as a condition in sexual

praxis, but it does free us to allow both the male and the female within us to grow to their full potential. Most sexual prejudices are irrational, and humans react emotionally to some possibilities of sexual variation. In fact, broad ideas as to what defines sexual deviation or abnormality are no longer tenable. Lesbian, gay, bisexual, transgender and intersexed individuals have always had a place in the humanity that informs the Tantric worldview.

Greg (Jewish): I don't see any reason why two men or two women who make a lifelong loving commitment to each other should not have that marriage sanctified in front of one's community, with the appropriate religious ceremony. There is nothing qualitatively different with my marriage to my wife and two men or two women marrying each other. There is nothing to say that theirs will or won't work any more than mine, apart from the patience, love and hard work that each couple puts into developing and maintaining their relationship over time. Religion is there to help us note holy moments, to sanctify time and space, and as such should have no qualms in embracing those who wish to commit to sanctifying their life choices together.

5: HAPPILY EVER AFTER?
Reflections on marriage and the Civil Union Act

Blissful complexities:
Black lesbians reflect on same-sex marriage and the Civil Union Act

Zethu Matebeni

Since the equality clause, also known the 'gay rights clause', was consolidated in the Bill of Rights in the 1996 Constitution, prohibiting discrimination on the basis of sexual orientation, groups of gay and lesbian people have pushed for equality on many levels of their lives. The most recent has been the recognition of same-sex marriages or unions, with the Constitutional Court taking a position in favour of same-sex marriages on 1 December 2005. Amid strong opposition, with high levels of homophobia, condemnations of same-sex sexuality and gay marriage as 'not traditional', 'evil' and 'unAfrican', the process moved through Parliament, and almost a year later, on 30 November 2006, the Deputy President of South Africa signed the Civil Union Act into law in Pretoria.

The Act came into being so that the law would be in line with the 'gay rights clause' in the Bill of Rights. While some have argued that this clause 'promotes' and 'strengthens' a sense of citizenship,[1] it has also been argued that the rights that accrue to individuals as a result are accessible only if a gay identity is claimed – that is, by 'coming out' as gay or lesbian, and/or by being openly gay or lesbian. Jacklyn Cock quotes activist Kevan Botha, who says, 'The clause is meaningless unless you're "out". In order to claim the rights you have to acknowledge and own the identity of being gay; furthermore, some argue that the clause is not useful for the 'masses' in lower-class positions.[2] It is undeniable that the activism around the battle for such rights is predicated on the identity politics of being 'out', but it could be argued that the Civil Union Act helps dissolve some of those distinctions, being inclusive rather than exclusive. It is also noteworthy that black lesbian views on the Act and its implications show a concern with larger social issues beyond simple identity politics.

In this essay, I engage with four black lesbians on their thoughts and experiences on: why they would marry, how they imagine their marriage or union taking place given the Act, and what the meaning of marriage or civil unions is to them and their relationships. Their stories highlight some of the joys, challenges and complexities of marriage. One informant, 'Linda', is preparing to get married and is saving up for lobola (bride price) for her partner of two years; another, 'Sibu', is in a relationship and thinking broadly about marriage;[3] and then there is a married couple, the MaseTshabas (Musa and Mantepu), who, when they got married, joined their surnames. In this essay, the MaseTshabas speak as a unit and not individuals. This is important for them as they feel that they have created their own identity and family.

Considering marriage?
Since the enactment of the Civil Union Act, many people in same-sex relationships have begun negotiating and discussing having their relationships officially and legally recognized. The idea of legalizing same-sex marriage has been joyfully accepted by many, who feel it has changed the nature of same-sex relationships. For the MaseTshabas, for instance, same-sex marriage is 'Beautiful, balanced and ideal – it is a better kind of marriage in that the marriage is seldom compromised to please family or friends, but is sincere.' For the MaseTshabas, this is clear in the way that they joined their surnames.

> We got married before the Civil Union Act was passed. We didn't want only one of us to give up their identity, that is, by joining the one family. We wanted to create our own family, our own identity and a new name for us and our offspring. So, we combined our surnames – Mantepu's surname was Masemola and Musa's surname was Tshabalala, thus we have MaseTshaba – meaning 'Mother of the Nation' in the Sotho languages and that is why the 'T' is a capital letter. This was a compromise agreement between the two of us. In doing this, we also wanted to exclude the Masemola and Tshabalala families from having claim on our family if something happens to one of us. It was for legal protection.

The issues of inheritance, property and protection of one's assets and family come across many times in discussions and writings about marriage. While it is clear that there is an economic relationship attached to marriage, for many people, marriage is seen as validating the relationship and showing that the two people are committed and love each other and wish to be permanently together. But these are not the only reasons why people marry. The informants here present a different dimension to marriage, one related to the social. Calling upon the social means that a married person is not only accountable to oneself and one's partner, but also to a larger community.

> **Sibu:** Marriage gives you responsibility, commitment, and, in a sense, ownership, in that you own the relationship and what the two people have made together. You say that this thing [the relationship] is mine and I cannot throw it away as easily as that.
>
> **MaseTshaba:** We had been living together with our child and thus decided to seal our relationship with a blessing from God. It also means we exclude any other from our relationship.
>
> **Linda:** I want to marry because also when you're married your social status changes. In my village, I am excluded from community meetings as an unmar-

ried woman. You get respect from people when they know and have witnessed your marriage.

Marriage also implies that one's behaviour has to change in the sense that one is no longer an individual but a unit (with another person). By being married you own and protect your relationship by excluding others from it and, at the same time, society regards you differently as your social standing is 'elevated'. This is emphasized by William M Hohengarten's understanding of marriage in the sense that when 'viewed functionally, legal marriage is essentially a binding commitment between two intimately related adults, a commitment which sustains the relationship between such adults by structuring their dealings with each other and with third parties. Conceived in this way, marriage is indifferent to the relative genders of its occupants.'[4]

Going forth – how do I say 'I do'?

The Civil Union Act has reshaped the way weddings and marriages are performed. Such a marriage can be solemnized by a religious marriage officer, who (if registered) will deal with the relevant authorities, but perhaps the simplest possible form that the marriage can take is that the two individuals concerned visit the Department of Home Affairs, with two witnesses, and sign the necessary documents to be together. The parties to the civil union may choose to have their union registered as either a marriage or a civil partnership, upon which a certificate will be issued. The MaseTshabas recount how they got married:

> We called in at our local Home Affairs on the 8th of January 2007. We were advised that one of us should come to the offices personally and set up an appointment, bringing along a green bar-coded ID Book. We went to the Germiston Home Affairs on the 9th of January 2007. We were given a date for the 11th of January 2007 at Edenvale. [Germiston did not have a marriage officer. They set up appointments based on the Edenvale office marriage officer's calendar.] We were advised to bring on the marriage date: ID books, two photos of each and at least two witnesses, one for each of us, with their ID books (no passports or driver licence cards). The appointment was for 9am, thus we had to arrive 15 minutes earlier as there is paperwork to be filled in, fingerprints to be taken. Then the marriage officer reads statements from the Act that you must comply with legally, and then we were pronounced married. Fingerprints and signatures of us and witnesses were taken afterwards. A certificate is then provided. I think we paid R10 or R12. We were also given an option of surname amendments, but because we already had one surname there was no need to amend it.

In African tradition, or a combination of African tradition with elements of Western tradition, the marriage ceremony for black people would usually be a lengthy process involving both families, negotiating lobola, organizing a church service or an equivalent service in some other space, and the slaughtering of animals. The whole community would bear witness. The celebrations would generally last at least two days. Under the Act, in the absence of traditional customs, things are a bit more relaxed, and for the married couple it is clear what the Act stands for and what it offers.

> **MaseTshaba:** It is an Act passed by Parliament to rectify the Marriage Act's 'only heterosexual marriage' clause. Anyone can get married under the Civil Union Act regardless of whether heterosexual or same-sex. One [same-sex couples] cannot however get married under both Acts.

Another level at which the Act intervenes is at a personal and family level. Families are always difficult to deal with, particularly when one introduces a potential new member of the family. For many people, it is still important to introduce one's spouse to one's family, although there is the possibility that the family may disapprove of the partner. In a same-sex relationship, introducing one's partner takes a different meaning: it may be necessary to 'come out' and disclose the same-sex relationship to the family. This is the situation in the case of Linda, whose partner would like a traditional marriage and to be declared as *umakoti* (bride), and for Sibu, whose family does not approve of her choices.

> **Linda:** From my side, I am not even 'out' to my whole family. Now, when I get *umakoti* I must tell everyone about myself and that I want to bring *umakoti* and formalize our relationship. In her situation it's different. Her mother and her whole family know about us ... My mother might agree to me marrying a woman, but my brothers will never agree to that. We'd even slaughter a cow to *ukungxengxeza to izinyanya* [appease the ancestors].

> **Sibu:** I don't think my family would want to be involved [when I get married] because they still have a problem with who I am. My younger sister could be there, but the rest would not come. They can't even tell people that I'm a lesbian – that's unimaginable. I don't think my mom can even say the word. She would be heartbroken even more than she is now – she'd say, 'This child is taking this further and further and there she is, signing her name on the first-class ticket to hell' – that's what it would mean to her.

For the MaseTshabas, the situation is different. They have support from their families of origin, and also have a sense that family can be a set of elective affiliations:

> We've always had supportive families from both sides and had already started our own immediate family by adding a son into our lives. Family is important as long as it is supportive and will not make you feel miserable. Family is not only your blood relatives but can be your own-described family of friends and acquaintances that love you.

When thinking about who would be involved in their marriage, Linda and Sibu have difficulties with the complications that may arise. Both of them feel that, when they get married, this should be a private matter that includes only close friends as witnesses. Yet, inevitably, they battle with the issue of involving family members.

> **Sibu:** I wouldn't tell my family about it – I don't tell them now what's happening in my relationships. We'd go to the court and just get married and sign. We'd just have a few friends that know about us.
>
> **Linda:** I'm comfortable with the Civil Union Act as it is, but I've realized that the person I'm with wants more. If it were by me, I would marry, sign and just call my friends. But now if I want to marry I must go the traditional route. In this case, marriage is not just about signing – you have to go back home and still do the traditional ceremony to finalize the marriage and lobola.

Meaning of marriage between two women

In the following section, I address some of the issues raised by Linda, Sibu and the MaseTshabas about women-marriage, an institution with a history in South Africa and other parts of the continent. This is important for two reasons: first, to show that women-marriages are not new in Africa and in our region, and, second, to show that women-marriages take different forms and mean different things to the people involved.

Saskia Wieringa notes that women-marriages, although to varying degrees and for different reasons, have always taken place in African societies. Many have been recognized through traditional and cultural forms. Vast evidence of traditional woman-to-woman marriages occurring all over Africa and in South Africa has been recorded: there are instances among the Venda, Balobedu (Lovedu), Pedi, Zulu and Narene peoples.[5] Such marriages or unions have been performed for two main reasons: one being that a woman marries another woman because of her powerful position (she has land and property), another because she is childless. In Kenya, for example, as Nancy Baraka and Ruth Morgan show, elderly women from certain tribes would decide to marry or need a female wife, not only for inheritance, but also as a way of continuing the 'female husbands' lineage.[6] The procreation would take place through a male genitor, in most cases an outsider selected by the female husband for the wife (although the partners in the women marriages cited in Baraka and Morgan made a joint decision regarding the choice of genitor).[7] The role of the genitor varies, but the female-husband remains the most important 'father figure' for children born to women marriages, and the sons would continue her lineage.[8] They add that in Kikuyu culture 'an older woman who is barren is allowed to marry a younger woman to give her children who could inherit her property. One of the motivations for marrying another woman is that the marriage enables the younger woman to improve her economic situation and inherit land. The older woman benefits by getting children who will inherit her property.'[9] In these types of marriages, sexual relationships between the women are either taboo or not recorded.

In South Africa, similar situations continue to take place, in for instance the case of the Rain Queen of the Balobedu tribe in Limpopo, who, like her mother and grandmother, can have numerous wives. Custom prohibits the Rain Queen from marrying, but she can have relations with men for the sake of procreation. She instead takes 'wives' – women who serve her and whose children are considered hers.[10] The Rain Queen has wives because of her powerful position as a queen and also for purposes of lineage.

Another case is that of a Pedi woman in Limpopo province who is known to have married a younger woman in order to have children.[11] Women-marriages also happen among sangomas (traditional healers). Nkunzi Nkabinde and Ruth Morgan elaborate on the relationship of the female-husband and the ancestral wife among sangomas in parts of KwaZulu-Natal and Johannesburg, where ancestral wives have roles and duties to perform for their female sangoma husbands. When a sangoma takes a wife, she or her family has to pay lobola for the ancestral wife. Wieringa notes that, in many of the studies of women-marriages she has encountered outside the Civil Union Act, every woman who has paid a bride-price (lobola) is called a 'female husband'. Yet not all women who pay bride-price can actually be considered to be playing the role of a husband. Some female husbands even take up the role of mother-in-law, or may be considered more as a senior women rather than as a husband.[12] Wieringa also shows that in some cases female husbands were seen as men, as was the case of the Balobedu Rain Queen, but this is not to say that all female-husbands are seen or see themselves as men. This issue is very real in the case of Linda:

> **Linda:** My partner and I are planning to get married and her mom is expecting lobola, so I'm starting to save. But then I think ... who should pay lobola? We are both women! In this case, what do we do? If I pay, she must pay. She's not willing to pay lobola for me. I'm the one who looks like a man. When it comes to who pays lobola, are we going to be looking at who behaves like what or whom?

The situation can get rather complex. Such traditions are firmly predicated on the idea of marriage as exclusive to a male-female partnership, with strictly designated roles for each. It requires one to engage with difficult issues of identity and address some of the frustrations that traditional marriage can bring:

> **Linda:** My partner wants to be *umakoti* [the bride]. She can't wait, she really wants to go to my village and wear those clothes that *umakoti* wears and do all the chores for my family. I will not do that [be *umakoti*]! If I don't, is it because I'm a man? I'm not a man; I don't feel like a man. I'm a woman! In our relationship we should be equal – we are women.

There are also duties involved in women-marriages. For example, among sangomas, ancestral wives have an important role to play in relation to ancestors as they help the sangomas with their healing work.[13] In these marriages sexuality is often taboo, although Nkabinde with Morgan's work shows the existence of secret sexuality and sexual relationships among certain same-sex sangomas.

The Civil Union Act goes beyond the parameters of tradition for women-marriages. It offers a Western-style pact that has more to do with the desires of the individuals concerned than with the structures of family and clan affiliation. Under the Act, partners can marry simply because they choose to be together, without the involvement of a male figure, and can have a sexual relationship. At the same time, while sexuality plays an important part in such unions, the couple can marry for emotional reasons such as love and commitment to each other, as well as for economic or social reasons. Under the Act, argue Vasu Reddy and Zethu Cakata, 'the benefit of marriage is the extension of citizenship rights that facilitate the assimilation of gay and lesbian individuals into the mainstream society'.[14] Although this broader concept differs from some of the reasons behind marriages given above, it shows that women-marriages are now part of a much wider sense of the possibilities of marriage in society as a whole. The benefits and complexities for same-sex marriage are now equivalent to those afforded to non-same-sex marriages. The following quotes are evidence of how women-marriages can be, in some ways, very similar to other marriages, while also engendering additional complexity. For example, when dealing with issues of inheritance or ownership, as well as certain elements of tradition, the same principles apply.

> **Sibu:** I think that paper will work as a legal proof, but, in all essence, if your families don't respect your union – even if you write it on paper – when their child dies it will always be their child. They will want her or his things and they'll tell you not to tell them about pieces of paper for gay people. Black people are worse in this regard – I don't know about white people. I think that what used to happen to widowed partners and how their in-laws mistreated them will continue to happen. The person left behind might be helped by that piece of paper so that the family doesn't take them for granted.
>
> **Linda:** Another thing, we as black people need family blessings. You can't just marry without blessings. Even if you won't pay lobola you need to ask the ancestors so they can say OK. Otherwise you will be calling for *ingqumbo yeminyanya* [the wrath of the ancestors].
>
> **MaseTshaba:** Official marriage has empowered our relationship further. For example, although we think our families [parents and siblings] appreciate our relationships and respect our spouses, when death or incapacity of the body or mind attacks; one needs the surety that the surviving spouse will legally have powers to make decisions without the families trying to take over.

While all informants show that marriages or unions under the Civil Union Act pose a number of challenges and complexities, they also make clear the joys and comforts it provides. There is a strong feeling that marriage under the Act will help stabilize such relationships and contribute to their longevity. It also means that both partners can access joint benefits.

> **Sibu:** A married person has this thing that is a commitment that says 'Let's try again' and they would try and try again rather than run at the first sign of trouble. As a result they would stay in that relationship longer than if they were not married ... marriage can give me that stability.
>
> **Linda:** The Act is good in terms of allowing us to access benefits, legal, medical, and buying a house together, etc, but traditionally and community-wise there's a gap. If you're in an urban area for example here in Johannesburg you can enjoy the benefits of the Civil Union Act, but if you go home it's a different story.
>
> **MaseTshaba:** We were in our seventh year together when we got officially married. Before the Civil Union Act was passed we had some legal domestic-agreement documents and wills in place. Because we had been 'married' before we got married, there are no significant changes.

While women-marriages under the Act show to have many benefits for the individuals involved, they also pose a number of challenges. Deciding to get married comes with a number of complexities including: how the couple should get married, family involvement, lobola and engaging with identity dynamics, as well as talking about the necessities and benefits of an official marriage. From the above interview quotes, it is clear that the Act can be beneficial, and complicated – as well as, for some, rather insignificant. It may not make much difference to how such unions are perceived in family and social terms.

Conclusion

Same-sex marriage, like any marriage union, requires careful consideration before one embarks on it. What is important to realize is that same-sex marriages do not take place in a vacuum. The individuals involved come from families, societies and cultures that may value relationships, tradition and cultural practices, but can also be patriarchal and even homophobic. Given all this, the individuals may also be challenged to negotiate their identities in relation to the partner they seek to marry and how they want their marriage to take place. While it is clear that marriage is complex, it nevertheless is something some lesbian women would like to achieve for themselves and their relationships.

For the informants in this piece, the complexities continue. Linda has not yet reconciled with her frustrations around lobola and the status of *umakoti*. She continues to save up for lobola and is contemplating telling her mother about the situation. Sibu continues to wonder if and how she would marry. She still battles with her family not accepting her lifestyle choices. The MaseTshabas sound a cautionary note:

> In any life-changing event, go for counselling. It is important to know each other's family backgrounds, beliefs, religion, culture, ambitions and goals and ideas on children. You must also understand the legalities of getting married in or out of community of property. Love alone is not a good enough reason to get married.

Notes

1 Jacklyn Cock, 'Engendering Gay and Lesbian Rights: The Equality Clause in the South African Constitution', in Neville Hoad, Karen Martin and Graeme Reid (eds.), *Sex and Politics in South Africa* (Double Storey, 2005); Vasu Reddy and Zethu Cakata, '"Even Animals of the Same Sex Don't Take This Route": Politics, Rights and Identity about Same-Sex Marriage in South Africa', *Sexuality in Africa* 4:1 (2007)
2 Cock, op. cit., 195
3 Pseudonyms have been used, by request, for 'Sibu' and 'Linda'. See page 105 (note 1), for a note on the usage of 'lobola'.
4 Archbishop's Committee, *A Report on Same-Sex Unions for the South African Anglican Theological Commission*, The Anglican Communion in Johannesburg, South Africa (2003), 1
5 Ibid., 5; Saskia Wieringa, 'Woman Marriages and Other Same-Sex Practices: Historical Reflections on African Women's Same-Sex Relations', in Ruth Morgan and Saskia Wieringa (eds.), *Tommy Boys, Lesbian Men and Ancestral Wives: Female Same-Sex Practices in Africa* (Jacana, 2005), 281-307
6 Nancy Baraka with Ruth Morgan, '"I Want to Marry the Woman of My Choice without Fear of Being Stoned": Female Marriages and Bisexual Women in Kenya', in Morgan and Wieringa (eds.), op. cit., 26-27
7 Wieringa, op. cit., 305-306
8 Ibid., 306
9 Baraka with Morgan, op. cit., 41
10 Dina Kraft, 'The Changing Role of Africa's Women', http://www.iol.co.za/index.php?set_id=1&click_id=68&art_id=qw107111754327B213, 11 December 2003 (last accessed 13 December 2007)
11 Archbishop's Committee, op. cit., 5
12 Wieringa, op. cit., 303
13 Nkunzi Nkabinde with Ruth Morgan, '"This Has Happened since Ancient Times ... It's Something You Are Born with": Ancestral Wives amongst Same-Sex Sangomas in South Africa', in Morgan and Wieringa (eds.), op. cit., 242
14 Reddy and Cakata, op. cit., 2

Lesbians and the Civil Union Act:
A critical reflection

Mary Hames

South Africa is the only country on the African continent to have ensconced the right to protection from discrimination based on sexual orientation in its Constitution. Through protracted litigation, homosexuals have been afforded significant rights, most recently the right to marry as legislated in the Civil Union Act, signed into law by Deputy President Phumzile Mlambo-Ngcuka on 30 November 2006. For many lesbian, gay, bisexual, transgender and intersexed (LGBTI) activists this Act represents the culmination of the process begun in the early 1990s with the lobbying of the African National Congress and other political parties to include the prevention of discrimination on the basis of sexual orientation in the equality clause of the Bill of Rights.[1]

Lesbians have played a key role in the litigation for rights that are otherwise automatically given to married heterosexual women. These include the right to a deceased partner's pension benefits; the right to immigration of foreign partners; the recognition of children born to same-sex couples by way of donor insemination; the right to non-discrimination in employment; full custody of children in instances of divorce; and the right to become joint, legal parents of adopted children.

The story of litigation for the right to marry ends in the Constitutional Court's *Fourie* judgment in 2006, but in the precedent-setting lead-up to the marriage victory there were significant cases in which lesbians also played a leading role. In *Greyling v Minister of Welfare* (1998) it was found that a lesbian mother could keep her child and not have to hand it over to its grandparents, and in *Mohapi v Mohapi* (1998) a lesbian woman gained full custody of her child.[2] In *Du Toit and De Vos v the Minister of Welfare and Population Development and Others* (2002) lesbian and gay couples were given the right to become joint, legal parents of adopted children. In 2002, Kathy Satchwell (a High Court judge) sued for her female partner's right to receive the same financial benefits afforded to a heterosexual spouse by the state. In the *Greyling*, *Mohapi* and *Du Toit* cases the issue of the 'shaping and recognition of an alternative parent-hood and family' was deemed to be of the essence. In this way, lesbians have contributed notably to a rethinking of marriage and the family as well as to the claiming of their rights. (See pages 55-57.)

These cases give an indication of how lesbian and gay activists have over the last few years successfully chiselled away at deeply patriarchal and sexist institutions. Marriage was regarded as one of the last remaining obstacles to full equality. It is undeniably important that all South Africa's citizens be afforded all the rights as set out in the Bill of Rights, but we need to ask what the meaning of same-sex marriage is for lesbians – in particular for black lesbians – and to locate such a question within the context of South Africa's present-day socio-economic realities.

The right to marry offers the promise of more substantive equality and inclusive citizenship. At the same time, it must be remembered that the state has consistently been the most ardent opponent in almost every precedent-setting case.[3] It can be argued that South Africa does not, in fact, have a benevolent state that embraces the diversity of all its citizens, but has to be forced to live up to its obligations in terms of the Constitution.[4] Furthermore, the right to marry may confer legal equality on LGBTI people, but we should not overestimate its importance or its efficacy in the battle against homophobic prejudice.

The pursuit of access to LGBTI rights is inflected by race and class. Much of the litigation for these rights has been conducted by privileged, white, educated middle-class lesbian and gay people, or has been driven by LGBTI organizations chiefly funded by foreign donors – although the foot soldiers, supporters and lobbyists came from across gender, race and class divisions. Thus race, class and education give some a distinct advantage in the claiming of constitutional rights such as financial benefits, the right to adopt, to take advantage of donor insemination, and so forth. By contrast, the claim of majority working-class black lesbians to their constitutional rights – and therefore to safety and security – are under the continuous threat of extreme violence, including brutal forms of 'curative' rape and murder.

Lesbian feminism and the problematization of marriage
'That black sister on radio must come here and I will show her what a woman is for' – this comment was made to Nonhlanhla Mkhize, director of the Durban Lesbian and Gay Community and Health Centre, during a radio debate on the Civil Union Bill in 2006. Two years earlier, an unknown lesbian testified to documentary-maker Lovinsa Kavumba, 'I was raped because they wanted to know whether I was a woman.'[5]

Even in a society where violence against women in general is widespread, the rape and murder of black lesbians is sinister. Very particular to South Africa is the 'curative' or 'correctional' rape of black lesbians – the bizarre belief, if it is a genuine belief, that such acts can convert a woman to heterosexuality. Over the last few years there have been several cases of rape and murder of black women who dared to live openly as lesbians. Many of these murders were first highlighted by the 'A Rose Has Thorns' campaign run by the Forum for the Empowerment of Women (FEW), an empowerment and support organization for black lesbians in Gauteng. Zoliswa Nkonyana was murdered in Khayelitsha in February 2006 by a group of young men because she dared to be a lesbian; her friend, also a lesbian, was stabbed in October of the same year. In April 2007, 16-year-old Madoe Mafubedoe, who was openly living as a lesbian, was raped and stabbed to death; on 7 July 2007 Sizakele Sigasa and Salome Masooa were brutally tortured, raped and killed in Meadowlands, Soweto, and their bodies dumped in a nearby field. Just over two weeks later, on 23 July 2007, another lesbian, Thokozane Qwabe, was murdered in Ezakeni, Ladysmith.

Such acts lead one to wonder about the hatred directed at black lesbians and why it is so deep-seated. Is it because these lesbians defy traditional heterosexual norms and challenge patriarchy, heterosexism, culture, religion and masculinity? Is it because they dare to live their sexuality without needing men to economically support or give them their identity? Certainly, lesbianism challenges patriarchal values – and marriage is one of those values. Alongside the strong resistance to the legalization of same-sex marriage from conservative religious bodies, one of its greatest opponents was Contralesa, the Congress of Traditional Leaders of South Africa.[6]

Feminism made it clear that the personal is the political, and this is no more obvious than in the cases mentioned above. There remains the conflict in our jurisprudence between laws that govern public activities and those that relate to private lives. Marriage is a public act that puts private, personal relationships on a social stage. It is important for lesbians to understand this paradox in our legal system if they decide that their lifestyle and sexual orientation is a private affair, because in such a case there is hardly any recourse for redress in cases of discrimination. There have been numerous undocumented narratives by lesbians who claimed that they have lost everything to their deceased partner's family because they could make no claim to a legitimate relationship

Although feminists have historically been proponents of the granting of liberal rights to ensure equality for women in both the private and public domains, some have also been antagonistic towards institutions such as marriage. Marriage, they contend, is a patriarchal institution that poses severe impediments to the freedoms women have fought for. As Ralph Smith and Russel Windes put it, 'The fundamental truth of marriage is that it is seen as a heterosexual institution: a union of one man and one woman as man and wife.'[7]

In her book *The Creation of Patriarchy*, Gerda Lerner[8] traces the systematic subordination of women through the ages and points to the fact that women's sexuality and reproductive potential held the capacity to acquire property and wealth for men on many different levels. Historically, a man's wealth could be measured in terms of the number of wives he had and the number of children he could father; women were thus seen as part of his larger material property. Paula Giddings mentions Plato, 'who placed women into three categories: whore, mistress and wife – the last of whom was expected to organize the household and provide 'legitimate' heirs to their husband's material acquisitions.'[9] Modernity has changed the means of wealth creation, but patriarchal ideas – which are deeply entrenched in our society – still see women as a the property of men.

Hence some feminists argue that marriage is essentially a patriarchal institution and its main purpose is to control women's bodies and sexuality. Marriage is firmly embedded in the 'private' domain, giving men power over a woman's reproductive rights, as well as unlimited access to unpaid domestic labour. As the anarchist thinker Emma Goldman observed, 'Marriage makes woman a parasite at best, a prostitute at worst.'[10]

Coming from within the broader feminist movement, it was lesbian feminists who tended to take this radical view. Some felt that the wider feminist movement failed to include the specific needs of lesbians, and in many instances were in fact hostile towards those needs. Because of this disillusionment with the exclusion of lesbian-specific concerns, lesbian feminists developed theories and strategies to emphasize their specific needs. Consequently they focused less on the extension of liberal rights and more on seeking to dismantle patriarchal and heterosexist institutions in general. One of their strategies was (and is) to promote lesbianism as a *choice* for women.

Lesbian feminists question the institution of marriage, which is traditionally based on the union between one man and a woman to the exclusion of all others – the common-law definition we had in the past. The radical lesbians of the early 1970s imagined a society free of oppression of any sex or gender, and in which the categories of homosexuality and heterosexuality would disappear. They were deeply suspicious of monogamy and saw it as part of the oppression of women. They also came out strongly against the butch/femme stereotype within lesbian culture, seeing it as a perpetuation of patriarchal and heterosexist roles.[11]

Adrienne Rich[12] contends that any form of feminist theory that considers lesbianism as simply an 'alternative lifestyle' or a mere 'sexual preference' is inherently flawed. She uses the terms 'lesbian existence' and 'lesbian continuum', indicating that lesbians have always been part of history and that there are a variety of women-identified experiences that do not necessarily focus on the desired genital sexual experience. These experiences include a myriad relationships of mutual support and love between women. Rich and other lesbian theorists questioned the assumption that heterosexuality is normal and natural, and indicated that honest feminist analysis will prove that many women are forced to live heterosexual lives and thus to marry.[13]

Sheila Jeffreys argues that such lesbian political theory transformed lesbianism from a stigmatized sexual practice into a political practice that challenges male supremacy and thus its basic institution, heterosexual marriage.[14] These interventions are important because they draw a connection between patriarchy and heterosexuality. From this perspective, it is important to identify lesbian identities and relationships as disruptive of the status quo. This analysis of marriage is crucial in considering its underlying social and ideological meanings. It means we need to think about the distinct political and social positioning of particular groups within the larger LGBTI community. We need to take into account the particular class-inflected, gendered and racialized ways in which certain groups, more than others, stand to lose from marriage as an institution.

Lesbian feminists felt excluded from the broader feminist movement, and black feminists experienced exclusion from white feminist discourse. Black feminists, amongst them Audre Lorde, Patricia Hill Collins and bell hooks, felt that white middle-class feminist theory excluded their realities, or, if included in mainstream theorization, their experiences merely became an add-on. They laid great emphasis on the intersectionality of race, class and sex.

This approach to intersecting identities and oppressions is clearly evident in the work of Barbara Smith: 'Feminism is the political theory and practice that struggles to free *all* women: women of color, working-class women, poor women, disabled women, lesbians, old women – as well as white, economically privileged, heterosexual women. Anything less than this vision of total freedom is not feminism, but merely female self-aggrandizement.'[15]

bell hooks takes this further, arguing that poor black women could hardly afford to seek social equality with black men, since the majority of black men are also exploited and oppressed.[16] Kimberlé Crenshaw also challenges the mainstream feminist view that the battle is about powerful men and powerless women: 'Black men and women live in a society that creates sex-based norms and expectations which racism operates simultaneously to deny; black men are not viewed as powerful, nor are black women seen as passive.'[17]

Even black women's experience of violence is different. Ien Ang uses the well-known maxim *'No means No'* as a poignant example. She points to the fact that when that slogan is used by a white woman it implies a certain culturally loaded context. The slogan belongs to a 'repertoire of rules for social interaction which prizes individualism, conversational explicitness, directness and efficiency – something that may not be available to 'other' women.'[18] This is a very important statement, as will become clear when we consider the environment in which black lesbians in South Africa have to negotiate their lives.

Black women's bodies have long been a site of sexual violence. Valerie Amos and Prathibha Parmar note that 'Black women's sexuality has been used in various oppressive ways throughout imperialist history. For instance, during slavery women were forced to breed slave labour force, raped, assaulted and experimented on; practices that still continue today under "scientific" and sophisticated disguises.'[19]

In South Africa, the sexual domination of indigenous women can be traced back to the beginning of the 1650s and European occupation of the land. It was common practice for settlers to have sexual relations with slave women, and the most valued slave was a child of a slave mother and white father. Thus women slaves were 'valued' in terms of their reproductive roles as well as their labour. As Giddings reminds us, 'The black woman alone could give birth to a slave. Blacks constituted a permanent labor force and metaphor that were perpetuated through the black woman's womb.'[20] Hence the necessity, even long after the demise of slavery and the dismantling of colonialism, for women to decolonize their bodies, as Cheryl Clarke puts it.[21] Lesbians – especially black lesbians – living out their sexuality may be the most radical form of such 'decolonization'.

What, then, might marriage mean to a black lesbian?

The meanings of same-sex marriage: A speculation

It is crucial to consider how lesbian women actually experience marriage, and what psychological, legal, social and emotional value they may derive from it. Exploring this topic in detail would require careful investigation. In the discussion that follows I will simply identify some important patterns that might be useful for further research. LGBTI people may be able to achieve important rights and social acceptance within the broader heteronormative society through their ability to marry, but by the same token they can actually validate heterosexist and patriarchal social norms by turning to marriage and entrenching gendered behaviours such as butch/femme roles in their relationships. At the same time, lesbian women and gay men, but especially lesbians, have crafted institutions that somehow transcend heterosexist ones and can use marriage to confirm their own social structures.

In South African townships the butch/femme stereotype persists, both for men and for women. The perceived necessary pairing is that of a masculine-seeming person with a feminine-seeming person. This is a form of assimilation to heterosexist norms. Rather than requiring friends and family to embrace their union on their own terms, many lesbian and gay people naturally want to 'fit in', to make their behaviour, their roles, and their conduct echo patterns evident in mainstream heterosexist society. Since marriage has been traditionally the union of a man and a woman, it may be that there is more pressure for lesbian and gay couples to indulge in roles that mimic such norms.

At the same time, the heterosexual institution of marriage may be disrupted, challenged and transformed by the addition of alternative perceptions and practices of marriage. Same-sex and heterosexual marriages are often seen to be alike, but there are many different interpretations of apparently similar values. The concept of sexual monogamy, for instance, is not as firmly cemented in same-sex marriage as it is in heterosexual marriage.[22] According to Josephine Mills and Leila Armstrong, same-sex marriage has the potential to create a social network of 'family' that is inclusive of past and present partners and children and couplings that challenge the historical notion of marriage.[23] Many non-heterosexuals, argues Jeffrey Weeks, strongly believe that they have greater opportunities than most heterosexuals to achieve egalitarian relationships.[24]

Over and above the desire on the part of lesbian and gay people to get married so that their intimate relationships can be publicly and legally recognized, legislation such as the Civil Union Act restructures families. Lesbians in long-term partnerships have long been adopting children, but previously the law only allowed for one member of the couple to become the legal parent. It was argued that to ensure that both are acknowledged as the legal parents of either the adopted child(ren), or of offspring through artificial insemination, marriage would be the best way to ensure legal parenthood. Procreation may or may not be one of the reasons why lesbian and gay people want to marry. Many lesbian and gay people have children already – from previous relationships, through adoption, artificial insemination, or, in many instances in South Africa, rape.

Black lesbians have always negotiated their socialization and their complex relationships within an extreme heteronormative, patriarchal and oppressive society. One of the first same-sex couples to publicly express their intention to get married under the new Civil Union Act was a lesbian couple from Soweto; they were aware that neither their community nor the broader society would accept their marriage.[25] If they went ahead one cannot but admire their courage. The statistics on same-sex marriages since the Bill was passed indicate that LGBTI people are using the institution of marriage as a means to gain acknowledgement of their relationships: between 1 December 2006 and 31 December 2007, 935 couples formed civil unions; 519 of those were lesbian couples.[26]

Because of South Africa's apartheid history, race still plays a divisive role even within the historically oppressed LGBTI community. Black lesbians tend to form intimate relationships within their specific 'race' groups. This can be ascribed to a variety of factors, among them the fact that many still reside in the historically black residential areas and attend historically racialized educational institutions. Race, class and economics play important roles in the formation of lesbian networks. Legal transformation has not translated into socio-economic transformation. During the apartheid years, the privileged middle-class homosexual could afford to pay for privacy and anonymity; in the post-apartheid era, such people can afford to pay for the acquisition of their constitutional rights.

For many lesbians the issue is still to be able to survive in an aggressively hostile world. Marriage includes legal contracts; marriage shifts the boundaries of commitment into the legal sphere; marriage also includes the possibility of divorce. So far same-sex marriage has not destigmatized same-sex love and relationships. It has, however, destabilized and challenged the notion of marriage as an exclusively heterosexual preserve, and thus the basis of heteronormativity. The wide public coverage given to the hearings around the Civil Union Act – and the opposition from religious groups and organizations such as Contralesa – indicates the degree to which it upsets patriarchal norms.

For a long time, lesbians have been in stable relationships and have raised families within the confines of conservative and prejudiced communities. Black lesbians, in particular, have, in spite of cultural and religious pressures, defied the constriction of normalized heterosexuality. As in many other areas of post-apartheid South African life, there has been gradual change in the level of acceptance of previously taboo practices; hence there is hope that same-sex marriages will lead to greater tolerance of alternative sexualities.

In the course of lobbying for the right to complete and inclusive citizenship, lesbians have already had a far-reaching effect on the transformation of South African society. The building of case law challenged religious morals, customary practices and patriarchal perceptions – and set precedents that transformed the law. Lesbians have brought about new transfigurations of the definition of conception and birth, and of family law; and they have introduced new dimensions to the Birth and Registration Act, the Children's Act and divorce law. Lesbians too have shaped inheritance law because by getting married they automatically receive the same inheritance privileges that heterosexual married women have been awarded all along, as well as the same financial benefits for same-sex partners. In fact, the field of jurisprudence has unequivocally been transformed. South African citizenship has acquired a whole new meaning. Lesbians in this country have upstaged the patriarchy and heterosexism like no other activist group has ever done.

The backlash against such advances may be read in the irrational fear that translates into violence against lesbians – as well as continued, everyday discrimination. A pertinent case would be that of a white lesbian who made inquiries at a hospital about fertility treatment and was turned away because of the hospital's exclusionary policy.[27] This kind of discrimination is still deeply embedded in our society. Members of the LGBTI community who belong to the working class, especially the black working class, are still struggling with issues of acceptance by family, community and religious structures; with matters of identity and empowerment of the self. As Supreme Court of Appeal Judge Edwin Cameron has said: 'There is rampant racism, rampant inequality and prejudice against gays and lesbians. We have a long way to go before the constitutional promises are translated.'[28] In spite of progressive laws such as the Civil Union Act, there is still a need for the education of the broader community in which we live to understand and accept the diversity that exists within it, and within the homosexual community itself.

Notes

1 Gertrude Fester, 'Some Preliminary Thoughts on Sexuality, Citizenship and Constitutions: Are Rights Enough?', *Agenda* 67 (2006), 100-11; Sheila Meintjes, 'Gender Equality by Design: The Case of South Africa's Commission on Gender Equality', *Politikon* 32:2 (2005), 259-75; Mikki van Zyl, 'Escaping Heteronormative Bondage: Sexuality in Citizenship', in Amanda Gouws (ed.), *(Un)thinking Citizenship: Feminist Debates in Contemporary South Africa* (UCT Press, 2005), 223-252
2 *Mohapi v Mohapi* (WLD 1998, unreported); *Greyling v Minister of Welfare and Population Development* (WLD case no. 98/8297, unreported), cited in Human Rights Watch, *More than a Name: State-Sponsored Homophobia and Its Consequences in Southern Africa* (Human Rights Watch, 2003), 184; http://www.hrw.org/reports/2003/safrica/safriglhrc0303.pdf (last accessed 10 December 2007)
3 Ibid.
4 Mary Hames, 'Sexual Identity and Transformation at a South African University', *Social Dynamics*, 33:1 (June 2007), 53
5 Lovinsa Kavuma (producer/director), *Rape for Who I Am* (documentary, DVD, 2004)
6 'Contralesa Slams Legalisation of Gay Marriages', http://www.africanveil.org/Southafrica084.htm (last accessed 10 December 2007)
7 Ralph R Smith and Russel R Windes, *Progay/Antigay: The Rhetorical War over Sexuality* (Sage, 2000), 158
8 Gerda Lerner, *The Creation of Patriarchy* (OUP, 1986)
9 Paula Giddings, *When and Where I Enter: The Impact of Black Women on Race and Sex in America*, second edition (Quill/William Morrow, 1996), 34
10 Quoted in Maria Bevacqua, 'Feminist Theory and the Question of Lesbian and Gay Marriage', *Feminism and Psychology* 14:1 (2004), 36
11 Radicalesbians, *The Woman-Identified Woman* (1970), Documents from the Women's Liberation Movement, Special Collections Library, Duke University, http://scriptorium.lib.duke.edu/wlm/womid/ (last accessed 13 August 2007), 1
12 Adrienne Rich, 'Compulsory Heterosexuality and Lesbian Existence', *Signs* 5:4 (1980), 632
13 Bevacqua, op. cit., 37
14 Sheila Jeffreys, *The Lesbian Heresy: A Feminist Perspective on the Lesbian Sexual Revolution* (The Women's Press, (1993), viii
15 Barbara Smith, *The Truth That Never Hurts: Writings on Race, Gender, and Freedom* (Rutgers University Press, 2000), 50
16 bell hooks, *Talking Back: Thinking Feminist, Thinking Black* (South End Press, 1989), 19
17 Kimberlé Crenshaw, 'Demarginalizing the Intersection of Race and Sex: A Black Feminist Critique of Antidiscrimination Doctrine, Feminist Theory and Antiracist Politics', in Joy James and T Denean Sharpley-Whiting (eds.), *The Black Feminist Reader* (Blackwell, 2000), 222
18 Ien Ang, 'I'm a Feminist But ... "Other" Women and Postnational Feminism', in Kum-Kum Bhavnani (ed.), *Feminism and 'Race'* (OUP, 2001), 398-399
19 Valerie Amos and Pratibha Parmar, 'Challenging Imperial Feminism', in Bhavnani (ed.), op. cit., 28
20 Giddings, op. cit., 39
21 Cheryl Clarke, 'Lesbianism: An Act of Resistance', in Beverly Guy-Sheftall (ed.), *Words of Fire: An Anthology of African-American Feminist Thought* (The New Press, 1995), 242
22 Elizabeth Peel and Rosie Harding, 'Divorcing Rights, Romance, and Radicalism: Beyond Pro and Anti in the Lesbian and Gay Marriage Debate', *Feminism and Psychology* 14:1 (2004), 590
23 Josephine Mills and Leila Armstrong, 'Commentary: Love and Marriage', *Canadian Journal of Communication* 31 (2006), 949
24 Jeffrey Weeks, 'Same-sex Partnerships', *Feminism and Psychology* 14:1 (2004), 162

25 'A Couple Wants First Wedding' (2006), http://www.africanveil.org/Southafrica064.htm (last accessed 11 December 2007)
26 Statistics supplied by the Department of Home Affairs, 14 January 2008
27 Helen Bamford, 'City Hospital Turns Away Gay Would-Be Mom', *Cape Argus*, 18 August 2007
28 Candice Bailey, 'Gay Rights Still Just a Promise, Says Judge', *Cape Argus*, 14 August 2007

De-gendering unions:
The Civil Union Act and the intersexed

Sally Gross

The Civil Union Act was signed into law on 30 November 2006, amid considerable controversy. Excoriated by partisans of exclusive heteronormativity, it also came under heavy criticism from many in the LGBTI community.

What is not in dispute is that the new statute is a significant milestone for same-sex couples joined in civil unions, or in marriages, in terms of the Civil Union Act. In contrast to the insecurity of the past, the Act affords the parties to such unions the kind of protections and rights that were the exclusive preserve of parties to heterosexual marriages until not so very long ago. The Civil Union Act may not be all that many same-sex couples would want it to be, but it is undeniably a significant improvement on the *status quo ante*.

In what follows, I propose to look at the implications of the passage of the Civil Union Act for people like me who are intersexed. The interrogation of the issues will be broad-brush: it will not involve close exegesis of the letter of the law, but will seek to tease out larger issues.

Historically speaking, marriage as a socio-legal institution in South Africa was an expression of the religious sensibilities and of the patriarchal character of the country's colonizers. It had its roots in the Christianity of the Patristic era, denying recognition in law until relatively recently to Muslim and Hindu marriages, as well as to marriages under African customary law. Although marriage law as such became increasingly secularized, and supplementary legislation was enacted by the post-apartheid Parliament to recognize Muslim, Hindu and customary-law marriages including polygynous marriages, the 'ad hoccery' which led to the passage of supplementary statutes governing marriage prior to the passage of the Civil Union Act suggests that South African marriage law was fundamentally deficient.

The biblical Book of Genesis contains two accounts of the creation of humankind. The account given first,[1] characterized by scholars as a priestly account, has it that the mythical first 'married' couple, were commanded first and foremost to 'be fruitful and multiply', that is to say, procreation was of the essence. The second (or Yahwist) account of creation,[2] which follows immediately after the priestly account in the biblical text, portrays companionship, rather than procreation, as the primary purpose of cohabitation. In Christian tradition, procreation seems, historically, to eclipse companionship completely in practice. Translated into law, this results in a notion of 'conjugal rights' that notoriously made intramarital rape legal in the past, and which made the failure to consummate a marriage sexually, and even the failure to conceive, grounds for the dissolution of marriages. In days before *in vitro* fertilization was even imagined, this model of marriage had no space at all for same-sex relationships which, because they were seen as thwarting the alleged exclusively procreative purpose of marriage as ordained by the Creator, were excoriated as contrary to the laws of God and of nature. Monogamy was another part of the package, once again an import from Patristic Christian tradition although it is most certainly not biblical in origin.[3] The model is thoroughly patriarchal: wives are chattels of their husbands and, historically, lacked many of the rights enjoyed by men.

Until relatively recently in the history of marriage in our country, part of the package as it were was the criminalization of sexual relationships which were not heterosexual. Acting on a sexual orientation which was not heteronormative was a breach of the law. It should be noted that women and men who were lesbian or gay were not barred from marriage as such even at that time, but gay men could marry only women and lesbian women could marry only men. Such women and men could benefit from the social rights and protection afforded by marriage by contracting into heteronormative marriages, albeit at what was often an extravagant psychological cost. With the decriminalization of lesbian and gay sex and protection from discrimination on the basis of sexual orientation, lesbian and gay sexual relationships and unions became licit in law, but the partners to such unions continued to be denied many of the rights and protection afforded to partners in marriage proper, which remained the preserve of the heterosexual.

In all of this, the intersexed – people who are not really determinately male or female – were largely off the map. Those whose appearance was 'passable', especially those whose genital anatomy did not appear particularly ambiguous whether by chance or as a result of genital surgery, would probably have been able to enter into marriages, but these would have been precarious affairs at best. Very few people who are intersexed are fertile, and this in and of itself would have been a potential ground for annulment. The very disclosure that a party to a marriage was born intersexed would itself have been grounds for a declaration of invalidity, the finding that there was not a marriage in the first place. In contrast with divorce, which involves the dissolution or annulment of a valid marriage, invalidity involves the finding that, whatever the appearances, there was never actually any marriage. Potentially, there was danger even if an intersexed person and his or her partner managed to negotiate these obstacles and if the marriage remained unimpugned until the death of the non-intersexed partner. The discovery at this stage that the surviving spouse was intersexed could constitute grounds for the denial to that person of all rights stemming from marriage on the grounds that the possession of such rights was conditional upon there having been a valid marriage, and that only someone determinately female and someone determinately male could be united validly in marriage. Additionally, in the days of criminalization of homosexual intercourse, sexual relations between an intersexed person and anyone else could have been construed as engagement in prohibited forms of sex, by reason of the fact that the sex of one of the partners was indeterminate, making the sexual act non-heterosexual. Much would have depended upon the willingness or unwillingness of officials to turn a blind eye.

Exclusion from marriage was perhaps not a 'big deal' for the independently wealthy, but it was a 'big deal' for most others in South Africa under apartheid in particular, and the lack of a framework offering the rights and protection afforded by marriage was a threat to the survival of those without such a framework even in post-apartheid South Africa. In the Yahwist story of creation in the Book of Genesis, God is portrayed as noting, with reference to the then Eve-less Adam, that 'it is not good that a person should be alone'. The Bible is absolutely right in this regard: companionship is fundamental to survival, in our urban jungles at least. There are contexts in which extended families and communal cohesion constitute a survival system for people who are not married or in a marriage-like union. Decades of apartheid and urbanization have eroded these social safety nets, and there are many people in the towns in particular whose links with their families are increasingly tenuous. Stigmatized as it is, a cost of being known to be intersexed in a rural context is often exclusion from the networks through which people survive. In an urban context, being intersexed also makes it far more likely than otherwise that one is on the margins, alone and desperately lonely. In these circumstances, being able to make a life in companionship with someone else is crucial to psychological survival and, at times of crisis or illness, can make the difference between surviving and going under.

The signing into law of the Civil Union Act undeniably changes a great deal for the better. It allows couples cohabiting in relationships which are not heteronormative to enjoy the benefits and protections afforded to the parties to heterosexual marriages. Civil unions entail a mutual duty of support, for example, something which can be fundamental to survival in our world.

The first draft of the Civil Union Bill (B26-2006) described civil unions in dichotomous terms which excluded the intersexed unintentionally – a couple one of whom is intersexed is neither a heterosexual or a same-sex couple. In a submission made in October 2006 with regard to the first draft of the Bill, the South African Human Rights Commission (SAHRC) drew attention to the fact that the Bill, as it then stood, excluded the intersexed by defining civil union and marriage in terms of determinate sex.[4] The definition of 'civil union' in the Bill and in the Act as passed is sex- and gender-neutral, defining it as 'the voluntary union of two persons who are both 18 years of age or older, which is solemnized and registered by way of either marriage or a civil partnership, in accordance with the procedures prescribed in this Act'. This is clearly to be welcomed. However, Section 8 (6) of the Act as passed states that a civil union 'may only be registered by prospective civil union partners who would, apart from the fact that they are of the same sex, not be prohibited by law from as the case may be, at any given time, concluding a marriage under the Marriage Act or Customary Marriages Act'. Given that the Marriage Act as it currently stands implicitly excludes the intersexed from marriage, given that they are not determinately male or female, Section 8 (6) also appears to exclude the intersexed by implication. This clearly requires amendment, given that the Promotion of Equality and Prevention of Unfair Discrimination Act (Act 4 of 2000; 'Pepuda') as amended by Section 16 of the Judicial Matters Amendment Act (Act 22 of 2005), stipulates that 'sex includes intersex', ensuring thereby that discrimination on the sole grounds of being intersexed is deemed *prima facie* to be unfair until and unless proved to be fair.

This must clearly be corrected to ensure that the language of the Act is gender-neutral and, by implication, that civil unions are open to the intersexed in principle as the amendment to Pepuda noted above requires. As matters currently stand, the offending section of the Act means that, as is the case in terms of the Marriage Act, even if a civil union or marriage in terms of the Civil Union Act is registered by the officers concerned, should one or both of the partners be intersexed (by which I mean objectively, that is to say, physically, notwithstanding notional classification of sex in identification documents), it can be argued to be invalid *ipso facto*. The fact that the opening definition of the Civil Union Act, in conjunction with an appropriate amendment to Section 8 (6), would open a possibility which was closed, in practice, to many people who are intersexed, nevertheless affords the intersexed with at least some reason to rejoice. Were the dichotomous language of Section 8 (6) of the Act to be amended to make it gender-neutral because it was pointed out that it excluded the intersexed by implication, there would be even greater reason to be glad.

What then of the complaints that the Civil Union Act does not *really* open marriage as such to same-sex couples, offering the possibility of something *called* 'marriage', under the rubric of a 'civil union' but lacking the religious imprimatur that many seek? Speaking personally, I find it difficult to understand why the possibility of entering into a civil union should not suffice. As I have implied in the previous paragraph, notwithstanding the misgivings of the SAHRC about the Civil Union Act as a whole, once Section 8 (6) is amended to render the Act unequivocally sex- and gender-neutral, I believe that the intersexed will have abundant reason to rejoice in the possibilities which already loom. As a legal institution, civil union as a form of cohabitation in this country should be viewed as a work in progress. It needs to evolve in order to meet social needs more adequately, and I do not doubt that it will evolve. Its inadequacies, as it currently stands, seem to me to derive not from its dissimilarities to the traditional institution of marriage, but rather from its having been modelled too closely on the traditional institution of marriage. Where there are those, including the SAHRC, who argue that there should have been no Civil Union Act at all and that existing panoply of marriage legislation should have been emended to allow for same-sex marriage instead, I would argue that it is marriage, as an institution in law which is fundamentally tainted by its patriarchal origins and rendered problematic by the lack of integration of the laws governing it in South Africa, which should be abandoned, leaving marriage as such to the religious. What I would like to see is a legal regime in which marriages are the exclusive preserves of religious denominations and in which every marriage has to be registered as a civil union to afford formal rights and protections in law. The scope of civil unions would need to be expanded sufficiently to allow for polygamous unions, but it would be ineliminably secular. This would make Section 8 (6) of the Civil Union Act as it stands, and any counterpart of it, wholly redundant, eliminating the multiplicity of marriage-like regimes, as it were, and preventing the lack of sex- and gender-neutrality in the pre-existing panoply of marriage laws from infecting civil unions.

This is predicated in part upon a suspicion that emendation of marriage legislation, which is riddled with sex- and gender-dichotomous language, would have excluded the intersexed in practice because of the history and nature of the institution of marriage. Some intersexed people are sexually attracted to men, others are sexually attracted to women, while yet others are sexually attracted to both. Still others, like myself, are asexual, natural celibates who are without a sexual orientation. I have never seen a survey, but I would guess that a larger percentage of the intersexed are asexual than the prevalence of asexuality in the population at large. Given that I am in my mid-fifties, my own chances of finding a life companion in a non-sexual civil union are probably around zero, and my lack of companionship is not something that I welcome as ill-health and age take an increasing toll. I know from hard personal experience that asexual people growing up now will need the possibility of life companions with whom they can live non-sexually in relationships which afford intimacy and the rights and protections of civil union. Marriage as an institution, almost inextricably connected as it is to procreation, seems to me unable to yield this. According primacy to civil unions in law, by contrast, allows this institution to be made far more sensitive to the diversity of our social and sexual needs than the patriarchal institution of marriage can be.

Growing up as a society involves recognition of diversity, be it cultural or physical, and the crafting of institutions which make the recognition of diversity into a source of strength and cohesion and not a cause of fragmentation and weakness. The equality clause of our post-apartheid Constitution is a triumph of this recognition. The passage of the Civil Union Act, deficient though it is as it stands, particularly in relation to the needs of the intersexed, should be welcomed as a legal instrument which affords opportunities for much finer recognition than previously. It acknowledges the needs that derive from our social, sexual and anatomical diversity, and for far more comprehensive satisfaction of these needs in a framework that respects the inherent dignity of all. It needs to be viewed as a work in progress, and vigorous efforts need to be made to make civil unions less like the patriarchal model of marriage. As a legal institution, civil union already has the potential to offer far more to the intersexed than can the traditional institution of marriage, which has helped to foster a blindness, only now beginning to be overcome, to the needs, and even the existence, of the intersexed.

Notes
1 Genesis 1:1-2:3
2 Genesis 2:4-24
2 Ibid.
3 The Hebrew scriptures permit polygyny (though they seem to be silent about polyandry).
  In the New Testament, II Timothy 3:2 is at pains to recommend that bishops (which, in the context of the text in question, might be a variant term for 'elders') be monogynous rather than polygynous. This suggests that there were Christian males not in positions of ecclesial leadership who had more than one wife. The passage mentions deacons, but does not require deacons to be monogamous.
4 SAHRC, Submission to Home Affairs Portfolio Committee, National Assembly on Civil Union Bill (B26-2006), paragraph 38. (See pages 117-119 in this book.)

Marriage, citizenship and contested meanings

Vasu Reddy and Zethu Cakata

The Supreme Court of Appeal in 2004 declared the common-law definition of marriage unconstitutional. This decision followed an appeal by Marié Fourie and her partner, Cecelia Bonthuys, which resulted in mixed public reaction. Phumlani Nxumalo (74) from Orlando West, not too far from Johannesburg, was appalled at the court's verdict: 'Even animals of the same sex don't take this route. We have lost *ubuntu bethu*'.[1] Unsurprisingly, a lesbian couple, Mbali Nkosi (19) and Joy Mbatha (18), said they were overwhelmed by the outcome: 'We were thinking of eloping because we always felt that South African law was insular and unfair to us. But now we are relieved because it is no longer only about the so-called straight people.'[2] The idea that *ubuntu* (humaneness or humanity) is lost through the accrual of rights for lesbian and gay people suggests that such rights, according to their opponents, should not be guaranteed. That the virtues of *ubuntu* are only morally sanctioned within a heteronormative model implies, in our view, a very limited perspective on equality and human rights.

Legal victories and policy reform have benefited the construction of lesbian and gay identities in South Africa. Such victories have progressively promoted claims to citizenship and nationhood. However, the struggle for identity is reinforced in the case for same-sex marriage. Elsewhere in Africa, Anglican Archbishop Peter Akinola of Nigeria objected vehemently to any legitimation of homosexuality when he claimed that 'the US Episcopal Church is creating a new religion in which God almighty has declared a sin is no longer a sin. He went on to add that 'we cannot go along with that kind of religion'. 'Our people are deserting the Anglican Church as a result' of [Bishop Gene] Robinson's election, the Archbishop said. 'We want to recover our people.'[3] Akinola's view that homosexuality is incompatible with his religion has seen increasing mobilization and support within the Anglican Church in Nigeria as a result of the US Episcopal Church's decision to elect Gene Robinson (openly gay) into the Church hierarchy.

Same-sex marriage connects two central ideas: first, the history and meaning of homosexuality; and, second, the history and meaning of marriage.

In most African states homosexuality is still criminalized and even actively policed. Such criminalization is fuelled by the notion of the 'unAfricanness' of homosexuality, despite overwhelming evidence of the historically traceable presence of African lesbian and gay people and of same-sex practices on our continent. The main issue about homosexuality in most parts of Africa is less its denial than the fact that it is viewed in hetero-patriarchal terms as a behaviour rather than an identity. Such a perception characterizes homosexuality as a 'perverse' desire associated with pathology, and signals a return to a biomedical and non-cultural understanding of human sexuality. The case for marriage in many African countries remains a distant ideal, given the prohibition of same-sex practices. Our sexualities, by no means representative of a uniform experience, confirm that pleasure, desire, and belonging reflect deep-seated political conflicts over identity, bodily integrity and morality.[4]

The far-reaching court judgments since the formal adoption of the South African Constitution have systematically advanced the administration of justice that facilitates identity-formation for lesbian and gay people. While the apartheid social and legal system criminalized homosexuality, the post-apartheid landscape has shown a progressive realization of the recognition of lesbian and gay identities.[5]

As an institution, marriage is an important property of the state. Such an institution is also accorded a special privilege by most religions. Viewed as an arrangement for procreation and the nurturing of children, marriage is seen by patriarchal structures and traditions as a part of the natural order requiring a mixed-gender relationship (man and woman). Marriage is not simply a symbolic institution that affords a legal status to a civil relationship, but also raises jurisprudential issues about the state's relationship to its citizens. In most countries marriage rights do not apply to gay and lesbian couples because same-sex relationships fall outside the scope of the legal definition of marriage.

The case for the redefinition of marriage in South Africa was in some respects a test for the post-apartheid state's recognition of lesbian and gay citizens as full members of the polity. The Constitutional Court decision of 1 December 2005 found South African marriage laws to be unconstitutional in that they undermined the equality and dignity of same-sex couples who may wish to marry. The law-reform process that followed, culminating in the passing of the Civil Union Act, has served to strengthen the development of lesbian and identities further, by securing rights that support citizenship. It is for these reasons that it is difficult to erase sexuality from its relationship to the law and citizenship.

The meanings attached to marriage revealed in the debates on marriage equality are important. A cursory review of public opinion suggests that reactions to same-sex marriage reflect basic attitudes towards sexuality and gender.

At the heart of the gay and lesbian lobby's defence is the right of everyone to choose the circumstances in which they live their lives. Marriage is one possibility of a full citizenship (which includes the right to equality and privacy). This view is underpinned by the conception of the LGBTI-rights movement as a public demand for respect of homosexuals (which includes the right to dignity).

Consequently, the primary benefit of marriage is the extension of citizenship rights that facilitate the assimilation of gay and lesbian individuals into the mainstream of society. Such a view does not imply that all lesbian and gay people endorse marriage; for many, the need for marriage is disputed, because it signals assimilation into a heterosexual model. Some feminists view marriage as an institution that regulates and controls sexuality (female sexuality especially) and strictly imposes a gendered division of labour (even though this is changing, the situation of many women in such relationships remains unchanged). The motivation for marriage, especially as advanced by many activists, is also informed by the strategy to normalize homosexuality in our society as an identity and not a behaviour that is viewed as a pathology.

In contrast, homophobic arguments mobilized against same-sex marriage are informed by patriarchal power related to reproductive relations, gender roles, and the role of children and adoption, and are usually voiced from a moral/religious vantage point. For example, Johanna Bonoko stated that 'first it was the abortion law, now same-sex couples can marry ... we're heading for disaster'. In the same interview, Carol Makhanya cautioned that granting of same-sex marriage rights reflected 'the signs of doom and corruption ... man has turned his face from God'.[6] These views underscore the opinions of many opponents who view same-sex marriage as a threat to the patriarchal order, because gay marriage does not result in two people producing children through heterosexual sex. More so, the absence of 'male' and 'female' parental roles (as in a heterosexual parental model), are often motivating factors for opposition.

The focal point of the social structure of marriage, for those in opposition, is a traditional understanding of the family. Underlining the animosity toward same-sex marriage rights is a moral panic that introduces the notion of the family into the dispute about marriage. To some extent, the debate about same-sex marriage slips into a moral argument about what constitutes a family. In the case against same-sex marriage, 'family' is conceived as a patriarchal, biologically determined institution, and the place for the moral development of heterosexual parents and their children.

Despite the ongoing public debate, South African lesbian and gay people woke up to new possibilities on 30 November 2006, when the Civil Union Act was signed into law. Despite its limitations, this parallel marriage law caters for lesbian and gay people and suggests an affirmation of identity through the development of rights-centred law. The institution of marriage implies a practical and symbolic guarantee of equality for two people of the same-sex to formalize their commitment to each other.

The legal recognition of a civil union for lesbian and gay people suggests a journey towards social justice. Marriage is a dynamic institution, always in transition, and is increasingly losing some of its sacred appeal and becoming secularized.

This, in our view, is not a sign of weakness in the institution but rather a reflection of its response to social change and growing inclusiveness. We have witnessed changes to the nuclear family, the advent of alternative family arrangements, and new ways of being in the world in the broad development of our sexualities.

The case for same-sex marriage reflects much contestation (most recently reflected in the Nigerian Bill to ban same-sex marriage). We must remain vigilant about the prospect that rights do not necessarily sustain justice. The victory in South Africa confirms developing freedoms for lesbian and gay people, but does not resolve the persistent threat of homophobia, prejudice, stigma and persecution, reinforced by religious and cultural intolerance. Patekile Holomisa, the leader of the Congress of Traditional Leaders of South Africa (Contralesa), stated at that organization's national congress in early 2007 that the Constitutional Court had erred in its ruling on same-sex marriage: 'We will continue to inform our people this is something we don't support ... It is taboo ... If you accept this [being gay], you might as well accept people having sex with their relatives or with animals for that matter.'[7]

Sadly, such views reconfirm the need to hold on to struggles for rights, to reinforce public education, and to challenge discrimination. The journey to justice means that democracy comes with risks, and that we must continuously fight to protect it. Views such as those expressed by Holomisa, that homosexuality and same-sex marriage are out of kilter with African values, customs and tradition, seem to be in contrast with the fact that South Africa is a constitutional democracy where the right to freedom, dignity and respect is guaranteed.

Notes

An earlier version of this essay first appeared as '"Even Animals of the Same Sex Don't Take This Route": Politics, Rights and Identity about Same-Sex Marriage in South Africa', *Sexuality in Africa*, 4:1 (2007), 1-4.

1. 'Same Sex Marriages', *Sowetan*, 1 December 2004
2. Ibid.
3. Sapa-AP, 'I Didn't Write the Bible', *Daily News*, 11 October 2004
4. Vasu Reddy, 'Sexuality in Africa: Some Trends, Transgressions and Tirades', *Agenda*, 62 (2004), 3-11
5. Vasu Reddy, 'Moffies, Stabanis, Lesbos: The Political Construction of Queer Identities in Southern Africa' (Unpublished PhD thesis, University of KwaZulu-Natal, 2005)
6. 'Same Sex Marriages', op. cit.
7. Christelle du Toit, 'Chiefs Bash Gays', *The Citizen*, 19 February 2007. See also 'Contralesa slams Legalisation of Gay Marriages', http://www.sabcnews.com/south_africa/general/0,2172,143964,00.html (last accessed 12 December 2007)

'Are our lives OK?' Reflections on 13 years of gay liberation in South Africa

Gerald Kraak

'Our lives are not OK.'

This was how a Ugandan lesbian activist summed up the situation of the LGBTI community in her country. She was speaking at a donor conference on sexual minorities in Nairobi, Kenya, in late September 2007. The object of the conference was to investigate how northern donors might begin to collaborate, to support emerging gay and lesbian organizations in East Africa.

Her observation was poignant. It described a situation of repression – in Kenya, Uganda, Rwanda, Burundi and other countries, where homosexuality remains outlawed, discrimination is legion, politicians randomly engage in homophobic hate speech and there are violent attacks on activists – that recalled South Africa, 20 years ago.

But it also resonated with a time when a small number of progressive northern donors in South Africa began to look at how the country's nascent gay and lesbian movement of the mid-1990s might be supported. Mainstream donors had never committed to supporting gays and lesbians, as part of a broader human rights agenda, and most have yet to do so.

It was not an optimistic environment. As in East Africa today, in South Africa then, LGBTI organizations were concentrated in urban areas. They were typically strapped for cash, crisis-driven, run by small, committed, activist staffs, sometimes lacked professional capacity to carry out their programmes and relied on one or two donors for support. There was little collaboration between them; the umbrella National Coalition for Gay and Lesbian Equality (NGCLE) was disbanded in 1999.

More problematically, the public face of the community was largely white, male and middle class. In a rapidly transforming, democratic South Africa, this historical anomaly inherited from the apartheid past was a particular challenge for donors contemplating support, in which the goal was to strengthen the voice and activism of the poor, black, queer majority. In supporting organizations in their current form there was the danger of preserving the relative privilege of the few. The problem was compounded by the fact that – although gay and lesbian organizations were beginning to emerge in townships and rural areas – they were not visible.

Together with the Joseph Rowntree Charitable Trust, the Dutch Humanistic Institute for Development Co-operation (HIVOS) and the Norwegian Agency for Development Aid (NORAD), the Atlantic Philanthropies, which I represent, funded the lobbying and advocacy activities of the NCGLE in the mid-1990s. This lobbying led to the inclusion of the equality clause (which outlaws discrimination on the basis of sexuality) in the Bill of Rights and Constitution adopted by the Constitutional Assembly in May 1996. These donors also funded litigation resulting in the abolition of the sodomy laws and a range of partnership rights for gay men and lesbian women for the first time. The culmination of such activism was the marriage campaign, which resulted in the Civil Union Act being signed into law in 2006.

The campaign for same-sex marriage fitted with new objectives for the Atlantic Philanthropies, which from 2003 had made human rights a key area for investment.[1] Five years later, what has been the impact of Atlantic's funding, which represented a significant increase in resources for the community, supplementing that of mainstays such as HIVOS?

The impact of the funding has indeed induced a sea change. It needs to be stated, however, that this has been less about an injection of cash into an impoverished sector than a synergy between targeted funding and imperatives within the movement itself. Atlantic's funding coincided with a strategic reappraisal within key gay and lesbian organizations, chiefly the recognition that the movement needed to represent the poor and marginalized, more forcefully. A new, younger generation of gay and lesbian leadership, in which black people and lesbian women claimed greater space, was also emerging. The willingness of organizations to partner with donors in a challenging and sometimes contested project of social transformation was evidence of this.

Gay and lesbian organizations have engaged in a period of critical self-reflection and strategic re-orientation towards the majority of the gay and lesbian community. For the white, often founding members and leadership of organizations, this has at times proved a particular challenge; it has involved stepping back and allowing new leaders and organizations to emerge; it has involved providing institutional support to new organizations and activists, as well as a complex negotiation of competition over resources; resolving competing needs and agendas of different constituencies, mediating race, class and gender differences, while at the same time continuing to advocate for rights and services.

The Joint Working Group (JWG), a national network of LGBTI organizations in South Africa, emerged in 2003. It was the JWG that represented the position of the LGBTI movement in the same-sex marriage campaign following the introduction of the Civil Union Bill to Parliament. Same-sex marriage proved to be an issue that disparate organizations could unite around because it traversed race, class and gender differences.

It is now some years later. I believe that in South Africa today we have a genuinely non-racial gay and lesbian movement, which has struck roots in townships and rural areas. It is a movement in which there is increasingly a commitment to the interests of the poor and black LGBTI people. It is better-resourced and -organized and more coherent than at any time in the past. The campaign for same-sex marriage is an example of this greater maturity. In achieving its goal, the movement also demonstrated that it has strategic acumen, making use of litigation to take advantage of a progressive Constitution to win rights and using advocacy to ensure the passage of the Civil Union Act through Parliament.

The campaign for same-sex marriage illustrates the value of an LBGTI agenda that focuses on issues that cross race, class and gender lines; builds links with other social movements and groups; and engages with homophobic arguments on the part of traditional leaders and religious bodies. One of its strengths was the clarity with which arguments were made to the African National Congress (ANC) leadership on the need to intervene and ensure the Bill was passed. But the campaign also points up one of the weaknesses of the current LGBTI movement: it still lacks a grass-roots constituency that can be mobilized around issues such as same-sex marriage – as shown by the public hearings.

While the success of the campaign is to be celebrated, the process does not end there. Ongoing work needs to take place to monitor the implementation of the Civil Union Act and to educate the public about the right of same-sex couples to marry.

So are we OK?

In many ways, yes. And we have been lucky.

In contrast to East Africa, say, the South African gay and lesbian community has benefited from the country's Constitution which provided a platform that allowed it to leapfrog into full citizenship. In many other countries this has taken (and will take) years of grinding activism to achieve. And the South African movement has also benefited for the experience and strategic acumen of gay and lesbian people who were activists in the ANC, the United Democratic Front and other formations of the liberation movement. At the outset of democracy a relatively sophisticated gay and lesbian movement was able to take advantage of democracy.

In other ways, we are definitely *not* OK.

For all the achievements of the past 13 years, the community remains divided and the fault-lines of race, class and gender persist. In the world of the commercial club scene, patronized by a mainly white and male clientele, there is little notion of solidarity or common experience with those seeking to find safe spaces in townships and rural areas. The differing aspirations of these two communities is replicated every year in the debate over the nature of the Pride parade, what its message should be and where it should be take place. The re-routing of Pride from the Johannesburg city centre to the wealthy northern suburbs of Johannesburg demonstrates this continued divide and the predominance of the interests of a privileged minority, at least in determining this part of the annual gay and lesbian agenda. It dispels the notion that people are united by the common experience of their homosexuality; class, race and gender remain greater imperatives and the progressive arm of the gay and lesbian movement needs continually to challenge these agendas and interests, while protecting its own constituencies.

Even some of the constitutional rights won by the gay and lesbian movement feed into this divide. Many of these, and I am thinking of recognition of partnership rights in terms of pensions, insurance and inheritance, have largely benefited employed middle-class people. Last year's seminal achievement – the recognition of same-sex marriage – is perhaps the one right that will have a more universal reach. Whatever one may think of marriage as a social institution, the recognition of gay marriage will allow people across cultures and classes to validate their relationships in a way that is universally understood and which has the greatest cultural resonance. It will almost certainly do more than any other reform to enhance gay visibility.

That said – and it may be precisely because a progressive and activist Constitutional Court has put in place a series of rights and entitlements, which are not supported by the population at large – the gay and lesbian community faces a backlash and a challenge to the rights it has won. This is manifested in the orchestrated violence against black lesbians and effeminate gay men that has become a feature of life in some townships. It is also manifest even in spaces where the community might expect allies. It should never be forgotten that senior leadership of the ANC had to intervene to force mutinous Members of Parliament to vote in favour of the Civil Union Act, which legalized same-sex marriages. This suggests that the ANC has not really engaged with the issue at a policy level (and historically the question of homosexuality almost never entered public political discourses during the liberation struggle and in the first decade of democracy). There is a progressive stratum within the ANC that is steeped in human rights, partly the influence of countries that hosted ANC exiles, and evidenced by the ANC government's inclusion of sexual orientation in labour legislation. But the ANC rank and file have certainly not embraced gay rights. This division within the ANC emerges in comments made by ANC president, Jacob Zuma a few weeks before the passing of the Act that same-sex marriages are 'a disgrace to the nation and to God'.[2]

The backlash against the gay and lesbian community is also manifest in the enhanced profile and voice of religious fundamentalists and the traditional leaders to whom Zuma's comments were calculated to appeal. Traditional leadership in South Africa is an essentially patriarchal and gender-discriminatory institution. Religious institutions are enormously influential in South Africa, where more than 80% of the population subscribes to one or other religion. In addition to shaping cultural values, religious institutions have significant political clout and have been a source of intense homophobia in South Africa. The ANC has worked to build and sustain alliances with religious institutions, and the passage of the Civil Union Act put this relationship under strain. Religious institutions were vociferous in their opposition to same-sex marriage and the Civil Union Act, perceiving it as a challenge to their cultural hegemony. (See pages 115-146.) One of the effects of the Civil Union Act has been – to some extent – to loosen the grip of religion on society and people are beginning to talk about marriage outside the context of religion. More than ever before, the Civil Union Act has opened up debate around sexuality and gay and lesbian rights.

In seeking full citizenship, the gay and lesbian community is confronting the deeply entrenched values and repressive institutions of patriarchy, as is the women's movement. The backlash is rooted in this and may be further encouraged by the current emergence of a populist political movement.

It is for this reason that the gay and lesbian community needs to begin building alliances with other social movements and groups that are marginalized in terms of access to rights (and progressive donors should back this). Until now the LGBTI movement has tended to confine its activism to the immediate imperatives of gay liberation. The campaign for same-sex marriage illustrated that successful campaigns depend on the existence of alliances between LGBTI people and other social movements and groups. Logical synergies exist, for example, between the movement against gender-related violence and formations of people with infected with and affected by HIV/AIDS. The issue of homophobic violence cannot be separated from that of gender-related violence more broadly. AIDS, once endemic in the gay community, now predominantly affects heterosexuals. In combating the spread of heterosexual HIV, latter-day activists have learnt much from the gay community.

The gay and lesbian movement also needs to engage with political parties, trade unions and mainstream faiths, not only in terms of advocacy, but as members. Where, for example, is the gay caucus within the ANC? Or the gay and lesbian chapter of the Congress of South African Trade Unions? These alliances can be extended into the arena of advocacy and activism for socioeconomic rights. In as much as black and poor gay and lesbian people experience the same poverty, joblessness, lack of housing and shoddy education and health services as their peers, there is common cause. The gay and lesbian movement needs to support these broader campaigns, not only as a political strategy to strengthen a rights-based political culture, but to make the community more visible.

Changing deeply entrenched public attitudes, values and beliefs that result in homophobia is the greatest challenge the gay and lesbian community faces. This cannot be secured through legislative fiat alone. It can only come about through greater visibility and community engagement, by moving out of the gay ghetto into broader social struggles, and by making common cause with others who still do not enjoy the full fruits of democracy.

Notes

1 We commissioned academics, government officials, activists and other experts to advise us on an appropriate strategy for our human rights programme. Our questions to them were: Which populations are most marginal in terms of their access to human and socio-economic rights in post-apartheid South Africa? And where could sustained and strategic investment on our part bring about demonstrable and lasting change? After several months of research our advisors identified the emerging gay and lesbian community as one such area, with an emphasis on making the black and poor component more visible and effective. Over the next five years, Atlantic would invest almost R70-million in the LGBTI sector and will continue to spend more over the remaining life of the foundation.
2 Sapa, 'Zuma Earns Wrath of Gays and Lesbians', http://www.mg.co.za/articlepage.aspx?area=/breaking_news/breaking_news__national/&articleid=285053 (last accessed 22 February 2008)

Queering marriage?
The legal recognition of same-sex relationships around the world

Craig Lind

The legal recognition of same-sex relationships has been a boom industry for several decades. Many people – on both sides of the debate – have been preoccupied with the issue and writing on the subject has increased exponentially in a few short years.[1] But why has this been so? Is it that there has been a shift in the moral centre of the Western world in the last century (or does it date even further back to the beginning of the Enlightenment)? Or is there something else at work?

In less than 50 years same-sex sexual conduct has, in the West at least, moved from 'odious crime'[2] to behaviour that is, if not completely respectable, at least an acceptable alternative to heterosexual sexual conduct.[3] Openness about same-sex sexual experience and orientation has become one of the touchstones of liberal openmindedness and the toleration of diversity. In much of the Western world – and in South Africa – it has become associated with the struggle for freedom from invidious discrimination. In short, it has become a banner for individual liberty.

If the sexuality that serves as the background to same-sex relationships has become acceptable in so short a space of time, it is no wonder that the reorganization of law to recognize the resulting relationships is following suit. These changes are inevitable. But the shape that law takes is much less inevitable. Given the way in which the (Western) world has moved on the issue in just two short decades, progress towards universal recognition of same-sex marriage in Western jurisdictions seems likely. And yet there are significant Western voices (and a myriad others) that oppose the recognition of same-sex relationships as marriage. Furthermore, the considerable pressures on marriage and its legal regulation must also affect our consideration of the available mechanisms for the recognition of same-sex relationships.

In this essay I trace international developments towards the legal recognition of same-sex relationships. I also reflect on the cultural consequences that both legal recognition and the process towards it has had, particularly in South Africa. But I hope to do more than just this. I will go on to reflect on the way in which the legal recognition of relationships beyond those celebrated formally might be influenced by the move towards legalizing same-sex marriage.

International progress
In this section I will trace the progress that has been made in various jurisdictions[4] around the world towards the legal recognition of same-sex relationships. Although Europe has the longest formal history of same-sex partnership recognition, and has (arguably) made more thorough progress in that respect, I will start this survey with North America. Overall, progress on this continent has been limited, but the USA, in the first instance, and Canada subsequently, have given us the most important practical legal and theoretical tools for thinking about a move towards the legal recognition of same-sex relationships. Thus, although these are not the jurisdictions in which same-sex relationships were first recognized in law, they are those in which the fight for recognition has the longest sustained history. For that reason, they demonstrate a level of legal engagement with the issue (and writing on the issue) unmatched in any other part of the world. And it should not be forgotten that Canada and one US state are among the few jurisdictions in the world in which it is now possible for same-sex couples to marry.

North America
The USA
The oldest formal evidence we have (in the modern Western state) of the struggle for state recognition of same-sex relationships are the cases brought before courts in the USA in the early 1970s. In *Baker v Nelson*,[5] two men asserted their legal right to marry each other. The state – Minnesota[6] – refused to sanction the marriage or to issue a marriage licence. The court dismissed the couple's challenge to the decision of local officials. Marriage, as traditionally understood and protected in law, was a heterosexual union. There was, the court found, no reason to alter that tradition. Indeed, in a parallel case in which Baker's proposed spouse (McConnell) was refused the job to which he had been appointed before the controversy over their marriage challenge arose, the court described the employers actions as reasonable. The action in seeking marriage demonstrated, the court said, his desire for 'employment on his own term[s]'. It was 'a case in which the prospective employee demands ... the right to pursue an activist role in *implementing* his unconventional ideas concerning the societal status to be accorded homosexuals and, thereby, to foist tacit approval of his socially repugnant concept upon his employer, who is, in this instance, an institution of higher learning.'[7] In effect, then, same-sex marriage, and the sexuality that gave rise to it, were 'socially repugnant'.

From those dark beginnings a litany of inauspicious attempts to create legally enhanced same-sex relationships arose. Initial (limited) successes were achieved at corporate and local-government level. When the state authorities would not recognize same-sex relationships (and were supported by the courts), activists turned their attention to their localities. By the early 1990s many local authorities and small and large corporations – even in conservative states where marriage at the state level seemed most fervently protected – offered local and corporate versions of marriage-like recognition to same-sex couples. Clearly these had no significant legal consequences. But they did affect rights which were in the power of local government and private business to allocate (local government services and employment benefits, for example; in the USA these can be significant).[8]

But the states were not to be immune from legal pressure simply because local government had taken up the cause of recognizing same-sex relationships. Individuals continued to assert their right to marry on the basis of their desire for equal treatment. And, finally, in Hawaii in 1993 a chink in the 'traditional marriage' armour began to appear. In *Baehr v Lewin*[9] the Hawaii Supreme Court upheld a trial judge's decision that the constitutional guarantee of equal protection, which prevented discrimination on the basis of sex, protected the individual's choice of spouse irrespective of sex.[10] This required the state to permit same-sex marriage unless there were 'compelling' state interests in refusing recognition. Most legal opinion was that establishing sufficiently compelling state interests to protect marriage as a different-sex institution would be an almost insurmountable task. And in *Baehr v Miike*[11] a trial court found it to be so; there were no sufficiently weighty reasons for refusing recognition to same-sex marriage.

Hawaii seemed set to become the first US state to recognize same-sex marriage. However, the state appealed the decision,[12] and while that process was pending it also set about altering the legal rules framing the decision; by referendum, the state amended its constitution to protect marriage as a heterosexual institution,[13] and it legislated for an alternative to marriage for same-sex couples (with a limited selection of marriage consequences available to them).[14] Victory for lesbian and gay activists had been short-lived. And yet defeat was not complete. The Hawaii case and its initial decisions had ignited massive nationwide debate in the USA (and around the world). The issue of same-sex marriage was in the public arena. Even though Hawaii failed to recognize same-sex marriage, it legislated for 'reciprocal beneficiaries', thus acknowledging the profound unfairness inherent in recognizing different-sex marriage without providing for the recognition of same-sex relationships.

The Hawaii experience gave activists hope and enhanced legal tools. The arguments and approach used in Hawaii and their short-lived positive outcome could be put to good use elsewhere in the USA – there were 49 other states in which the challenge could be brought, and it was more than just feasible that some judges in some of these courts would respond as the Hawaii judges had done. In every state in which court battles were pursued over the next decade emotionally charged public debates were ignited, always spreading beyond the borders of the state in which they took place. Same-sex relationships would be pushed further and further out of the closet until their recognition became inevitable. It was always likely that activists would keep fighting until the marriage battle had been won.

The knowledge that these political battle lines were drawn inspired two important reactions in the USA. The first was at the level of federal regulation. The US Congress passed the Defence of Marriage Act in 1996. This legislation set out to protect marriage as a heterosexual institution by allowing the federal government and individual states to refuse recognition to the legal same-sex marriages of those states that, in time, would come to recognize them. In this legislation there is an ironic recognition that same-sex marriage would become legal in some places (in the USA and probably around the world) and that that recognition should be pre-empted.

The second reaction inspired by developments in Hawaii was a trend in other US states to legislate against recognition of same-sex marriage where those marriages were celebrated outside the relevant jurisdiction. There seemed to be a fear that same-sex couples married in one state would infiltrate the many other states that refused to allow such marriages and demand legal recognition of their relationships there. If no defence were available, those marriages would have to be granted legal status everywhere.

Despite these counter-currents, however, the activist struggle for same-sex relationship recognition carried on unabated.[15] By the time of the Hawaii decision, challenges to the inherent heterosexuality of marriage had already been launched in several states[16] and more would follow. In the USA, where public opinion on sexuality is, for a Western nation, remarkably conservative, it was always likely that some battles would be won, but most would be lost. What remained significant was that these struggles took place in state institutional forums that gave public platforms to, and fed, debate on the issue. Even where the particular cases were lost, therefore, the increasing tendency for these matters to be aired outside the closet and inside the most hallowed sanctuaries of state governance was bound to lead to some revision of law that had previously excluded same-sex couples from its scope. State legislation recognizing alternatives to marriage for same-sex couples (other ways of formalizing legally acknowledged relationships) began to proliferate. Hawaii's Reciprocal Beneficiaries legislation (1997)[17] and Vermont's Civil Unions legislation (2000)[18] were the earliest examples of this kind of regulation. But other states – including California (2003),[19] Connecticut (2005),[20] and Oregon (2007)[21] – have followed suit. And more will do so.[22] Each of these legislative devices gives same-sex couples access to some (usually most, if not all) of the legal privileges from which they have, traditionally, been excluded.

Perhaps the most significant single development in the ongoing American same-sex relationships saga has been the steadfast, principled stance of the Massachusetts Supreme Judicial Court on the issue of same-sex marriage. In two opinions – one on a challenge to the ban on same-sex marriage, and the second on the state's proposal to create a civil union[23] alternative to marriage for same-sex couples – the court insisted that only marriage for same-sex couples would do. In *Goodridge v Department of Public Health*[24] the court found that the state could not refuse recognition of same-sex marriage without offending the state's constitutional protections prohibiting discrimination on the grounds of sex. In a separate opinion to the state's senate, the Court held that a parallel institution would remain fundamentally offensive to those anti-discrimination provisions. Only marriage for same-sex couples would be constitutionally compliant. So far the road to constitutional amendment in Massachusetts has not been taken successfully. Attempts have been made to amend the constitution to rescue the heterosexual character of marriage in Massachusetts, but nothing can happen until November 2012 (when it will, for the first time, be possible to put a constitutional amendment to a referendum).[25] Same-sex marriage will have some real life in that state – but that life may be impeded in time. The politics of same-sex marriage in the USA are volatile.

Because the recognition of same-sex marriage was always likely to increase over time, opponents of same-sex marriage have sought an entrenchment of the heterosexuality of marriage. The most secure way to accomplish this end is to amend the US Constitution. President George W Bush proposed such an amendment. Congress, however, has not (to date) taken up that proposal. But similar proposals in many states – including Hawaii – have succeeded.[26] Yet calls for the recognition of same-sex marriage will not go away. The combination of international[27] and domestic pressure[28] – from both institutional (courts) and cultural sources (television, film, and real-life weddings) – will, it seems, inevitably, bring some form of recognition to same-sex relationships in many (if not all) states in the USA. Some will follow the lead established by Massachusetts (opting for marriage).[29] Others will go the way of Hawaii (formal same-sex union separate from marriage). And the debate will rumble on.

Canada
Although Canada came to the issue of legally recognizing same-sex relationships later than the USA, it has progressed much further on the issue and now recognizes same-sex marriage. Unlike US family law, Canadian family law is regulated in part by the federal government under the federal constitution and in part by the provinces.

The advent of the Canadian Charter of Rights and Freedoms in 1982 (a Federal Charter of Rights) gave impetus to this process. Section 15 of the

Charter provided for the equal protection of all Canadians from discrimination on a number of stipulated grounds. These did not include sexual identity or orientation, but in 1995 the Canadian Supreme Court – in *Egan v Canada*[30] – took the view that sexual orientation was an 'analogous' ground upon which discrimination would be unconstitutional. The aftermath of that momentous decision was bound, eventually, to include the extension to same-sex families of the full panoply of family rights and obligations enjoyed by different-sex couples. Progress was initially patchy (some provinces moved on the issue more quickly than others) but the federal government did, quite early, decide that the battle was not worth fighting. In 2003 it decided not to appeal against an Ontario Appellate court ruling[31] requiring that same-sex marriage be recognized if the state were to comply with the Charter of Rights. Instead, the government announced its intention to legislate for same-sex marriage. In July 2005 legislation was passed confirming the court-based process towards the recognition of same-sex marriage. Canada was now firmly in the group of states opting for the legal recognition of same-sex marriage.

Europe

European progress towards the recognition of same-sex relationships has been very different from the North-American experience. It is possible that our attention has been diverted by our inability (because of language barriers) to follow developments in Europe in the way in which we follow them in the English-speaking world. But it is probably accurate to say that Europe's progress has not been based on court challenges founded on notions of fundamental rights to the same extent as North American challenges have been. European legal changes – although influenced by human-rights norms – have been waged more powerfully (and successfully) in political and not legal forums. Civil law jurisdictions seem more attentive to political compromise on issues of social, moral and ethical controversy, and legislatures seem more willing to address controversial issues. European progress therefore starts with limited partnership recognition framed as compromise in legislatures, and then moves to full marriage recognition, again through legislative action.

Formal progress started on the continent with the Danish Registered Partnerships legislation of 1989. For the first time in the world this gave a legal status to same-sex couples who had been denied marriage and had sought legal recognition elsewhere. By this time Sweden had already extended its (generous) provisions for unmarried cohabitants to same-sex couples,[32] but formal marriage relationships were still exclusively heterosexual. Within a few years, all the Scandinavian countries (Norway in 1993, Sweden in 1994, Iceland in 1996, and Finland in 2001) had followed the Danish lead by creating registration schemes for same-sex relationships that provided most of the legal benefits of marriage.

From its early outing in Denmark, the idea of domestic-partnership registration filtered into the rest of Europe. But two of the Benelux countries and Spain took the matter further. The Netherlands has the distinction of having been first in the world to complete the transition to same-sex marriage.[33] In 1998 it set up a partnership-registration scheme and, after a very short interlude, enacted legislation to recognize same-sex marriage in 2001.[34] Belgium followed a similar path, but was slightly slower than its neighbour: its registration scheme came into being in 2000 and it enacted legislation recognizing same-sex marriage in 2003 (but only completed that process by recognizing gay adoption in 2005).[35] Luxembourg remains the conservative Benelux country, with only a registration scheme, which came into effect in 2004. Spain is one of the two European Mediterranean states to have formalized its recognition of same-sex relationship, and it is the only one to have progressed all the way to same-sex marriage (which it did in 2005).[36]

France and Germany followed a more cautious path. In 1999 France created an alternative status to marriage for anyone who wished to enter it. The Pacte Civil de Solidarité (PaCS) provided a limited range of marriage-like consequences for those who could not marry (including same-sex couples) or wished for something with fewer legal consequences imposed upon the partners than marriage would impose. Although the shared rights and obligations were, initially, fairly limited, over the years the PaCS has grown into a formal status very close to marriage.[37]

Germany's Life Partnership Act of 2001 followed a similar trajectory. It started as a fairly limited registration scheme granting limited marriage-like rights and obligations, but has grown into something approximating marriage. Politicians were of the opinion that the protected status of marriage under the German Constitution required that any alternative to marriage have less serious consequences than marriage; it would have to be a secondary institution, clearly marked out as such. However, the German Constitutional Court found that the constitution would not stand in the way of same-sex partnerships equivalent to heterosexual marriage, and a 2004 amendment to the legislation enhanced the legal consequences of same-sex relationships so that they are now much closer to marriage.

Some European countries have taken an interesting approach to the recognition of same-sex relationships. Essentially, they have recognized same-sex relationships as part of another family phenomenon that has grown in significance in the last half century and requires resolution: unmarried cohabitation. In 1996 Hungary's civil code was amended to provide state recognition (for limited purposes) of unmarried relationships; these provisions applied equally to same-sex relationships (Hungary went on to pass civil-partnership legislation in December 2007).[38] Portugal followed this trend in 2001,[39] legislating for an extension of the consequences of unmarried cohabitation to same-sex couples. Croatia[40] and Austria[41] did something similar in 2003 (although Austria may have been induced to take this action by the European Court of Human Rights decision in *Karner v Austria*[42]).

The United Kingdom started its progress towards the recognition of same-sex relationships in a similar fashion. From the mid-1990s, legislation applied to unmarried heterosexual cohabitants was gradually extended to same-sex couples (culminating in the *Fitzpatrick* and *Mendoza* decisions in the House of Lords[43] and in the Adoption and Children Act of 2002[44]). But it was also clear that some formal recognition was required. In 2004 the British Parliament finally passed the Civil Partnerships Act, which recognized the registered relationships of same-sex couples as the equivalent of marriages. They had almost all its consequences, though such registered relationships were available only to same-sex couples. If different-sex couples wished to have the same rights, the government explained, they had only to marry. The UK had created gay marriage, but without using the language of marriage.

A number of other European states have recently introduced partnership-registration schemes. These include Switzerland (2005, by popular referendum),[45] Andorra (2005),[46] the Czech Republic (2006)[47], Slovenia (2006)[48] and Hungary (2007).[49] Several other states are in the process of considering registration schemes or have done so, but have not yet implemented them. These include Ireland, Italy, Lichtenstein, and Poland.

The rest of the world

Except, perhaps, for Australia and New Zealand, the rest of the world is not as obviously Western in its cultural composition as Europe and North America are. It ought, therefore, to be no surprise that Western states were the first to provide formal recognition to same-sex relationships.[50] The sexual identity upon which such legal demands are made, is, after all, a phenomenon of Western cultural history,[51] and has extended to the rest of the world because of colonial history and, more latterly, globalization.

I will, therefore, start this section of my analysis with a look at developments in Australia and New Zealand. The analysis will then roam through the haphazard collection of other states around the world in which progress has been made towards the formal recognition of same-sex relationships, whether or not those relationships are celebrated formally.

Australia and New Zealand

Australia's legal attitude towards same-sex families is complicated by its federal system, which, like Canada's, leaves some family regulation to the states and some to the federal government. The state-based systems in Australia have been fairly progressive in their recognition of and allocation of rights to *unmarried* families; same-sex couples were incorporated into these programmes fairly early on. Furthermore, some same-sex partnership registers have been created at the local and state level, allocating a few additional formal consequences to same-sex couples.[52]

But federal regulation (in particular, its jurisdiction over the regulation of marriage) has been (until the recent change of government) much more conservative, and there has been very little progress towards same-sex marriage in Australia. Ironically, the incorporation of same-sex relationships into *unmarried* family regulation may be partly to blame for this slow progress: because there are legal avenues available to same-sex couples to claim family status, there has been no pressing need to push for same-sex marriage. That and the fact that the federal government was in one of the most sustained periods of conservatism in Australian history tell us why progress has not been made.

Because of its cultural similarities with the Anglo-American world, however, it is likely that these problems will be progressively addressed and resolved. The new Prime Minister has already indicated his preference for legislating for same-sex partnership registers and recent polling suggests that most Australians favour same-sex marriage recognition.[53]

New Zealand – like South Africa – is a unitary jurisdiction. There is no separation of family regulation between central and regional governments. This has meant that same-sex couples have, as in the UK, benefited from the gradual extension of family benefits to them. Two developments worthy of note are the extension of unmarried cohabitation rights to same-sex couples and the creation in 2005 of a civil-union status to which same-sex couples have access,[54] giving them the rights and obligations of marriage.

South and Central America, the Middle East, and South Africa

Uruguay approved same-sex civil unions at national level in January 2007, becoming the first South American state to do so. Brazil, Argentina, and Mexico each have provinces and cities that provide civil recognition to same-sex unions, but only to the extent that they have the power to do so. Local government rarely has power to define marriage or determine its legal consequences. There are, however, local consequences (locally administered welfare benefits, housing, etc) that depend upon a local recognition of the status of claimants, and here same-sex relationships are recognized. But there is no national recognition of same-sex relationships in these countries. Israel also provides limited recognition to same-sex (unmarried) relationships.[55]

Because South Africa is the subject of this book, no detailed analysis of that jurisdiction will be offered here. But I do have two comments about the Civil Union Act passed in 2006. In the first place, it allows same-sex couples to marry or to form a civil union – but the consequences of each are indistinguishable from one another. In this respect it is full marriage and it is a civil partnership or union like those celebrated in places like the UK, Connecticut, or New Zealand. In the second place, it is an Act inspired by a court process that compelled its existence. This isn't democratic legislation in the ordinary sense. It is legislation passed by a majoritarian democratic process after a court decision required that the interests of a minority, protected by the Constitution, should be dignified with an appropriate status. In this respect, it is the culmination of a process that resembles those in Hawaii, Massachusetts and Canada (although with different outcomes in each of those jurisdictions). And it is unlike the process in most European jurisdictions where reform was (largely) based on debates in legislatures and in other political forums.

Two further observations are necessary. First, in this jurisdiction, unlike many of the others reflected in this overview, unmarried cohabitation has no significant legal consequence.[56] Those who cannot marry are, therefore, not family for the purposes of many of the rights and obligations of family law. There is no other way to acquire these than by marriage. Second (and related to this point), the South African state makes only the most rudimentary welfare provision for its people. In these circumstances family relationships are like American family relationships in providing the source of fundamentally important material support to people living in relationships which have no legal status. There were, therefore, pressing social reasons for the need to recognize same-sex relationships as family relationships in South Africa.

Queering family law?

Same-sex families and the recognition of same-sex relationships are moving family law in the direction of diversity,[57] but I take the view that this does not, in any profound sense, 'queer' family law.[58] Still, moves like those described in this essay do make us consider other family norms and familial needs. Institutionalizing these will bring us closer to a queer (or queerer) family law.

The debate about and (in some places) recognition of same-sex relationships has reminded family lawyers that marriage itself is not a uniform tradition, despite the assertions of some of its traditional defenders. Its rules and consequences differ from place to place and have changed over time.[59] The adventure we are on – promoting the legal recognition of same-sex relationships – is an adventure in discovering the variety of relationships that family law around the world can recognize. Changes in the status of relationships, and differences in legal recognition across different countries,[60] will, in time, cause us to rethink the very bases upon which we recognize family relationships. At present we look for formality; my suspicion is that in the future we will look to something else: function, perhaps.

Perhaps the closest we will get to really 'queer marriage' will arrive in the guise of unmarried relationship recognition.⁶¹ Legal authorities will impute a marriage-like status to relationships that satisfy a large variety of objectively verifiable relationship criteria. Formalities celebrated in one country may be sufficient to have a marriage recognized in another – but so too might other extraneous characteristics (child rearing, familial caring, interdependence, long standing cohabitation, etc.). These 'marriages' will only be queer to the extent that there might be a greater variety of relationships recognized by the state. But I think that a more profound queering of family law must be sought elsewhere than in the formal recognition of same-sex relationships.⁶²

Parenthood might provide fruitful analytical terrain.⁶³ Historically, in Western societies at least, parenthood was intrinsic to marriage. Childbearing outside marriage was socially taboo, leading to severe legal disadvantage for children and legal and social ostracism for mothers. But the Western world has, again, changed quite dramatically in the last half-century. The growing concern for the rights and well-being of children and our changing moral ethos have meant that unmarried women frequently have children without risking (traditional) moral opprobrium.

Because our concern has shifted from the marital relationship to the relationship between adults and children, the state has had to alter much of the law relating to children. To promote their welfare the law has been adapted to – and become supportive of – the many unorthodox ways in which children are reared. Before same-sex relationships were formally recognized, it was clear that rearing children was a way in which some family recognition would accrue to same-sex couples (even in the USA, where progress on adult relationship recognition has been slowest). This concern for children encourages the promotion of stable relationships. Because Western societies regard married-type relationships as more stable than unmarried relationships, it is necessary to pursue an ideal of formal relationships for those raising children. The rearing of children, therefore, has had an important impact on the promotion of formal same-sex relationships. But again, this is only the mildest queering of family law.

Something more important than the recognition of formal same-sex relationships may be happening in the family laws of the jurisdictions I have considered. That something relates to unmarried cohabitation. People who fail to formalize their relationships create difficulties for lawyers and policymakers. When such informal family relationships end, many are left with an uncomfortable feeling about what the consequences of those relationships should be. The problem is that, where no family-law remedy exists, resolution will rely on ordinary law. But law that settles the consequences of intimate relationships as if they were business (or other 'stranger') relationships, where there is no familial intimacy, seems misapplied. Family relationships – including unmarried family relationships – deserve law of a different order.

Yet recognizing the problem does not provide a solution. At its simplest, the problem of providing rules to govern unmarried cohabitation is that, because people fail to marry for a great variety of reasons, solutions must necessarily be various. Trying to work out a single (family) pattern of consequence for the very different relationships in the category of unmarried cohabitation is almost impossible.

An eventual solution to the regulation of unmarried relationships is likely to give us a much clearer idea of how we might successfully promote diversity in the legal recognition of family relationships. When we have managed to set up a fair process that operates a fair set of rules to deal with the consequences of all family relationships – from marriage and civil unions to the great variety of unmarried relationships – we will have come as close as we ever will to creating a legal framework for the real admiration of diverse families.[64]

Notes

1 See, for example, Robert Wintemute and Mads Andenaes (eds.), *Legal Recognition of Same-Sex Partnerships: A Study of National, European and International Law* (Hart, 2001); Andrew Sullivan (ed.), *Same-Sex Marriage, Pro and Con: A Reader* (revised edition, Vintage, 2004); Patricia A Gozemba and Karen Kahn, *Courting Equality: A Documentary History of Same-Sex Marriage in America* (Beacon, 2007). There are hosts of other books and many more articles in learned journals across disciplines dealing with this subject. Any academic library search will yield a wealth of literature on the topic.
2 Taken from the title of Stephen Cretney's book, *Same-Sex Relationships: From 'Odious Crime' to 'Gay Marriage'* (OUP, 2006), which borrows the expression from the view of same-sex sexuality adopted in some English cases: see, for example, *Russell v Russell* [1897] AC 395 (Cretney, 3).
3 The fact of the Civil Union Act of 2006 (and similar legislation in countries around the world) demonstrates the extent to which this must be so.
4 By jurisdiction, I mean a geographic area with a single legal system and a fairly uniform set of legal rules. Calling the United States – and some others – 'a' jurisdiction for these purposes is, therefore, problematic. For the purposes of the recognition of same-sex relationships the USA consists of 51 (significant) jurisdictions: there are the 50 states, each with its own family laws, and there is the federal state which, although it has no role in the regulation of the family, does have a peripheral role in allocating federal legal consequences to family relationships (like, for example, federal taxation which offers spouses some privileges). There are, of course, other authorities which exercise (particularly cultural) power in relation to family recognition (like, for example, local government) which will not be considered here: for more on local government in relation to same-sex relationships see Craig Lind, '"Pretended Families", Law and the Local State in the UK and the USA', in *International Journal of Law and the Family* 10 (1996), 134-158.
5 191 NW 2d 185 (Minn. 1971); 409 US 810 (1972), appeal dismissed. There are a number of cases which follow this lead: another early example is *Singer v Hara* 522 P 2d 1187 (Ct App. Wash., 1974), 84 Wash. 2d 1008 (1974), review denied

6 It is interesting to note that Minnesota did not have a gender-specific definition of marriage. It is not alone among US states in this category.
7 *McConnell v Anderson* 451 F 2d 193 (8th Cir. 1971), 405 US 1046 (1972), cert. denied
8 See Lind, op. cit. This trend towards the more localized recognition of same-sex relationships was followed around the world, especially in countries in which there was (and in some, still remains) no appetite for the full legal recognition of same-sex relationships (outside of North America and the UK, parts of Spain and France also adopted this strategy before national schemes of recognition were established. Brazil and Argentina are examples of states still in this category).
9 *Baehr v Lewin* 852 P 2d 44 (1993)
10 One of the clearest proponents of the view that discrimination on the grounds of sexual orientation is a form of sex discrimination prohibited by sex-discrimination statutes is Robert Wintemute. See, for example, Wintemute, *Sexual Orientation and Human Rights* (Clarendon Press, 1995), especially 199ff.
11 Judgment of Chang J in the Circuit Court of the First Circuit Civil, Case 91-1394: 1996 WL 694235 (Haw. Cir. Ct Dec. 3, 1996)
12 See *Baehr v Miike* (1999) 994 P 2d 566
13 1997 Haw. Sess. Laws HB 117 § 2, at 1247
14 Hawaii's Reciprocal Beneficiaries legislation – Haw. Rev. Stat. § 572C-1 (2004) – allocated around 60 rights previously exclusive to married couples to be extended to those who were prevented in law from marrying (including same-sex couples).
15 Even school rules on the partners of pupils (and ex-pupils) were challenged: see, for example, *Engel v Worthington* 23 Cal. Rptr 2d 329 (Ct App. 1993), where it was held to be unlawful sex discrimination to refuse to include a photograph of a same-sex couple in a high school reunion memory book, and *Fricke v Lunch* 491 F.Supp. 381 (RI US Dist. 1980), in which a schoolboy successfully challenged his school's refusal to allow him to take his male partner to the school prom.
16 Examples include Alaska (*Brause v Bureau of Vital Statistics* 1998 WL 88743 (Alaska Supr. Ct 1998), Vermont (*Baker v State*, 744 A 2d 864 81 ALR 5th 627; Vt 1999) and Washington DC (*Dean v District of Columbia* 653 A 2d 307; DC 1995).
17 Hawaii Revised Statutes § 572C
18 Vermont Civil Union Act, Act 91 of 2000 (26 April 2000)
19 Domestic Partner Rights and Responsibilities Act, Chapter 421, 2003 Cal. Stat. 2586
20 Public Act 05-10 (SB 963): An Act Concerning Civil Unions (passed 20 April 2005, effective 1 October 2005)
21 Family Fairness Act 2007 (passed 9 May, effective 1 January 2008)
22 Movement is quite erratic and can be fairly quick. I know there is talk of similar legislation in New York and New Hampshire at present, and probably in much of the rest of the north east. But other states are also bound to follow in time.
23 In this essay I have used 'civil union', 'civil partnership', 'reciprocal beneficiaries', and similar expressions to describe a type of gay 'marriage' that allocates some (sometimes almost all) marriage rights to same-sex couples, but does not wish to see same-sex couples simply regulated under the ordinary laws of marriage.
24 440 Mass. 309; 798 NE 2d 941. It is, perhaps interesting to note that Chief Justice Marshall, who authored this ground -breaking opinion, was born and raised in South Africa and graduated from the University of the Witwatersrand in 1966. See the website of the Supreme Judicial Court of Massachusetts: http://www.mass.gov/courts/sjc/justices/marshall.html (last accessed 15 October 2007)
25 Pam Belluck, 'Massachusetts Gay Marriage Referendum Is Rejected', *International Herald*

Tribune, 14 June 2007; available at http://www.iht.com/articles/2007/06/15/america/15gay-web.php (last accessed on 31 January 2008)
26 So far at least 11 states have amended their constitutions to inscribe heterosexuality into marriage. Even more (almost all) specifically define marriage in their statutes or their common law heterosexually: see Paul Axel-Lute, 'Same-Sex Marriage: A Selective Bibliography of the Legal Literature', http://law-library.rutgers.edu/SSM.html (last accessed 31 January 2008)
27 See below, for developments in other (principally Western) nations around the world – which would, in time, begin to affect the way in which the debate was framed in the USA.
28 Activism on the issue continues unabated in the USA. Most (if not all) states have significant community organizations dedicated to achieving same-sex marriage in their state and across the Union.
29 Iowa has just followed suit in a trial decision that is on appeal to the Iowa Supreme Court: see Associated Press, 'Judge Overturns Iowa Ban on Same-Sex Marriages', *New York Times*, 31 August 2007. See too Arthur S Leonard, 'Iowa Trial Courts Rules for Same-Sex Couples in Marriage Case', http://newyorklawschool.typepad.com/leonardlink/2007/08/iowa-trial-cour.html (last accessed 31 January 2008).
30 Canada (1995) 2 SCR 513. Despite this finding the court did not find that the creation of heterosexual family benefits denied to same-sex couples was unconstitutional discrimination. In 1993 a court had already dismissed a claim that prohibiting same-sex marriage contravened the constitutional guarantee of equality free from discrimination in *Layland v Ontario* (1993) 14 OR (3d) 658.
31 *Halpern v Toronto* (2003) 65 OR (3d) 161. A series of court decisions in Canadian provinces had paved the way for same-sex marriage recognition in those provinces by this time. The legal and community politics on the issue were similar to those experienced in the USA, but with less of the conservative and religious vitriol that frequently accompanied debate about the issue in the USA.
32 The Swedish Homosexual Cohabitants Act 1987
33 It is possible that Canada had, in effect, recognized same-sex marriage first by virtue of its provincial court decisions. But because there was some doubt about the status of those decisions and the relationships they created, Canadian same-sex marriage is reliably traced to the federal legislation on the issue. This is the problem judging legal developments in countries in which courts make decisions changing legal status. Those decisions must be allowed to settle into legal certainty before that status can be relied upon confidently. And this sometimes takes time. A retrospective judgment may, therefore, one day be made that the first legal same-sex marriages celebrated in the world were celebrated in Canada. Or elsewhere in the world, where they have yet to be tested in courts of law.
34 'Dutch Legalize Gay Marriage', *BBC News*, 12 September 2000, http://news.bbc.co.uk/2/hi/europe/922024.stm (last accessed 31 January 2008); 'Gay Marriage Goes Dutch: World's First Same-Sex Marriages Under Law in the Netherlands', CBS News, 1 April 2001, http://www.cbsnews.com/stories/2001/04/01/world/main283071.shtml (last accessed 31 January 2008)
35 See Danny McCoy, 'Belgium's Parliament Backs Gay Adoption', 6 December 2005, http://www.pinknews.co.uk/news/articles/2005-234.html (last accessed 31 January 2008). See too 'Gay Marriage around the Globe', *BBC News*, 22 December 2005, http://news.bbc.co.uk/2/hi/americas/4081999.stm (last accessed 31 January 2008)
36 'Spain Approves Gay Marriage bill', *BBC News*, 1 October 2004, http://news.bbc.co.uk/2/hi/europe/3706414.stm (last accessed 31 January 2008); Jennifer Green, 'Spain Legalizes Same-Sex Marriage', *Washington Post*, 1 July 2005, http://www.washingtonpost.com/wp-dyn/content/ article/2005/06/30/AR2005063000245.html (last accessed 31 January 2008)
37 It may be that the 'growth' of the significance of the PaCS was a deliberate political strategy

designed by activists and politicians to take the sting out of a full-scale public battle for same-sex marriage recognition.
38 'Timeline of Gay and Lesbian Marriage, Partnership or Unions Worldwide', *UK Gay News*, 28 December 2007, http://www.ukgaynews.org.uk/Archive/2005dec/0502.htm (last accessed 31 January 2008)
39 This occurs despite the conservative attitude of the Portuguese state evidenced in its action before the European Court of Human Rights in 2001: *Salgueiro da Silva Mouta v Portugal* (2001) 1 FCR 653 (in which a gay father challenged the decision of a Portuguese Court of Appeal to remove his child from him because he was gay).
40 'Timeline of Gay and Lesbian Marriage ...', op. cit. (note 38)
41 Ibid.
42 *Karner v Austria* (2003) 38 EHHR 528 (in which the court found that preferring different-sex couples to same-sex couples for the purposes of succession to tenancies amounted to discrimination contrary to Article 14 of the European Convention on Human Rights).
43 *Fitzpatrick v Sterling Housing Association* (1999) 2 FLR 1027 and *Ghaidan v Mendoza* (2004) 2 AC 557. In these cases same-sex partners were extended the right to inherit a tenancy from deceased partners. Initially, in *Fitzpatrick*, this was done on the basis that the legislation permitted such property transfers to members of the 'family' of the deceased. But later, in *Mendoza*, the court treated same-sex couples as cohabitants in the mould of heterosexual cohabitants who had to pass a 'spouse-like' test.
44 This Act allowed same-sex couples to adopt children as couples for the first time in English law.
45 'Timeline of Gay and Lesbian Marriage ...', op. cit.
46 Ibid.
47 This legislation was passed by the Czech legislature, then vetoed by the president, and finally reinstated by a parliamentary override in July 2006. See 'Timeline of Gay and Lesbian Marriage ...', op. cit.
48 Ibid.
49 Ibid.
50 Of course, it is possible that same-sex sexual conduct has given rise to patterns of family life which are recognized in other parts of the world. But the little anthropological writing on the issue – such as Will Roscoe and Stephen O Murray (eds.), *Boy-Wives and Female Husbands: Studies in African Homosexualities* (Palgrave, 1998) – does seem to problematize the issue. For that reason, I continue to take the view that pressing for same-sex marriage is a predominantly Western concern.
51 See Michel Foucault, *The History of Sexuality, Volume 1: An Introduction*, translated by Robert Hurley (Penguin, 1978); Jeffrey Weeks, *Coming Out: Homosexual Politics in Britain, from the Nineteenth Century to the Present* (Quartet, 1977); Weeks, *Sex, Politics and Society: The Regulation of Sexuality since 1800* (second edition, Longman, 1989); and Randolph Trumbach, 'The Birth of the Queen: Sodomy and the Emergence of Gender Equality in Modern Culture, 1660-1750', in Martin B Duberman, Martha Vicinus and Jeffrey Chauncey, Jr (eds.), *Hidden from History: Reclaiming the Gay and Lesbian Past* (Penguin, 1991), 129.
52 See, for example, the legislation in Tasmania and the Australian Capital Territory.
53 Michelle Paine, 'Registry Wins Gay Support', *Mercury*, 17 December 2007, http://www.news.com.au/mercury/story/0,22884,22935535-3462,00.html (last accessed 31 January 2008); Angus Reid Global Monitor, 'Australians Back Same-Sex Marriage', 28 June 2007, http://www.angus-reid.com/polls/view/australians_back_same_sex_marriage/ (last accessed 31 January 2008)
54 By the Civil Unions Act 102 of 2004.
55 For immigration purposes, unmarried same- and different-sex couples can apply for the same kind of immigration status, governed by the same conditions.

56 See *Volks v Robinson* 2005 (5) BCLR 446 (CC). Although unmarried same-sex couples were given significant rights before same-sex relationships gained recognition in the Civil Union Act, we cannot, it is submitted, be certain that those rights will survive the enactment of that legislation.
57 See William N Eskridge, 'The Ideological Structure of the Same-Sex Marriage Debate (and some Postmodern Arguments for Same-Sex Marriage)'; Janet Halley, 'Recognition, Rights, Regulation, Normalisation: Rhetorics of Justification in the Same-Sex Marriage Debate', both in Wintemute and Andenaes (eds.), op. cit.
58 I use 'queer' in this piece to reflect an idea of disrupting 'norms' of family behaviour and family formation. Although I understand that the law is not the best place in which normalization might be challenged, it seems to me possible to argue for a queerer law if we could argue for a more open recognition of unsettled and various family forms. See Valerie Lehr, *Queer Family Values: Debunking the Myth of the Nuclear Family* (Temple University Press, 1999).
59 Western culture sometimes demonstrates an incredibly short memory with respect to the nature of marriage. The advent of (easy) divorce is the clearest illustration of how dramatically 'marriage' can change in a fairly short period of time.
60 See *Wilkinson v Kritzinger* (2006) All ER (D) 479, in which a same-sex couple married in Canada tried (and failed) to have their marriage recognized as a valid marriage in the UK (and not simply as a civil partnership under the Civil Partnership Act of 2004).
61 Something like the tradition of common-law marriage, in which marriage was imputed to people who did not satisfy the requisite formalities for marriage but demonstrated other extraneous characteristics that allowed their societies (especially historically) to presume them to be married in the full legal sense (and so inescapable except by divorce).
62 For an excellent critique of moves to queer marriage through a political strategy aimed at achieving same-sex marriage see Davina Cooper, 'Like Counting Stars? Re-Structuring Equality and the Socio-Legal Space of Same-Sex Marriage', in Wintemute and Andenaes (eds.), op. cit.
63 See Alison Diduck, '"If Only We Can Find the Appropriate Terms to Use the Issue Will Be Solved": Law, Identity and Parenthood', in *Child and Family Law Quarterly* 19 (2007), 458; Sally Sheldon, 'Fragmenting Fatherhood: The Regulation of Reproductive Technologies', in *Modern Law Review* 68 (2005), 523
64 I have left out of this account a discussion of the appropriateness of Western family norms and values in cultures that are not Western. That discussion would also have to engage with the problematic nature of (Western) homosexuality that has led to calls for and the development of Western-style family structures for same-sex couples in non-Western states (like South Africa). See Craig Lind, 'Unanswerable Dilemmas? – Legal Regulation for Cross-Cultural Family Norms', in Penelope E Andrews (ed.), *Comparative Constitutionalism and Rights: Global Perspectives* (forthcoming).

'We first need to be recognized'
Activists reflect on same-sex marriage and LGBTI rights in Africa

In May 2007 more than 60 LGBTI activists from 15 African countries gathered in Johannesburg, South Africa, to discuss ways in which to consolidate the LGBTI movement and make further progress in self-organizing at a regional level. This first-ever pan-African LGBTI conference was organized by the International Lesbian and Gay Association (ILGA), along with African partner organizations. The editors of this book took the opportunity to talk to some of the delegates about the passing of the Civil Union Act in South Africa and its implications for their own countries and activism. Their responses were collated into the following discussion.

The participants are:
- Linda Baumann works for The Rainbow Project, an LGBTI organization in Namibia.
- David Kato is from Uganda, where he works with Integrity, a faith-based organization that deals with homosexuality and religion. Integrity is a member organization of the LGBTI coalition, Sexual Minorities Uganda.
- The Reverend Rowland Jide Macauley is the founder of the House of Rainbow Metropolitan Community Church in Nigeria. The church is an LGBTI-affirming congregation.
- Lourence Misedah is from Kenya, where he works for a community-based organization called Ishtar MSM that works on identifying the health needs of men who have sex with men in Kenya.
- In 2002, Naome Ruzindana formed an organization in Rwanda called Little Sisters of Rwanda. It later developed into the Horizon Community Association (HOCA), which aims to raise awareness of LGBTI issues.

How did you get involved in lesbian and gay activism?
David (Uganda): I was working in Uganda, but when they discovered I was gay they chased me from the job. I managed to come to South Africa, where they were a bit more open about being gay. It was the early 1990s and the National Coalition for Gay and Lesbian Equality was working on the equality clause. I became involved with the National Coalition. We used to meet with Edwin Cameron and Simon Nkoli in the Skyline bar in Hillbrow. This is when I picked

up this activism work. I realized people in South Africa were fighting for their rights. When I left South Africa and went back to Uganda I realized that we, the gay people of Uganda, were also being discriminated against. I dreamed of doing the same as South Africa. But I was got by the police and put in police custody for a week because I had some gay literature with me. So I gave up for some time. But I realized that I really had to do something to take care of the young ones who are just coming out. I'm a Christian, so when I heard that the Ugandan Bishop Senyonjo had formed a group for gay and lesbian Christians called Integrity, I joined. Our bishops and our clergy are very conservative and Senyonjo was then excommunicated from the church in Uganda when it became public. Integrity tries to help people who have been marginalized because of their sexual orientation.

Linda (Namibia): Activism has always been part of me. But it was internal homophobia that started off my gay and lesbian activism. I was always curious to read magazines about LGBTI people, but I did not want to be associated with them. In the end I realized this was because of the set up that I grew up with in Namibia where homosexuality was seen as abnormal. I ended up in The Rainbow Project, where I was a volunteer for three years. I am now employed by them, and I am working with issues of sexuality and human rights. We celebrated our tenth anniversary of achievements in 2007.

Naome (Rwanda): I'm an accountant by profession and I worked in a bank. I was already a lesbian, but I thought I was alone. Then I came to know my neighbour, a lady I worked with at the bank, who was very rough and built. There was one time that we went out and she told me that she was a lesbian. I told her that I was as well, and we started a relationship. We began meeting other girls who were lesbian while we were going out, and each year we would discover more girls. When we found out that there were many of us we decided to form a group. We formed it in 2002, and we named it Little Sisters of Rwanda.

Rowland Jide (Nigeria): I think the purpose behind setting up the church in Nigeria is because I have gone through experiences in my life where I have been marginalized. And I thought it was wrong. It's not a political move to have a church. I think that it fills the gap for the spirituality of sexual minorities in Nigeria. The Nigerian president and religious leaders said that there are no homosexuals in Nigeria. I took a stance to say, 'Hello, I am a Nigerian and I am gay.' I called myself a 'happy holy homosexual'. Which I think for me is a liberating slogan.

What is the situation for lesbian and gay people in your country?[1]

David (Uganda): Right now the authorities are still harassing us and arresting us. But we are encouraging and sensitizing the LGBTI people in our country not to give in to blackmail from the police, but rather to take the case to court so that we can ask the government why Uganda is not acting in accordance with the international covenants it has signed. Uganda is one of the signatories of many international covenants that talk about non-discrimination. But when they come back from signing, the Constitution is not changed. One of the objectives of Integrity and Sexual Minorities Uganda is to fight the legal system and the discriminatory laws. We are trying to advocate and lobby organizations and decision-makers to fight these laws. We need to remove the idea our leaders have that this is a white thing. They are always saying that it is the whites who are spreading this homosexuality. They forget that we are born gay.

Linda (Namibia): Namibia's population is 1,8-million, which is about the same size as that of Soweto. But the level of homophobia is high. I live in a township where I still face homophobia. I am told to be careful – *'Jy moet oppas, ons gaan jou kry'* ['You must watch out, we're going to get you']. The hate crimes are also high. Last year The Rainbow Project started documenting some of the hate crimes, including two gay men who were killed. We also have a lot of lesbians and gay men who are experiencing 'correctional rape'. But people do not speak about it. That is why The Rainbow Project campaign for this year [2007] is to raise awareness of the importance of documenting hate crimes. There is no law in Namibia that explicitly says homosexuality is illegal. Chapter 3 of the Namibian Constitution speaks about the fundamental human rights of people in the country and that gives LGBTI people some room to manoeuvre. But the Labour Act, which was the only Namibian law that protected LGBTI people, was changed in 2004 and the clause about sexual orientation was removed. While we have backbenchers in Parliament who support the LGBTI struggle, I feel most of our politicians do not really want to sit down with the LGBTI community in Namibia and talk about their issues. It is already often said that homosexuality is 'unAfrican'. Somewhere, somehow, the rights of LGBTI people in Namibia will be recognized. I believe in that, and am committing my life to it.

Lourence (Kenya): Currently it is illegal to be gay or lesbian in Kenya. But people are being charged with public indecency and not for being gay or lesbian. We took a petition to the Kenyan Human Rights Commission who agreed to help us. They said that no-one should be discriminated against because of their sexual orientation. We are trying to work out legal systems to ensure this. We are also trying to use health as an entry point, and we've been included in the National AIDS Control Council (NACC) Strategic Plan. The NACC is a governmental body. If the government accepts the health bit of it, then we will use that to get them to accept the legal bit of it. There are some gay and lesbian people who are publicly out in Kenya. But this involves risks. During the recent World Social Forum held in Kenya, the Gay and Lesbian Coalition of Kenya (GALCK) hosted a discussion that aimed to raise gay and lesbian issues. We were tired of politicians in Kenya saying that we do not exist, and that homosexuality is 'unAfrican'. We felt it was important to put a face to the issue and so some of us agreed to talk to the media. But the media had just found out that South Africa had passed the Civil Union Act and what they did was to misrepresent us and said that we wanted to do the same in Kenya. The interview was shown on TV. I had problems with my family after that. They disowned me and said that they did not want to associate with me. I was thrown out of the place where I was staying, and I didn't have anywhere to go for a time.

Naome (Rwanda): The Constitution of the Republic of Rwanda does not consider homosexuality. But – how ever much they pretend we are not there – it still says in the penal code of Rwanda that whoever is discovered and found guilty of homosexuality is supposed to be put in prison. A while back they announced they are going to change the penal code, and said that since Rwanda is a democratic country they must include us. We are waiting for that to be finalized. When people in Rwanda hear of homosexuals they regard them as irresponsible people who are not educated and dress as others cannot. If we homosexuals are in a bar, they will get out of that bar. If we lesbians are in a church, we will not be allowed to sit next to a girl. Society does not allow us. Even our families do not like us. But it also gives you the courage to work hard to please the people in your family and to challenge them, so that they can believe in what you are doing. One of the challenges we're facing is that although I'm out it is difficult for me to identify other lesbians apart from the ones I formed the organization with. Even if you know someone is a lesbian and you approach her and tell her about yourself and your activism, she tells you, 'No, I'm not a lesbian.' They think you are spying on them.

Rowland Jide (Nigeria): The Nigerian penal code stipulates that carnal knowledge is prohibited between a man and a woman and also between men. Same-sex relationships are prohibited and this is the law that is enforced against homosexuals. Of course the chances of enforcing it against heterosexuals are very slim. This law was inherited from the colonial era, and it has remained on Nigeria's statute books up to today. In 2006 the Nigerian government introduced the Same-Sex Marriage (Prohibition) Bill. The Bill is an attempt to ban homosexuality and gay marriage, and it seeks to push away the issue of homosexuality or any association with it – including gathering literature, attending lectures, or anything to do with same-sex relationships. The legislation has a history in that the government said there are no homosexuals in Nigeria, and that homosexuality is 'unAfrican' and unbiblical. Now obviously when activists globally, including myself, spoke out that we are Nigerians and we are homosexual, the Nigerian government introduced the Bill. To me it is telling me that they are now acknowledging that there are homosexuals in Nigeria but they want to outlaw them. They want them to become outcasts under the law. There is homophobia on every street in Nigeria. Because if you are gay and it becomes public knowledge, people are going to taunt you, they are going to verbally abuse you. It's even more difficult for people who are effeminate, or people who are transsexual. They get picked on quite easily. And people have suffered homophobic attacks and violence.

What are the possibilities for lesbian and gay law reform in your country?
David (Uganda): If we begin asking for marriage now our mission will backfire. They will think we're just looking for sex. What we need is to be tolerated and to have the same rights as other people. What we need now is to break down discriminatory laws.
Linda (Namibia): South Africa has got a lot of LGBTI organizations, and that is where the power is. South Africa has networks that are already up and running and it has voices from all corners of the country. That is a process that we can learn from. But you need a continuous support system in place in order for your advocacy and lobbying work to continue. In Namibia, success will depend on how much support we get from other human-rights funders and non-governmental organizations. The Rainbow Project has grown stronger over the years, and the visibility of our organization has also grown. But one of the challenges that we face is that people are afraid to be seen. You can count on your hands the strong gay activists in Namibia who are out and proud and able to speak.
Naome (Rwanda): Rwanda is a sensitive country. This is true even of the human-rights defenders who are there. When we go to them with a problem and ask them to react or to assist with a case they say, 'No. First deal with this yourself and then give us a call.' They fear the government, and they have not helped us at all. Is there potential for these kinds of changes to the law to happen in Rwanda? I think so. Maybe in ten years!

How do you feel about the fact that same-sex couples can now get married in South Africa?
David (Uganda): Since Integrity is a Christian organization, love has no barriers for us. Love can be between a man and a man, or a woman and a woman. If the couples are of the age of consent we do not see why they should be prevented from marrying. Some people think marriage is just about getting children out of it. But not all heterosexual couples produce children. They forget that marriage is also about companionship and love for one another. In South Africa, gay marriage is going to help many gay and lesbian people take their relationships more seriously because they know that the relatives accept, the community accepts, the government accepts. They do not have to worry about getting raided by the police, or put into captivity.
Linda (Namibia): I am proud that at least one African country has achieved this. South Africa is really far in front in terms of their systems and laws, and is

setting an example for the whole African continent. But what is happening at the grassroots in South Africa? The laws have been passed but the people are not benefiting from these laws.

Lourence (Kenya): It is OK for me that same-sex marriage is legal in South Africa. But the situation we have right now in Kenya is that we first need to be recognized before we can reach that point. For example, I can be chased out of school because of my sexual orientation, or thrown out by landlords. This is what we want to address first before we start talking about marriage. I also think one of the main priorities in Kenya now is in terms of health.

Naome (Rwanda): In December 2006, I was listening to the radio in my room when I heard about the same-sex marriage law being passed in South Africa. The listeners were all reacting, and saying that this news should not even be announced on the radio in Rwanda! But I think it was good for those Rwandans who wanted to hear about the same-sex marriage laws in South Africa. I know that same-sex marriage is difficult for some to understand, but there are some people who got the message and discussed it.

What impact do you think the legalization of same-sex marriage in South Africa will have on your own country?

David (Uganda): The day that we heard that same-sex marriage was OK in South Africa gay people in Uganda were very excited. They said, 'Now we are coming down to South Africa. We are going to make marriages.' Some people in Uganda are being harassed because they tried to copy same-sex marriage, forgetting that in Uganda we are still a long, long way off. For example, there is a couple who has been together for some time. When they heard about the same-sex marriage laws in South Africa they really tried to celebrate it. But the local council can always poke their nose into your business, and they did that here and wanted to arrest the couple. The couple had to go into hiding and move to another place. Sometimes we become too excited. We don't think of the consequences of what we are doing.

Linda (Namibia): The Civil Union Act made headlines in Namibia. We made sure that people were aware of what had happened. But there was not much public discussion outside of our LGBTI communities. When we got the news we immediately assigned our lawyers to look at what our Namibian Marital Act says, and they felt that we have room to manoeuvre around that. The Namibian Marital Act recognizes all marriages in South Africa. So if two gay or lesbian Namibians come to South Africa and get married they can go and file for recognition in Namibia [this possibility has still to be tested in a Namibian court of law]. If our judges are people who uphold the principles of human rights and respect the laws that are in place, they will get their recognition. But if someone tries to do that our ministers might try to ban same-sex marriage.

Lourence (Kenya). After the news reached Kenya, people were saying that we are trying to copy what South Africa has done with same-sex marriage. So we do not want to use the South African context. We want Kenyans to see things in our context and know that we are Kenyans and not South Africans. If they do that, then they will not see gay and lesbian rights as an imported thing.

Naome (Rwanda): When people heard about South Africa's same-sex marriage law in Rwanda, people said that South Africa is the first African country that is doing that because it is a country dominated by whites. They tend to think that homosexuality is a Western practice and that it is not African. Personally, I don't think this is true. It was there even in the Rwandan hierarchy. Kings used to do these things.

Rowland Jide (Nigeria): When we talk about same-sex marriage in Nigeria we say that our sister, South Africa, now has a law that protects same-sex people. There are laws in South Africa that give rights to gay and lesbian people. Nigerian legislators are very slow to learn about the changes in the world and to take on board things that would benefit sexual minorities. How many lesbian and gay Nigerians are going to have to leave the country so that they can live their lives properly? But having said that, it [same-sex marriage in South Africa] is having an impact on the way that the law is being debated, and on society itself. It's actually creating a sense of homophobia in the country because ordinary people are becoming more aware of that.

Note

1 In 2007, no fewer than 85 member states of the United Nations still criminalized consensual same-sex acts among adults. Of these, 38 are African governments. For more information see ILGA's report 'State-Sponsored Homophobia: A World Survey of Laws Prohibiting Same-Sex Activity between Consenting Adults', by Daniel Ottosson, 2007, available at http://www.ilga.org/statehomophobia/State_sponsored_homophobia_ILGA_07.pdf (last accessed 2 March 2008). For more information on LGBTI issues and experiences across Africa, visit the website Behind the Mask at www.mask.org.za.

'The traditional model of marriage is oppressive'
Feminist perspectives on marriage

The editors asked a group of woman activists to discuss marriage, and the Civil Union Act, in relation to feminism. It began as a round-table discussion, and was supplemented with a follow-up interview. This is an edited version of these discussions.

The participants are:
- Pumla Dineo Gqola is a feminist writer and associate professor of literary, cultural and media studies at the University of the Witwatersrand.
- Zethu Matebeni is a PhD candidate at the Wits Institute for Social and Economic Research (WISER) and is studying same-sex sexualities among black women in South Africa.
- Dawn O'Reilly is director of the Forum for the Empowerment of Women (FEW), an organization that works to advance, promote and defend the rights of black lesbian, bisexual and transgender women.

How do you identify in relation to feminism?
Dawn: I am a feminist, no apologies, no qualifications. I understand feminism to be a way of thinking about the world that has women at the centre. It makes visible male domination in society and it seeks to eradicate that.
Pumla: I am a feminist. I disagree with some feminists on quite fundamental things, but I am not willing to surrender the term because it describes enough about me. I am fine that there are feminists using the same term to describe themselves when we have little in common politically outside of a basic understanding that patriarchy exists in the world.
Zethu: I don't identify with feminism. Never have. I grew up feeling that feminism did not capture everything I experienced in my life and context.

What is your view of marriage as an institution?
Dawn: I have quite strong views on marriage. I was married myself for many, many years, to a man, many years ago. So some of it is linking the personal and the political and my own concerns with the institution of marriage. I think marriage is a harmful thing for people and if I had my way I would abolish it as an institution. From a feminist perspective, it is one of the institutions that

oppresses. It is set up to limit, regulate and control. A person's intention when they marry might be to celebrate the commitment to another human being, but often it is about setting boundaries, limiting autonomy, limiting freedom, and limiting the right to make decisions about yourself and your own life. I think we need to separate marriage from the need that many people have to commit to a particular person. I think we tend to conflate them. When I hear somebody is getting married I say, 'What is the point?' They say, 'It's because I love her and I want to commit to her,' and I say, 'Then commit to her and love her. Why do you need this particular institution to help you do that?'

Pumla: The traditional model of marriage is oppressive. But it seems to me there are ways in which you can have relationships within marriage, across sexual orientation, that are not traditional or hetero-patriarchal. I'm often frustrated by feminists who get married, and who are very apologetic about it. I assume that married feminists 'do' marriage differently. I think there needs to be more recognition that people do not have to have a conventional patriarchal, heterosexist marriage, and that there is room to manoeuvre. Yet that argument is often quite muted. It is also important to remember that a lot of the patriarchal nonsense in marriage is found in heterosexual relationships of a certain kind outside of marriage. It shouldn't be assumed that if you are in a relationship outside of marriage that you have a relationship that is equitable simply by virtue of its not being marriage.

To what extent do you think the campaign for same-sex marriage in South Africa challenged ideas around marriage as an institution?

Dawn: It's unfortunate that the campaign was conducted in a pressured way. The pressure was about human resources, financial capacity and a range of other issues. The legal process took precedence from start to finish. I don't think there was much space for debate and dialogue about the notion of marriage within the Civil Union Bill. The main thing in activists' minds was to win the legal battle. That was the focus of the campaign. But I think we got the best product that we could under the circumstances. We have to accept that this is where we are now, and look at how to make the most of it. I don't think it is too late to have those debates around marriage. The challenge is there for the LGBTI community and for feminists, and I am hoping in the next year or two we start those conversations and get people to think more critically about marriage as an institution.

Pumla: I would love to just have a revolution and get it over and done with. Unfortunately I have to deal with the fact that change is gradual. I think same-sex marriage is continuing to shift ideas around marriage. But I do not think that as soon as the Bill was passed we had a different sense of what marriage is. But we're getting to a point where the more same-sex couples choose to go the marriage route, the more the face of marriage will change. There's obviously still a lot of resistance. But the fact that it's legally an enshrined right slowly changes the character of marriage. Other feminist challenges to patriarchy have been slow, but more and more people are coming around. I suspect the same thing will happen with marriage. Do I think marriage is what it was 200 years ago? No, I think something has shifted. Do I think there'll be another shift in 50 years? I do think something very exciting is happening, but unfortunately it is slow. I would love to live to be 200 to compare.

Zethu: The same-sex marriage campaign definitely challenged our conventional understandings of what marriage is and what kind of relationships people are living in. I think the backlash to same-sex marriage points to just how much of a threat was felt by a number of conservative South Africans. I still cannot figure out the point of the public consultations. This is legislation to bring us in line with our Constitution. I was struck by the hatred that came out during the public consultations on same-sex marriage. I do not think those discussions challenged ideas around marriage. Instead people were challenging us as gay and lesbian people: 'How dare you enter an institution that has no space for you?' The whole backlash against same-sex marriage also challenged notions around majority decision-making in a democracy. If we based our laws on public consultations on a range of issues – such as the death penalty – we would be back in the Stone Age.

What about the dilemma that some feminists have voiced: supporting same-sex marriage as a human rights issue, but at the same time opposing marriage as an institution because it is patriarchal and oppressive?

Dawn: That's the position I personally was caught in. I was thinking this is just such a horrible thing and that I wish we did not have to look for this kind of equality. It is about wanting to be the same as heterosexual people. I took the pragmatic position that if those benefits and opportunities are available in society for one group of people then they should be available to all. I think that is the dilemma for feminism. We talk about choice, but is it really a choice? Or is it a subtle form of coercion? Often there is societal pressure to conform to the norms of society and that's what people do when they get married.

Pumla: I wrote publicly in support of the Civil Union Bill in several of my columns in the *Mail & Guardian*. The reason I supported the Bill was because I supported the rights of people to choose whether to enter into the institution of marriage or not. It's all very well for heterosexual women to sit back and say marriage is a fascist institution, so nobody should have access to it. But when you are saying that a group does not have access to that position where you can make that choice, that's something fundamentally oppressive and you need to get rid of that. The second thing is that marriage and all its manifestations is always more than just the physical ceremony and the physical piece of paper. It has a certain currency that is about taking people's lives seriously – that is about validation. We can problematize that, but you do not problematize it by gate-keeping and not giving people access, by taking it upon yourself to bar people access to all those other things that come with having your relationship validated. Is it a problem that relationships are placed in a hierarchy? Of course it is. But how do you say 'Well, I have access to this hierarchy, but I have a problem with the hierarchy'? I felt that we can either abolish the institution of marriage altogether, in which case nobody has access to it, or we can all have access to it, and all have an equal role and choice to keep it fascist or make it revolutionary. But we can't gate-keep.

Do you think that the process of getting same-sex marriage in South Africa has any lessons for feminists?
Dawn: Feminist voices, or feminist thinking, was absent in the debate on same-sex marriage. I think as feminists we really should have ensured that those voices were heard. I would say a key lesson from the campaign is about being responsive to the different advocacy-activism processes that are happening in the country at any given time and ensuring that our voices are heard and that the debates happen. In terms of LGBTI activism, I think that our political analysis needs to be deepened quite significantly. Our thinking is often scattered and we don't bring our thoughts together as activists in the LGBTI sector. We need to make space for debate and dialogue and take very clear political positions and articulate them more clearly.
Pumla: One of the things that annoy me about the women's movement in South Africa is the overwhelming silence around issues that pertain to lesbians. I think the South African women's movement is still deeply homophobic. How many of us in the women's movement said anything in support of the Civil Union Bill? I do not see how homophobia or heterosexism or heteronormativity is ever *not* a feminist issue. I think the same-sex marriage campaign is a painful reminder of how the legal-rights framework is both incredibly useful but also very limited. It is useful because, slow as it is, it can put certain frameworks in place quicker than other approaches to change society and bring about equality across the board. But the legal-rights framework is also a double-edged sword. The legal protections don't necessarily make you safe. Legislation falls so far short of what we would like it to do. It is useful to the extent that it can enable certain things and open things up. And sometimes, as with traditional leaders, this is needed. Otherwise, 150 years from now traditional leaders are still going to be saying women should not be inheriting and same-sex marriages shouldn't happen. We constantly have to deal with this nonsense that often comes couched as culture or as religion. But why do

traditional leaders own culture? There are LGBTI people in all those communities who equally own the culture.

Do you think same-sex marriage will transform the institution of marriage?
Dawn: I don't see the point of transforming marriage. I don't think it is necessary. Inequality exists in both heterosexual and same-sex relationships whether you are married or not. Same-sex relationships are often unequal and I think that same-sex marriage will just solidify that. It will institutionalize that inequality unless you make a bold and conscious attempt to work on inequality within that marriage. I don't have grudges against people who are going ahead and doing it. It would be lovely to see people interpreting marriage in progressive and creative ways and showing that it can be different. But I wish the level of debate was a lot deeper before we got ourselves stuck in this kind of institutional mess.
Pumla: I do think that you can negotiate marriage. For example, I do not see why, if two lesbian feminists or a heterosexual feminist man and woman enter into a marriage, it has to be in the traditional, conservative, patriarchal sense. We often act as though we are helpless in the face of some institutions, and do not engage with them. I think that what makes conventional heterosexist marriage so deeply patriarchal is the same thing that makes a lot of heterosexual relationships deeply patriarchal. We deflect dealing with the way that heterosexuality is constructed in ways that violate people who are gay and lesbian because it is everywhere. It is convenient to say that marriage is an institution. But heterosexuality is also an institution, and we are not dealing with it when we pretend that the problem is only marriage. Heterosexuality is flawed as lived, and that translates into marriage. I also know that there are same-sex relationships that are exploitative. There are exploitative people regardless of their sexual orientation. It seems to me that we need to deal with the extent that heterosexuality is often premised on patriarchal exchange between man and woman.
Zethu: Marriage is about a woman being oppressed, not necessarily the man. So if, of two men, one is a 'woman' – which is possible – then we're not changing the institution. But there are ways in which the institution can be changed. Marriage has its functions – the function of procreation, the function of being spiritual, of being together. You know those things can happen anywhere, with any two people, or five people. So we can transform the institution of marriage by not trying to copy heterosexual relationships.

What impact do you see same-sex marriages having on LGBTI relationships?
Dawn: I think that being married imposes another layer of expectations on you. There might be a 'positive' impact for people who are looking to be sanctioned by their families and society. But there is a negative spin-off to that. Do I have to

then go the route of obeying rules that do not make any sense to me in order to be accepted? That isn't acceptance. I don't think people are going to get acceptance from family by being married. There is also a set of practical impacts that people are going to go through, and it is going to be about what it means to be married on a day-to-day basis, and to have these rules that determine how you live and act out your life.

Will same-sex marriage have an impact on how ordinary people perceive gay and lesbian people and their relationships?
Dawn: I think one of the things that is going to happen with LGBTI relationships is that we will be seen as wanting to be like heterosexuals and to replicate their relationships. Maybe most LGBTI people just want to get on with their lives, but there is a political identity to being a LGBTI person. My identity as a lesbian is both personal and political. From a political point of view, it is really bad in terms of public perception if we are viewed as wanting to be like heterosexuals. From an ideological point of view, it is sad if they think that what we are doing is trying to live up to standards set by someone else, when we are actually trying to be who we are and to defy their norms when they do not work for us. I also worry that because we are now going to feel more accepted that emotional things are going to become hidden. Is it really a gain to say that we can marry? Are we really addressing homophobia and discrimination?
Zethu: It was interesting to see in the media coverage on same-sex marriage the usual boring heterosexist projections on same-sex desire and marriage – people saying things like 'Which one is the woman?' when it is two men. Why do they want there to be a woman? The media was making a clear, concerted effort to make marriage between two people of the same sex and the same gender look as much as possible like a heterosexual marriage, and be classified as such.

Now that we have same-sex marriage, will it mean that other kinds of alternative relationships and families will be devalued?
Dawn: When we are talking marriage we also have to start confronting the oppressive ways that family operates. Often the pressure to marry is coming from traditional ways that family is acted out and lived. This is often very rigid. It is pushing for majority practice. Now more people will be married and it becomes the norm of what heterosexual people and LGBTI people do. It is broadening the mainstream and marginalizing those who choose not to do that, who then take on that pressure of rejection because they are not conforming. I wish we could get to a place in society where there are different ways to organize your day-to-day life with other people.
Pumla: We have made marriage accessible to certain types of people, but we have not dealt with the core issues. When we say that anybody, regardless of

their sexual orientation, can access the institution of marriage, we do more than just open it up. We also strengthen that institution even as we convince ourselves that we are changing it. One of the ways that oppressive systems, such as homophobia and patriarchy, stay alive is by taking bits that are radical and challenging and co-opting these. Also, one of the feminist criticisms of traditional marriage is that monogamy is patriarchal. It privileges lifetime coupling and enforces a regime of intimacy on these relationships. A lot of feminists are critical, at least at an ideological level, of the locking of intimacy to two people. You find some feminists who say that polyamorous relationships are not necessarily negative or harmful. If you legalized polyamorous relationships or marriages between gay men or lesbians then that might be the ultimate challenge to the marriage institution. The problem I have with polyamory as an intimate arrangement is that I am never sure that you actually have buy-in by all the people involved. I have anxieties about people compromising themselves in those contexts.

What do you think about the Civil Union Act?
Pumla: I am in a relationship with a man, and we said for years that there was no way we would even consider marriage until everybody could get married. Now that this is the case, I am anxious about beginning to think about whether to consider marriage or not. Everybody has to have the right to choose to go into marriage or not. But I remain unconvinced that there is anything that happens in marriage at the level of exchange between the two people involved that doesn't happen in a relationship leading up to marriage. I worry about marriage being the ultimate validation for anybody who is in a relationship. We know that at different times we have relationships that are incredibly meaningful and affirming [but aren't marriages].

Zethu: I felt the courts passed the buck on same-sex marriage. I do not understand why it gave government time to think about it and then maybe pass a law. I thought the courts should have effected the change. I am scared of the Civil Union Act. You fight for it, but you do not necessarily want it. Now I find myself in a situation where I still believe I do not want marriage or anything close to it. But I find that it has destabilized me extremely in the way that I think about myself and about my own political stance.

6: TYING THE KNOT
Marriage in action

'They knew we were serious'
Interview with Charles Januarie and Hompi Januarie

Charles Januarie and Hompi Januarie (formerly Ndimande) have been in a relationship since 1995. They had a wedding ceremony in 2002. After the passing of the Civil Union Act they got married for a second time, so that their relationship could be legally recognized.

What was it like to grow up gay in the townships?
Hompi: I grew up without knowing who I am. I did not know that I was gay. I used to be accused at school most of the time for hanging out with girls. They used to call me *stabane* and I did not know what it meant. I grew up with foster parents and as the only child I was dressed like a girl. I used to feel comfortable dressing up like that. When I was in Standard 4, I had friends who understood what it meant to be gay. These are the people who told me that it means I am attracted to men. I knew then that I was gay and so did my family. My family was understanding because they knew gay life from the mines. In the mines men like me were called *abo-madlamini*. The *madlamini* men were often Zulu migrants coming from KwaZulu-Natal, and they were known for plaiting hair and for wearing aprons. So my family did not have any problem because I was then understood for being *u-madlamini*. I told them that should I marry they should not expect a bride but a groom coming into the family, and the message of my identity was sent to the rest of my family, including my foster parents, and they all at least knew about my status. However, my biological mother did not understand and I think I humiliated her in our community.

Charles: I grew up with foster parents and people have been calling me 'moffie' all the time. They said I was talking like a woman and always concerned myself with woman affairs. At school I used to play with boys and kiss them. But at school I did not get lots of problems – it was only when I was at home that my straight friends called me 'moffie'. I had been gay all the time but I did not let people know about it. I was in the closet. It was before the marriage that I had to tell my stepmother, but before I did not talk about it.

What was your experience of getting married to each other in 2002?
Charles: My father passed away a few years back, and I did not know where to stay. Hompi asked me to come stay with him. I was concerned about his HIV

status so we decided to get married so we can look after each other and progress with life. We got married in a church because we wanted to do things in front of God.

Hompi: I wanted our marriage to be blessed by God. I wanted to do it in a religious way because I think we are all religious. We got married in a church for straight people in KwaThema and the pastor used our wedding to educate the members of the church. Our other church is called Hope and Unity. It is a church that accepts gay and lesbian people. But there are no such churches in the townships, and that is why we had to travel to Jo'burg for the wedding.

Charles: In Hompi's family, because of the traditional things, they demanded lobola. With my family we are Christians so there was nothing like that. I had to do it for the sake of Hompi.

Hompi: I am a woman and I come from a cultural background – *ngiphuma esintwini*. I wanted Charles to say that I have paid lobola for him and be proud about it. For my family it was more like, despite the fact that he is gay, we would go through lobola and release him into the Januaries. It was important for me.

The community was amazed about our wedding. Such a thing never happened in their lives. They wanted to see how would such a wedding take place. Gay people are newsmongers. They go around telling everyone they know, even straight people. So the wedding raised lots of curiosity in the community, with people wanting to see a man in a wedding dress and so on. Some people attended our wedding just to see what was going to happen. We met with the ward councillor and he accepted our wedding in his territory. I think he allowed us to get married because he always knew me and I was always with Charles. He blessed us and encouraged us to work together as a couple.

Can you describe your wedding day in 2002?

Charles: I was more man-like. I was wearing a suit and Hompi was wearing white – it was his desire. I was surprised when I saw all these people and some I did not even know. The time when we had to make our vows I realized, Charles, now you have to be sure what you are doing. That was my special moment.

Hompi: When I first realized that I was gay, I said to myself, 'I want to get into a white wedding dress.' It was my dream and it so happened that God answered my dream, and hence the white dress on my wedding day. I put on my dress and I was suddenly scared just taking to the street. But after I was given marital advice by my family I felt very strong and courageous to face the onlookers. Lots of people were surprised because I left my home as a real woman. Even Charles was taken by surprise. I think he was expecting a drag queen, but I looked like a real woman in my style and make-up. It was my dream to wed as a woman. My entire extended family was there. With Charles, it was only immediate family members, and his sister was there. My stepmother saw Charles as an addition to our family. She was very happy. I was the second child after my brother to get married and all our sisters were not married.

Charles: My sister was the only one at my wedding. I was scared to inform the rest of my family because they did not know me very much. We were never close.

What are your thoughts on the campaign for same-sex marriage?
Charles: At the time of a GLOW [Gay and Lesbian Organization of the Witwatersrand] march, I was rejoicing because doors were going to be open and as I was gay I felt that there is going a foundation laid for me. I remember there was court case. We followed it on national TV.

Hompi: After the case at Constitution Hill [when the *Fourie* judgment on same-sex marriage was handed down], we were told that we are going wait for another year. I was not happy because a year was too long for me. We were told on the radio and television that our marriage was null and void because the law was not yet passed. It felt like we were just playing games, although that is not the way I felt personally, because, like I said from the beginning, the first marriage was the most important one.

When the law was passed I was happy that I was going to be recognized and lots of things were going to change, like for instance my last name would be Januarie. I think the majority accepts and the minority does not accept [same-sex marriages] due to lack of knowledge. We need to conduct more workshops, educate people about gay marriage. Some people still maintain that a man is man and woman is a woman. Some people see our government as rotten for legalizing gay marriages and they see it as the end of the world. I think now, as the lesbian and gay community, we are going to be stable. Before, gays did not plan for the future because there was no future for them. With these new laws I think they will able to plan for the future and be more stable. I am also grateful especially for the gay and lesbian organizations for fighting for our rights and to enable all other gays to come out and claim their future.

What was your experience of getting legally married in 2007?
Hompi: I think our marriage was by far the best compared to straight marriages. It was excellent. It was glamorous, and straight marriages are not glamorous. My wedding was divided into two. I first did a traditional wedding, and after the church service we got on to a civil wedding to accommodate Charles's coloured background.

Charles: Why we got married the second time was to make it legal, so we can plan our financial matters, and in case something happens to either one of us. But the real reason we got married the second time was because we wanted it to be legally binding.

Hompi: It was important because I wanted Home Affairs to recognize my marriage status. During my first wedding I was not recognized by Home Affairs, but now I am recognized. I think the first wedding was important for recognition in church and before God and for the rest of the community to bear witness that I was married. The second one was more about recognition from Pretoria that I am a married individual.

I think the second wedding was less difficult than the first one. The first one was overwhelming due to the experience I have been through in my community. I had to expose myself to the community and declare that I am getting married, while with the second one I only had to go to Home Affairs for a wedding date. With the first wedding I wanted all the people to know that I am married, and with the second one I wanted to have a marriage certificate.

Charles: The first marriage did not give me much hope because it was not legalized, but the second one was great because it was legal and important. I did not plan a lot in the first wedding.

Hompi: On the 28th of March 2007 we went to Home Affairs like straight people and we were told to bring photographs, identity books, two witnesses, and we were given a date. Home Affairs treated us with support and they encouraged us. They even asked us how many years we were together and they knew that we were serious about it. We brought everything and proceeded with our wedding. We were wed by a white woman and we were the first gay couple to be wed by her. She said I can now change my surname.

Charles: We did not even discuss anything about changing our surnames. It was Hompi who came up with it. I was more concerned about getting our marriage legal. I think everybody calls him Mrs J. It was our decision and it was after we had done that we let our families know. They have come to terms with it and have accepted it. It is a relationship and they respect and accept it. They do see our relationship as a marriage.

'Why is it okay when they hold hands, but not us?'
Interview with Nozipho Ngcobo and Thulile Ngcobo

Nozipho Ngcobo and Thulile Ngcobo (formerly Gasa) were married in a civil ceremony at the Home Affairs office in Pietermaritzburg on 26 September 2007 and then in a religious ceremony at the Kismet Hotel on 29 September 2007. They were the first same-sex couple in Pietermaritzburg to have their wedding featured in the local newspapers. Shortly thereafter they were the victims of a homophobic attack. Nozipho works for the Pietermaritzburg Gay and Lesbian Network and Thulile is training as a counsellor through LifeLine. They are both 28 years old.

How did you meet each other?
Nozipho: We met at a party in 2006. Thulile was sitting there quietly, so I went to sit next to her and we started talking. I asked for her number but she refused. I eventually got it from a friend of hers.
Thulile: I had never had a woman partner before. I did not understand when Nozipho said she loved me, because she is a girl! I refused to take her calls. But she was persistent and full of love. We ended up being in a relationship.

What is the situation for lesbian and gay people in Pietermaritzburg?
Nozipho: In Pietermaritzburg people still have the tendency to say negative things when they see gay and lesbian people. They say things like, 'You think you are a boy?' and when Thulile and I are walking down the street holding hands people say negative things like calling us *izitabane* ['hermaphrodite'; insulting term used for homosexuals]. Especially the taxi drivers! Why is it okay when they hold hands, but not us? It is our right to hold hands.
Thulile: We just carry on walking. We do not mind them.

How did your families feel about your relationship?
Thulile: I told my sister first. When we went to visit my place, my mother could see there was something between us and asked me. I told her Nozipho is my friend, but when I left I asked my sister to tell her. My mother did not like it in the beginning, but she ended up accepting it.
Nozipho: My family knows I am a lesbian. They were fine the first day I came with Thulile. They were just going on about how many girlfriends I come with.

When I told my family I was getting married they said if I am sure and serious they would support me. Our families are supportive because they know we love each other. They know it's a way of life.

Why did you decide to get married?
Nozipho: I wanted to marry Thulile because I love her, and I wanted to be committed, and in a stable relationship. I used to have many girlfriends, but when I saw Thulile everything changed. I told myself I was going to stop all that and stick with her. The other women I was with were troublesome. Thulile is respectful. I can see that she loves me. She is caring and always supportive. And she is beautiful.
Thulile: I love Nozipho, and I thought that for us to stay together we need to get married. Nozipho is different from the men I had relationships with before her. Men are troublesome. They give you headaches. Since I met Nozipho everything has been fine. We understand each other. She is quiet and full of love. She is patient, and when I do not understand things she is able to guide me.

Can you tell us about getting married?
Thulile: We first had our marriage registered at Home Affairs. Then we had a religious wedding. The two of us planned the wedding, and we did everything ourselves. We invited our families and friends and they came. My mother and sister were not sure we were serious. They did not think it would be a real wedding. They were surprised when I had a veil on.
Nozipho: Everyone in the community was looking forward to the wedding and curious about it.
Thulile: The hall was so full, and some people could not get in. We had a priest to bless us. He said we should not be late, and then we were late! The priest did not want it to be public; it should just be the two of us and our witnesses. We did that part, and then we continued with the programme and the reception.
Nozipho: Thulile's grandfather phoned during the wedding. He was ill and could not come, and he wanted to find out if everything went well. My sister made a speech. She said they are welcoming *makoti* [bride or daughter-in-law] and I must take care of her, and she must take care of me. At home they call Thulile *makoti*, especially my brothers. She is the first daughter-in-law in my family.
Thulile: My family calls Nozipho *ndodakazi* [daughter]. She is just like me.
Nozipho: The traditional part of the wedding is still to happen. I am paying lobola to Thulile's grandfather and grandmother. My family represents me, and I go with them and just sit in. I had to send a few cows. I haven't finished. Once I have paid what is left, Thulile's family will burn *mphepho* to welcome me as part of the family and Thulile's grandfather will do the traditional wedding.

What impact has getting married had on your relationship?
Nozipho: Now that we are married I feel a hundred percent safe in our relationship. She is mine. She is the only one. I am glad that we have been able to practice what is our human right.
Thulile: I feel like any other married woman.

After your wedding was featured in the newspapers you were the victims of a homophobic attack. Can you tell us about that?
Nozipho: On the 31st of October I accompanied Thulile to the clinic, and on our way back suddenly three boys appeared. One of them wanted to talk to Thulile. I heard them saying, 'How can a girl go out with another girl?' One boy grabbed Thulile and they started beating us.
Thulile: I did not know the boys, but I think they knew us. They might not have known us by name, but they knew us by sight. I think they had bad intentions from the beginning. As they were beating us a van pulled over and they ran away.
Nozipho: I was scared because Thulile was badly injured. But before we went to the doctor we went to the police station and laid a charge of assault. We told the police we were lesbians, and some of them recognized us from the newspapers.
Thulile: The police helped us, but they said they weren't able to do anything. They said we should report immediately if we see the boys again.
Nozipho: Since the incident we still walk the streets. Thulile always walks me back from work.

'Saying to our children we are a unit'
Interview with Lael Bethlehem and Emilia Potenza

In 2000 Lael and Emilia felt it important to have a ceremony where they publicly declared their 'commitment to each other and our intention to be faithful, loving and supportive'. In 2007 they chose to get married under the Civil Union Act. Lael is CEO of the Johannesburg Development Agency and Emilia is a consultant at the South African Apartheid Museum.

How did you meet?
Lael: It was 1994, before the democratic elections. I was a member of the ANC Yeoville branch choir. I love singing and I especially enjoyed being part of the choir in that incredibly exciting time. Emilia's brother and sister were choir members and one day Emilia came along. I was mesmerized by Emilia, although I knew very little about her. I just had such a strong knowledge that this was the person for me. She was funny and gorgeous. She was politically active and did such interesting work. I just fell in love.
Emilia: Until I met Lael at the age of 35 I thought I was heterosexual, although I had always fantasized about having a sexual relationship with a woman before I died. Then when I met Lael I fell in love with *Lael*. In that sense my identity was already formed. I am in a lesbian relationship with Lael, but I don't define myself first and foremost as a lesbian. I am one of those who can, and has, gone either way.
Lael: In gay-activist circles there is still an insistence on a strong homosexual identity, which I don't think either of us feel that strongly. For me, and more certainly for Emilia, sexuality is much more of a continuum.

Can you tell us about your commitment ceremony in 2000?
Lael: It was on our own terms. I know a lot of couples who have struggled with their weddings because of the strong expectations of their communities and their families. We were released from all of that.
Emilia: We had space because of the unconventional nature of the ceremony, so we could do whatever we liked. And we did. We put together a ceremony with our families, our friends, and our choir. It was outside on Langermann's Kop in Kensington. It's a beautiful ridge, and has a spectacular view of the city. It's one of Jo'burg's best kept secrets. You walk up to the top of the hill where there is a natural amphitheatre. We set up chairs and a wooden platform which one of

our friends built. We even took a piano up there. Another friend's gift to us was to hire a bottle-green 1930s Rolls-Royce for us to arrive in.

Lael: The driver was a very adventurous guy. He drove the car up this very uneven and bumpy path right on to the koppie, with the engine doing the maximum effort. There was a cloud of dust …

Emilia: And this Rolls-Royce. Our friends had put sunflowers all over. We emerged at the top of the hill as these two goddesses. We had beautiful dresses. Someone had made garlands for us. We stepped out into a beautiful Jo'burg evening with all our friends and family looking on.

Lael: We invented our own rituals. We put together an amalgamation of different things. We had Jewish elements, Hindu elements, Buddhist elements. We had a meditation in the middle of the ceremony. The important thing was our choir, because we met in the choir. The choir sang throughout the wedding in English, Hebrew, Latin, Xitsonga, and isiZulu.

Emilia: We made up our own vows and we said those to each other. Then Lael's parents came and gave us a blessing in Hebrew, which was an incredible thing for them to do in front of 250 people, including their friends and relatives. So everyone went the extra mile. After the ceremony, we had drinks on the koppie, before we went to the reception. It had started to thunder. Just as we were leaving the koppie the heavens opened. There was a shower of rain which everyone said was a blessing.

Lael: But we should not feel as if we are the first people to transform marriage. Though marriage has often been about enforcing a gender hierarchy, it hasn't been so in every heterosexual relationship. Maybe the left-wing critique of marriage as oppressive and conservative has been a rather partial view all along. Maybe there have been a lot of heterosexual people that have had liberating marriages. Maybe it has been there for the taking all along.

Since your commitment ceremony in 2000 you have adopted two daughters. Why did you decide to become parents?

Emilia: I think we both always wanted to parent. I always imagined that I would have my own child one day. Then time passed, and by the time we decided to have a child I was already in my forties. Lael could have had a biological child. We decided to approach an ex-boyfriend of hers who now lives in Australia, and in fact met with him to talk about it. Somehow all three of us reached the conclusion that we could not go through with it. You start to realize the enormous implications of what you are doing. Legally the biological father would have had more rights to the child than I would.

Lael: It would have introduced an inequality in our relationship that felt wrong. The child would not have been legally Emilia's, whereas with adoption the child is legally both of ours.

Emilia: I did feel slightly uncomfortable about the idea of Lael being pregnant, Lael breastfeeding. About its being her baby in that sense and not mine. I would have been like the 'auntie' whereas adoption has been such an equal thing for both of us. I think we made the right decision for our relationship. It's been such a blessing to have Lulu and now Thembela.

Why did you decide to get married under the Civil Union Act after having had a commitment ceremony in 2000?
Emilia: The step between the commitment ceremony and the civil union was adopting our daughter Lulu. When we adopted Lulu we could not adopt as a same-sex couple. I had to adopt her as a single parent, even though I was in a long-term relationship with Lael. But we were aware of the *Du Toit and De Vos case* [see pages 57 and 258], which was then making its way through the courts. As a result of that case, the law changed quite soon after our adoption. It had immediate implications for our lives. We went back to court to re-register Lulu not only as my child but as Lael's child too. We got a letter from the Department of Social Welfare saying 'Lulu is your child as if she was born to both of you.' There is something very profound about that. Then when we adopted our second daughter, Thembela, the issue of marriage came up again.
Lael: If you are a heterosexual couple you have to be married before you can adopt together. For same-sex couples there was a loophole because the *De Vos* court battle had been won. So in adopting Thembi this year the social worker said, 'Since you can get married now, we are asking you the same question we ask heterosexual couples: If you want to have children together why don't you get married?' We said, 'Well, we consider ourselves married.' She said, 'That's all very well, but legally that is not true.' I said, 'We just haven't got around to it.' I thought that was so lame. So we got around to it. I think for children in a family where there are two adults in a loving relationship, the prospect of that relationship falling apart is very threatening. Marriage sends a signal that the two individuals want to be together on an ongoing basis. Marriage is a way of saying to our community and our children that we are a unit. We intend to live our lives together. If you have that intention then it helps your children to know that and to rest easy.

Can you describe the process of getting married under the Civil Union Act?
Lael: I had heard from a friend that she and her partner experienced difficulty. They arrived at a Home Affairs office and the marriage officer refused to marry them on the basis of conscience. So I decided I had better get organized. I did that classic thing where you phone Home Affairs, forgetting the fact that Home Affairs do not answer their phone. I tried dozens of times. I phoned David Bilchitz, and he said Home Affairs in Edenvale is the place to go. He gave me the name of this woman called Mrs Horsten. I got there and she said she had

very few appointments left until the end of the year but there was one available on Tuesday at 8am. A less romantic prospect than getting married at the Department of Home Affairs in Edenvale at eight in the morning has not been invented! But we took the appointment and arranged for Emilia's sister and our friend Steve to witness our marriage. We took our two girls and we got ourselves to Home Affairs in Edenvale.

What was your experience of getting married at Home Affairs?
Emilia: The marriage officer, Mrs Horsten, was wonderful. She told us that she had completed a course so she could perform civil unions, and that she had done 62 in the last year. She had a lovely way about her, extremely warm and kind and not intrusive. She had all the admin completely under control. There was this sense of pride in her office. She had created a wonderful space in this horrible government building. She just made us feel special. Then she gave us a bit of advice about marriage, which involved bringing God into our relationship.
Lael: Which in itself is an interesting thing for her to say. She was a Christian, but she was telling a lesbian couple to bring God into their marriage. She told us what she thought marriage was about, and a bit about her own marriage. It was as if it was completely normal for two women to be getting married. I was so impressed with her and Home Affairs.
Emilia: And it cost R10 to get married!

How did your daughter Lulu feel about your getting married?
Lael: She was pleased. We had told her about the wedding in 2000 and shown her the pictures. She always seemed quite put out that she wasn't there. I took her back to school after we got married, and we told the teachers, who were very supportive.
Emilia: Lulu enjoyed it. We resurrected our wedding dresses. It was quite an affair, to traipse through Home Affairs past all these queues of people sorting out their IDs in our wedding dresses, with our kids and our witnesses.

What do you think about the Civil Union Act itself?
Lael: I am an ANC member. I was disappointed that the ANC did not just change the law proactively as the Constitution clearly required. But I think we must give the ANC government credit, because once the Constitutional Court made its ruling it got the process together and made the changes. The ANC was the only political party to vote for the new law *en masse*.
Emilia: We are grappling with the fact that our Constitution is way ahead of the views of a lot of people in our country. That is a dangerous situation. If people lose confidence in the Constitution, it undermines the power of the Constitution. This is one of those moments. It is challenging those very fundamental

Christian values. You can only push that so far so fast. From that point of view, I think the Civil Union Act was an enormous victory. It pushed further than I thought we would actually be able to go as a society.

Do you think the debate around same-sex relationships in South Africa has had any impact on how ordinary South Africans see same-sex marriage?
Emilia: Let's assume that Mrs Horsten is an ordinary South African. It has certainly shifted the way she understands marriage. She actually enables and organizes same-sex marriages as a government bureaucrat.
Lael: The security guard who let us in assumed that our witness, who was male, was there to be the groom. We said, 'No, there are two brides.' At first she was a little taken aback, but then she said, 'Don't worry, you are not the first.' So the bureaucracy is adapting and hopefully that signals something about our society as a whole.

'The marriage ceremony was turned into a training session'
Interview with William Stewart

Since the inception of the Civil Union Act, many couples have approached the Department of Home Affairs to get married. In some cases, couples have been met with negative attitudes by Home Affairs officials. In other cases the response has been positive, as described in the previous interview in this book. Here William Stewart talks about the experience that he and his partner Richard Holden had of getting married under the Civil Union Act. The couple had had a commitment ceremony to formalize the relationship in August 2002, then got officially married at Home Affairs in Johannesburg on 29 January 2007, with Richard's three sons as witnesses.

William: After the Civil Union Act was passed Richard and I went for the marriage ceremony at the Home Affairs office in Johannesburg. It was quite amazing, although the actual ceremony was a horrible experience. The appointment was for one o'clock, but Richard likes to be early so we were at the Home Affairs office at twelve o'clock. There were no chairs, and we were pacing up and down the passageway. When one o'clock came, there was still nobody at the marriage office, and the marriage office was locked.

We were lucky that a freelance photographer, who was not part of the staff, took pity on us and got the key to the office. He said we must sit down and just be patient and they would be there to help us. He went downstairs to get a marriage officer. While we waited, there was this fear that we might be discriminated against. I think gay people tend to feel insecure if they have lived through the times when you could be shot if you were caught having sex with another guy and tried to flee. You come from that background of fear, that it should be a secret, and that you are supposed to be quiet, and then moving to the point that you can be legally married and recognized by the state and society.

The photographer found a marriage officer and she came upstairs to marry us. But when she realized that we are a gay couple she started shouting in a language we didn't understand. That was a bad experience because it felt as though she did not want to marry us because we were gay. You start feeling more and more insecure. The old feelings of unworthiness resurface. I think that part of the reason is also that she did not know how to marry us. The Civil

Union Act requires different forms, and the department did not have enough people to do it. The marriage ceremony was turned into a training session.

We had waited an hour and a half before it eventually happened, and then the ceremony itself was muddled. It was not done properly in the sense that important parts of the ceremony were not read out or presented properly, and the lady performing the ceremony could hardly fill in the forms. But we managed to get through the paperwork and we eventually ended up getting the certificate and were married.

You felt very vulnerable, because you were dealing with a government department. You were in a situation were you knew that you had the right to a service, but the department was not able to deliver it. You were in the hands of an incompetent department, and there was nothing you could do. You were totally disempowered. You could not scream and shout because that would not change anything. You could not plead, because who could you plead to? You just felt helpless and powerless. It was very disappointing for me, because it did something to one's self-esteem.

But after you got past the disappointment of the ceremony there were other experiences that made it worthwhile. I did not expect marriage to change the way Richard and I felt towards one another, but it has tended to make the relationship much stronger and much more settled. We feel a lot closer to each other than we did before.

'Making the box bigger'
Interview with Robert Hamblin and Sally-Jean Shackleton

Robert Hamblin is a photographer and transman who has made the transition from female to male. He is on the board of Gender DynamiX (an organization focusing on the transgender community, providing related support and information to transgender people and the wider public), but says, 'I'm a provocateur, which I suppose is an activist. But more through my art.' Sally-Jean Shackleton is the chair of Gender DynamiX, an organization she was introduced to by Robert. She says that working with Gender DynamiX, and as an activist, 'has meant that I get to be part of transforming something so fundamental, which is gender itself'.

How do you identify in terms of your gender and sexual orientation?
Robert: I am a transman, meaning I am a female-to-male transsexual. I'm busy with my transition. I am 38 years old. I prefer women sexually, although if I really have to state my absolute sexual preference it would probably be bisexual because I find men sexually interesting too. But I partner with women. Necessarily up to now I have led the life of a lesbian, which I'm happy about. I always say 'I used to be a lesbian'. But now I am supposedly male – 'supposedly' because I'm very interested in alternative identities. I am transsexual, but I like the identity of transgender because transgender people do not run after the binary – they kind of do interesting things with it. I think I identify as queer. But a lot of people would see me as like a heterosexual man. This is where interesting dynamics come in with partners.

Sally-Jean: Gender-wise I am happy with my femaleness. Sexual orientation – I identify as a dyke. Which means more than just my sexual orientation to me. It's a political orientation. It means that I place myself in a realm of alternative sexualities and identities. Politically I am also a feminist. All of these things cause me to say that I am a dyke. I believe women need empowerment, and that society is fundamentally unequal. That is why I call myself a feminist. I've had a lot of questions from very good friends about how I can identify as a dyke and be involved with Robert. Some people say to me that I *can't* identify as a dyke.

The lesson I have learnt in being with Robert, and in previously being Robert's friend, not his lover, is that identities are fluid. You can inhabit different spaces at the same time. Often our identities are more about our alliances – who we choose to align ourselves to. I choose to align myself to a dyke identity. I know that a lot of my friends, as well as strangers, would disagree with me. But I welcome that debate.

What are your thoughts on marriage as an institution?
Sally-Jean: I think that there are lots of problematic associations with marriage. But then there are lots of problematic associations with relationships in general. Marriage is an institution which has a historical context of women being subordinate to men, of women not being able to make decisions about their lives. I think I have a healthy disrespect for the institution. But there has been a lot of progress, and I think that that needs to be acknowledged as well.
Robert: With Sally, and also because I am a transgender person now and living my life as I want, I totally allowed myself to feel the romance that I'd suppressed before, ironically, as a woman. Marriage for me is a romantic thing. I like its family context – the fact that we're announcing it to her parents, to my family. Now the world is free to me and I can have any kind of marriage I want. I can have the good old-fashioned marriage, or we could have the Civil Union Act. I would have probably been really frustrated if I didn't have the option of making that kind of civil statement.

How was the subject of your marriage approached?
Robert: I asked her in a very romantic moment. It totally made her go quiet and non-responsive. I thought, 'Oh my God, what did I do?' So we just ignored it. And then later Sally kind of squeaked through the side of her mouth, 'Would you ask me again?'
Sally-Jean: The subject of marriage was unexpected. I've also always been a dyke, so I hadn't ever thought I would be confronted with that question. My immediate response was to think of all of the stereotypes about marriage. Then I thought, 'This is the person that I love. This is the person that I would choose to spend the rest of my life with. And I want my family and my friends to see my relationship in that way too.'
Robert: We had watched a film where a character asked, 'Why is marriage so important?' The answer was: 'Because it's almost like one's life is only real if someone witnesses it.'
Sally-Jean: Ja, she said, 'Every life needs a witness, every person needs a witness.' She wasn't saying that it's better, but that you are living life in the gaze of others. And it's a good thing to spend your life in the gaze of someone that you love, and who loves you back.
Robert: I think that moment it really fitted in with what I was going through. My life had always felt like some kind of an act. I realized how much I loved Sally. I thought, 'What a terrible tragedy it would be for humanity if no-one witnessed

this incredible person's life.' And that seems like a calling to me. I mean, that's my job. I am an artist, I am a photographer, I document people's lives, interpret people's lives.

Sally-Jean: I was reading one of those bridal magazines and it was truly frightening – 'The best day of your life', 'Your big day'. Those were really scary things. I do not want this to be the 'best day of my life'. I have a whole life. I like every day to be OK. And all the hype about marriage and the pressure – I don't know how heterosexual people manage it. When you're thinking about it in your own life, and your own definition of what it might mean to your life, it's pretty good. But when you start thinking about how other people see it ... I started thinking about 'Mrs' and how scary that thought is. And that it's assumed that I would take Robert's name. It's a really frightening encounter with society.

Robert: Sally's aunt came to the rescue. She lives in Canada, and she just said, 'You find ways to make it have meaning for yourself, and not in the light of everybody else's ideas about marriage.' It's very important for us to make it our own. We have the option of getting married under the old Marriage Act or under the Civil Union Act. We see the traditional Marriage Act as something for fundamentalists, whether traditional Africans or religious fundamentalists. I think everybody should use the Civil Union Act.

What responses have you had from friends, family and strangers to the idea of your marriage?

Sally-Jean: We have a bit of a complication. We are not a straight or a same-sex relationship. Robert is a transman. So, we first have to deal with my long-time good friends being a little taken aback because they think that I am leaving the 'club', the safety of being lesbian. I do not think I am doing that. I think it is interesting for me because I realized how much we rely on our friendships and our community for safety. I think a lot of people felt a little afraid, or a little unsure about where my identity was going to go. But I think they're working through it. And they are all unequivocally, completely happy about us getting married.

Robert: I think it helps that they can also get married, otherwise we would have been under attack politically. It seems heterosexual people get much more excited because they have it ingrained in them that marriage is special. It's been a transgender confrontation for them. I've had three older heterosexual women say to me, 'Will there be men at the engagement party?' I was like, 'Well, I will be there!' They still see us as living in this Amazonian community of women. Now there is one that has less breasts.

Sally-Jean: My family has been great, they've been very supportive.

Robert: Sally's family has always been there. I come from a very conservative family, and the men in my family are not accepting my transition. I've only invited the two matriarchs in my family to my engagement. Their vibe is they just want me to be happy, though it's going to take them a long time to see me as a heterosexual male. But I was just insistent. They are now coming to the party, and they are all excited about what to wear and that kind of thing. This is why events like this are important. It's because it will be an affirmation. It's ritual. Somehow it makes you less of a human being if you do not have those rituals where society is participating and affirming with you.

What are the main issues for transgender people and marriage?
Sally-Jean: Transgendered people are often married as heterosexuals before their transition, and then it becomes a same-sex relationship. They have to get divorced [under the Marriage Act] and then marry again under the Civil Union Act. I would like to see that changed. I would like to see people be able to continue their relationships in the way that they choose.

It's ironic, because people who are transgendered, who are in marriage relationships, sometimes are able to be married for a very long time until the transgendered person decides to change their ID. It also makes fun of this idea that we're all purely heterosexual people and we all behave in heterosexual ways in our marriages. It's a complete myth. People have diverse sexual practices. They have lots of different kinds of ways of being in their relationships that aren't heterosexist – even if you are heterosexual. I like the idea of the Civil Union Act being a place where transgendered people, straight people and gay people can come together and celebrate their relationships in the diversity that really exists in reality.
Robert: Since we've brought in the Civil Union Act, I would like to see the Marriage Act be made something cultural and not a legal, civil thing. It must be something you do in your church or in your *dorp*, and that it is not the official thing that happens between one man and one woman.
Sally-Jean: When the Civil Union Act was first passed, I was really disappointed. I wanted one law that would govern all relationships. I was really disappointed that this is the route that our government chose to take. It shouldn't surprise me, though. I think in general our government is backtracking on a lot of the things that I had thought we could take for granted that they would support us on. But despite that disappointment I am glad that it is there. I hope that heterosexual people will choose to use this piece of legislation, and that the Marriage Act will become redundant.
Sally-Jean: What's great is that if we change marriage, we'll change an institution that is very old, very conservative. Women benefit from changing those stereotypes and making the box bigger. I'm looking forward to seeing that.

'I didn't marry the body, I married the person inside'
Interview with Christelle Delport and Raven Delport

Christelle Delport is a computer programmer and transwoman who has made the transition from male to female. Raven Delport is a homemaker. Christelle and Raven were married under the Marriage Act in 2000 when Christelle was still a man. Following Christelle's transition in 2004 the couple were obliged to divorce in order for Christelle to be able to change the description of her sex to female. The couple plan to remarry under the Civil Union Act. Christelle and Raven are the co-founders of The Budding Roses, a support group for transgender people and their families in Gauteng.

Can you tell us about yourselves?
Christelle: I was born male, but I identify as female. I was six years old when I told my stepdad, 'I'm supposed to be a girl.' I got the beating of my life. So I decided I'd better keep it to myself. You get to a point where you feel guilty about your own feelings, and you try and fit into this role of what society wants you to be. Puberty was hell. Your body grows into something that is the opposite of what your brain tells you that you need to be. There wasn't the information available that there is now. It wasn't until I was in my thirties that I came across the story of a transsexual in *You* magazine. Suddenly a light went on. Suddenly it made sense. I was already married to Raven at that time.
Raven: I was born and raised in rural Kentucky in the USA. I grew up at a time when a woman was supposed to marry and have kids. I did that. I didn't like it. The biggest thing I ever did, besides have kids, was to meet Christelle and move to South Africa.

Christelle, how did you come out as transgender to Raven?
Christelle: Two years after I married Raven I told her I thought I might be a cross-dresser. I felt so comfortable with Raven. That's ultimately why I came out to her. I felt I could trust her with my secret. I had been through a bout of severe depression before that. Raven thought it was her fault. It got to the point where I thought I had to be honest with her.
Raven: When Christelle first told me, we were both more afraid that the other person would want to leave. Once we had a heartfelt talk and said that we did not want to be without each other we were able to move on.

Christelle: Raven saw that I was researching transsexuals on the internet, and one day she came to me and said, 'Listen honey, if you feel you have to go all the way I'll be behind you 100%.'
Raven: I went to her and told her that. She didn't ask. I was sceptical at first, but when I started reading the information and I saw how Christelle felt I thought it would be awful selfish of me not to support her. I didn't marry the body, I married the person inside. I don't consider myself lesbian, but I would never leave Christelle.
Christelle: I started seeing a therapist, and he helped me to start recognizing my own feelings. Raven joined me at sessions and we spoke about how we felt and what the process would be. Over the next six months we worked through our feelings. Once I decided that I was transsexual then it was full steam ahead.

How have your families responded to this change in your lives?
Christelle: I have a son from a previous relationship. I always kept myself at a distance from him. It was only after my gender change that we really connected. Initially it was really hard. He felt that he was losing a father. I think the rest of my family thought it was just a phase that would pass.
Raven: It wasn't until we were actually going to fly to Thailand for Christelle's final gender-reassignment operation that they realized this was serious. Everyone tried to change her mind. And then they blamed me for not stopping it. My own father has no problems with our relationship. He loves finally having a daughter-in-law. My daughters love their two moms. But my mother is closed-minded. She won't speak to me because I didn't leave Christelle. She's afraid of what people might think.
Christelle: When I grew up I was taught family was a mother, a father and children. In our family you still have two adults and the children. It's just that we changed the 'mother and father' part. Now we have two parents. We still have the same functions. I'm still head of the household. We've just taken gender out of it.
Raven: Our roles in our family didn't change. Christelle is still the career person, and I'm still the homebody who takes care of the home and the family. Family is about unconditional love. There is no 'I will love you if you do this.'

Christelle, can you tell us more about your experience of transitioning?
Christelle: I went to a doctor in Thailand who specializes in gender-reassignment surgery, and has perfected the procedure. When I came back to South Africa I had to get the description of my sex changed to female in my ID book. My male ID book caused problems. For example I would go into a bank and withdraw money and the teller would look at my ID book and then say, 'I need to call my supervisor.' You have to stand in front of all these strangers at the bank and explain your situation. It's embarrassing. To do that I had to get the

supporting documents together. The official said, 'Everything looks fine. I just need a copy of your divorce certificate.' I said, 'Divorce certificate?' Suddenly I discovered Raven and I had to get divorced. It was either that or I had to stay with a male identity. So we got divorced.

Can you tell us about that experience of having to get divorced?
Christelle: We could not stay married under the Marriage Act because we would be two females. So we were forced to divorce even though we didn't want to. That was very traumatic for us. You are in this safe cocoon, and all of a sudden you get yanked out of it. All your protection gets taken away. All your surety gets taken away. All the dignity that your relationship is provided with is taken away. This was in 2004, before the Civil Union Act was being spoken about.
Raven: One of the things we were concerned about was whether I would be taken care of if something happened to Christelle.
Christelle: I had to make double-sure that if anything happens to me Raven is taken care of. That she's not going to lose the house. She won't be kicked out on the streets. In that regard it was stressful.

Do you plan to get married again under the Civil Union Act now that it has it has been passed?
Christelle: We plan to get remarried on our wedding anniversary on 4 February.
Raven: We didn't want to change our anniversary date by getting remarried on a different day. We want to carry on as though the divorce never happened.
Christelle: The divorce decree is just a piece of paper that we have to rectify. They say we got divorced, but in our minds we never got divorced. People ask, 'Are you married?' and I say 'Yes we are.'

How do you feel about the Civil Union Act itself?
Christelle: You feel as though you get treated as a second-class citizen. We were good enough for the Marriage Act as a man and a woman. Now we're no longer good enough. There has to be something separate for us. Instead of being treated like everyone else, you get treated differently. If you take it from Raven's point of view, she gets punished for loving me. That's not fair. All we want is to be together and to be married to each other. Having said that, the Civil Union Act gives us the same protection that we had before.

'The guts to get married'
Interview with Sadia Kruger and Zukayna Kruger

When Sadia Kruger and Zukayna Kruger (formerly Leonard) were married on 3 February 2007 in Cape Town, they became the first same-sex Muslim couple to do so publicly under the Civil Union Act. The pair met and fell in love 15 years ago and have lived together for nearly 12 of those years. Sadia and Zukayna both grew up in Muslim homes and are active members of the Inner Circle, an organization providing support and services for lesbian and gay Muslims. Sadia works as a driver in the male-dominated transport industry, and Zukeyna in food preparation.

Can you tell us about being lesbian and Muslim?
Sadia: Both of us are Muslim. We say our prayers at home, and we fast, and we go to mosque. We do everything that Muslims do.
Zukayna: I know a lot of Muslims don't like gay people, because they think it is a sin. They treat people as if they will never accept gays in the Muslim religion. Sometimes when I was younger I felt like this is something wrong that I do. Especially when I went to mosque, people made me feel that it is wrong. This is a free country now, so why can't we be free?
Sadia: It doesn't make sense to me. I was born a Muslim and no-one can change me. They are not God and only God can punish us. If it was a sin God would not give me breath. Who are they to judge me?
Zukayna: If you're not acceptable in a mosque, or you don't feel free to go there, you can still say your prayers at home. That's how it is for me. At night, when I go to be bed, I can say my prayers. God can see and hear you anywhere.

How do your families feel about your sexuality?
Sadia: My family knows my life. My mother was a bit unhappy when she first saw me with a girl. She said we mustn't go out together. But one day she saw lesbians on TV and she phoned me and said, 'Sadia, there are lesbians on the TV,' and after that it was fine. My father was excited. He was a woodcutter, and he always wanted me to go cut wood with him in the bush.
Zukayna: My mother is very supportive, as is my whole family. They've known us as a couple for so long, they don't have a problem with it.

Do you know many other gay and lesbian Muslims?
Sadia: Oh, there are a lot of them! You get to know people by their nicknames,

but when you find out the person's real name you realize they're Muslim. Now why hide? And we know more through The Inner Circle, a community organization that stands behind gay and lesbian Muslims.
Zukayna: They're scared to come out as gay and Muslim, because of people's reaction.

How did you decide to get married?
Sadia: I bought Zukayna a wedding ring every year, hoping to make her my wife. We followed the marriage campaign on TV and it just got us so excited. I asked Zukayna to marry me the same week the law was passed.
Zukayna: The law was passed on a Thursday and on the Saturday we got engaged. There was no doubt in our minds. It meant a lot when the Act came in. It was such a relief for us. We had been waiting for this for such a long time. Now we could do it!

Why was marriage important for you?
Zukayna: You can have a commitment ceremony, and you commit to the person, but still anything can happen. Marriage is different. It says, 'You belong to me, and I belong to you.' You have that respect for your partner at all times. You feel proud about yourself, because you are now a married person. When people ask about us I don't have to say, 'We are just partners.' Other people respect your relationship more.

Tell us about the wedding itself.
Sadia: We got married at Home Affairs in Mitchell's Plain on the 3rd of February 2007.
Zukayna: It was the first wedding that the Home Affairs official did. She was proud, that day, to marry us. I arrived an hour late – I was still busy dressing. I had someone make a dress for me – I didn't want to be married in someone else's dress. The wedding itself was hectic. We did it very fast, and on our own. There was a party afterwards at the Alliance Française in Mitchell's Plain.
Sadia: The party was a gift from my friends and working colleagues. I felt so happy on the day. I felt like I'm a big man now! Thanks to Thabo Mbeki!

What has been the response of the Muslim community to your wedding?
Zukayna: People thought we wouldn't have the guts to get married as two Muslim people. People are *mos* scared to come out. At first I didn't even want the people to know I was getting married. I thought, 'Keep it quiet.' But then I said to myself, 'Why not?' People know that although I'm a Muslim I'm also a lesbian. If they want to say something they must say it to my face. They are not God. They can't judge me. When I meet someone new and they ask me, 'Are you

married? Do you have someone?' I say, 'Yes. I'm a lesbian. Feel free to be my friend or not be my friend.' That works well for me. When someone gets closer to me, some of them start asking me different kinds of questions, and I feel free to talk about being a lesbian. People mustn't be scared to come out, or get married. Because you know in yourself who you are.

Sadia: I am with these people every day, and no one has insulted me. For our wedding, the people said we must marry again because they'd never seen a wedding like it in their lives! They still talk about it. My customers all cut out articles about our wedding after it appeared in the newspapers.

Did you go on honeymoon?
Sadia: There was a friend who offered us a room in a hotel in Cape Town the night of the wedding. But we refused. We wanted to be alone in our own house. Our house is important to us.
Zukayna: The first place we stayed together was a caravan, and we rented a yard to put it in. But you know how people are if you're two women living together in a gay relationship. Not everyone was happy. So we moved the caravan to another yard.
Sadia: We had also applied to the council for a house, and after a few months they phoned us: 'You must come fetch your keys, you've got your house.' It's almost 12 years now that we've been staying at that house in Delft.

'Rejoicing in merit'
Interview with Wayne Sampson and Vajradhara

Wayne Sampson cuts hair and Vajradhara (his ordained name) teaches meditation and Buddhism. Vajradhara is one of only two order members of the Western Buddhist Order in Africa; the Order was founded in the 1960s to create a form of Buddhism accessible to the West, and now has centres throughout the world. Wayne is in training to be ordained into this Order. Wayne and Vajradhara are based at Shantikula, a Sanskrit name which means Peaceful Tribe. Shantikula is a Meditation and Buddhist Centre; Wayne also has his studio there. They were married on 24 March 2007, three and a half years after they met.

How did the two of you meet?
Wayne: I was interested in deepening my meditation experience. I typed in 'meditation' and 'Buddhism' in the search engine on Gaydar and it came up with his profile. I saw a photo of him, and then we met, and he was quite fantastic! In fact, it had been his birthday a few days before, so I was like a belated birthday present. Prior to meeting Vajradhara, my idea had been to move from my salon in Hyde Park, which was very expensive to rent, pay off all my debts, simplify my life. I was going to sell my flat, save money, maybe go and do a long silence. I wanted to have a more monastic lifestyle. Now it's all in one place and this makes a difference in terms of accessibility for people interested in meditation and Buddhism. I work here, I've got my studio here, I live here, I grow vegetables here.

Vajradhara: I was not interested in a monogamous sexual relationship. That was the basis on which Wayne and I got involved. As it has turned out, now I am only involved with Wayne, but we didn't get married on that basis. Our loyalty to each other is of a different kind. The commitment to each other is more about what we're trying to do in the world than it is about the mode of our sexuality.

At the beginning, I wanted to get married for financial reasons, because I had put a lot of money into a pension scheme and I wanted the money to go to projects that I believed in, and you don't get the full benefit if you don't have a surviving spouse. But what also happened was that the Buddhist representative on the National Religious Leaders' Forum asked the Buddhist groups in this country for their views on same-sex marriage, during the process of that year between the Constitutional Court ruling and the passing of the Civil Union Act, so I made a submission to him. He obviously didn't present only my view – he decided to neither support nor oppose the Bill. But that made me think about marriage, and in the meantime my personal situation in terms of relationships changed and deepened. I like to do things wholeheartedly, so I thought quite seriously: 'Why am I doing this?' And in the end we had quite a big wedding, where family and friends came and witnessed and celebrated that.

What does marriage mean to you?
Vajradhara: Marriage is not a Buddhist concept. It can be seen as a contradiction of Buddhist principles, because one is making a very strong commitment to something that you could say is a barrier to the spiritual life. It ties you up. But the romantic attachment is a very strong pull – it comes from the human need to be loved, and from the fact that we have a body with the biology of sex. On the positive side, you can argue that it simplifies your life to make such a commitment.

Traditionally, in Buddhism, you have a split between monks and nuns, and laypeople. What is unhelpful about this split is that the monks and nuns are considered to be the serious spiritual practitioners, and the laypeople serve the monks and seek blessings on various occasions such as marriage, birth, death and so on. There would be some kind of marriage ceremony in a socio-legal setting, and then they would go for a blessing, depending on the particular cultural or ethnic situation where people were Buddhists.

The Order in which I am ordained seeks to transcend this polarity between monastic and lay. This polarity is unhelpful for many people who seek to commit themselves to the spiritual life but don't wish to become celibate or are not ready to become celibate. Premature celibacy has contributed to much suffering, for example among Roman Catholic priests and those who have somehow come within their sexual ambit. So I'm ordained but I'm not celibate. Some members of my Order are celibate. It's the same ordination, but they take a different precept in terms of sex. They take a precept abstaining from sex, whereas those who are not celibate take a precept abstaining from sexual misconduct.

This polarity has an effect which is in some ways similar to the problem that can arise when people hold to the idea of God as an authority figure who, if they do wrong, is going to withdraw love. It's the same with parents, teachers, friends – the feeling that they could withdraw love. That leads into a whole arena of low self-esteem. It constrains us from leading a wholehearted and emotionally positive life. So, in some ways, I'd argue against marriage because it's not a spiritual construct. It can subsume the individual into coupledom. Buddhism starts with the individual, it's the expression of one's own aspirations to become enlightened. It's a conundrum – our wish and intention to be altruistic, to be kind and compassionate, comes about more effectively through seeking to transform ourselves, by understanding the true nature of how things really are.

So we didn't have a Buddhist wedding. We had a wedding in a Buddhist context. We just decided what we wanted to do. I've done some blessings for heterosexual weddings, so we had some ideas. At the beginning, everyone at the wedding did a loving-kindness meditation. That was half of the whole ceremony. We did a variation of a common loving-kindness meditation practice. Everyone first cultivated positive feelings towards themselves, then wished Wayne and myself well, then cultivated kindness towards everyone at the wedding, before expanding outwards to wish all beings well.

Then we each spoke about what marriage meant to us, and why we were getting married to each other, and then the magistrate did the legal bit. He's a magistrate who comes to the Buddhist centre. He doesn't normally do weddings, but any magistrate is entitled to conduct a marriage ceremony. We signed the papers before we went in, and later he stood up and did the three lines that you've got to say, and we shook hands. By law, you've got to join hands.

We had supper afterwards, but because we don't drink alcohol we didn't want to have toasts, so we had what we call in Buddhism a 'rejoicing in merit'. People speak about what they like and admire about you. They rejoice in your positive qualities. An old friend of each of us stood up and spoke, and then it was open to everyone else. A number of people got up and spoke – friends and family. And then Buddhist blessings were chanted. It was lovely. People told us afterwards they were very moved.

Wayne: A friend who was at the wedding said it was the first time he'd understood meditation. What was nice for me about the wedding was that it didn't follow any format that was traditional. It wasn't trying to make a comparison with a heterosexual wedding. There were no rings – we didn't have any jewellery. We had scarves, and a friend's mother gave us beautiful garlands to swap. The combination of the meditation and the blessings made it feel like a very natural thing. No big fireworks. Afterwards there was a dinner.

What are your thoughts on the Civil Union Act itself?
Vajradhara: In our ceremony, we used the 'marriage' wording, not 'civil partnership'. I was opposed to the idea that it should be 'separate but equal'. In the European countries where there are civil unions or partnerships, I understand it was better to get it through than not at all. But where you've had it for a long time, like in Holland, people eventually want to make a legal challenge, and it moves from being a civil partnership to being a marriage – the same words. In South Africa, the law is leading social attitudes. In Europe, certainly in the UK, the civil-partnership law for same-sex couples has *followed* social attitudes – I think people are ahead of the law.

Gay people want to be acknowledged, for their emotions to be given valid expression in the social situation. I can't say that's why I did it, because I have no difficulty expressing that in my life normally, but I felt that when I was doing it.

Has marriage changed your relationship?
Wayne: When I spoke during the wedding ceremony about what marriage meant to me, I gave the analogy of two leaves drifting downstream, coming together, then moving apart. There's nothing that's forced. It's a subtle change in energy. If you want to define what the energy of being married is about, it's like the two leaves touching. They're just somehow brought together by this dynamic.

Vajradhara: There was a funny incident the other day at the Garden Shop. I went to pay and the cashier said, 'Have you got your Garden Shop card?' I said, 'No, my husband always has it. Can you give me my own one?' She said, 'No, as long as you've got the number of his card, it's OK,' and then she searched for it on their computer and entered it into my cell phone. On a subsequent visit to the shop when we were there together, she said, 'Now I can see you're here with your husband!' It was a very lovely moment. I could see that when I first told her I had a husband she was a bit disconcerted, but it was an opportunity to engage in a way that was entirely natural. That's the small details of the Constitution of this country finding expression in our day-to-day lives.

'A living tradition'
Interview with Margaret Auerbach and Liebe Kellen

In March 2007, Margaret Auerbach and Liebe Kellen became the first Jewish lesbian couple to be married in a Jewish religious ceremony recognized by the state. The newspaper The Citizen *ran a story on their marriage under the headline 'Lesbians Make it Kosher'. The couple met in 1984, and at the time of the interview had been together for 23 years. Margaret works as a puppeteer and Liebe is involved in social work.*

Why did you choose to be married in a Jewish religious ceremony?
Liebe: The ceremony itself was about showing our connection to the faith that we were born into. My grandfather was a rabbi. I grew up in a strict Orthodox Jewish household in a small town – the Reform movement was a 'no-go'. Margaret also grew up in an Orthodox family, although hers was more liberal. But there was a long period in which we had both moved away from the Jewish religion, and, in fact, had felt quite alienated from it. We tried to locate ourselves spiritually by exploring other religious options, like Buddhism. But we found that the religion you are born into has a much stronger impact than you realize. We came to understand that, spiritually, we needed to start where our roots are.
Margaret: We were looking for spirituality, and we found that within the Reform movement in Judaism. We joined a *chavurah* [community of friends] that meets at Temple Emanuel in Johannesburg.
Liebe: It was an important realization that Judaism did not need to be what we had grown up with, that there was room for change.
Margaret: I approached our rabbi to bless our marriage. He said that he would only do the blessing for us in the synagogue if it was me and Liebe on our own. Otherwise he was willing to do it in his office with our immediate family, or he would do a house blessing. I said, 'Thank you. Goodbye.' We worked with David Bilchitz from [the LGBTI organization] Jewish OutLook to plan the wedding. When it came to planning the ceremony we realized that there are lots of elements in a traditional Jewish wedding that don't sit very comfortably with us. We wanted a wedding that would affirm us as Jewish and as lesbians and feminists. The wonderful thing about being a lesbian is that it forces you to redefine a lot of things, to look at traditions in a new way. We realized that we would have to change some of the rituals so that they reflected our lives and our

sense of who we are. David helped us do that in a way that we felt still honoured the traditional meaning that the rituals held. On the day itself David officiated over the religious part of the ceremony, and Pastor Janine Preesman [a religious marriage officer under the Civil Union Act] took care of the legal part.

How did you go about reinventing the traditional Jewish wedding ceremony?
Margaret: We looked at the specific practices that are available, so we didn't have to try to invent things from scratch. We were able to make use of things that had been there all along. So, we included traditional elements such as the *chupah* [wedding canopy], circling seven times, and the breaking of the glass, but we tweaked or adjusted these practices. For example, we used the feminine in the Hebrew blessings in the ceremony; also the word Shekhinah, or divine presence, instead of God. The *chupah* was dyed in rainbow colours. These things made a big difference to us.
Liebe: Also, instead of the *ketubah* [traditional marriage contract], which can be a sexist document, we put together a Covenant of Love. There is a moment before the traditional ceremony where the groom puts a veil over the bride – the idea of a protective garment. There was no way we were going to do that, so instead we both exchanged scarves. The breaking of the glass symbolizes sorrow at the destruction of the Temple in Jerusalem. In our ceremony we both broke a glass, and for us the breaking was also a reminder that in our time of joy we should still remember the gay and lesbian people who are experiencing the oppression of the closet.
Margaret: It was important that we find a way to incorporate these traditional elements so that Jewish people could recognize what we were doing and feel that our wedding fell within the bigger tradition of Judaism.

Why get married after having been in a committed relationship for so many years?
Liebe: It was partly about pushing the envelope. The Reform Jewish movement had not made a decision about whether it was going to allow same-sex marriages or not. It felt as though that decision had been put on hold, and that it would remain that way unless a sense of urgency was created. We thought that in getting married in a religious ceremony we could help to create that sense of urgency, and open the way for other Jewish lesbian and gay people who also wanted to get married.
Margaret: And it worked – a month or two after our marriage the South African Union for Progressive Judaism decided to allow marriage between Jewish gay and lesbian couples. Of course there were also personal reasons for us to get married, in addition to the political reasons. It was also about publicly acknowledging that we are a loving couple who have been together for a long time.

Liebe: The change for me came when I watched the development of the same-sex marriage legislation and took part in some of the discussions around same-sex marriage. Margaret and I had been very critical of marriage as a patriarchal institution in the past. I realized that marriage could be turned on its head and transformed. We also had practical reasons for getting married – protection in the event of illness and death, for example.

Margaret: I did not feel initially that we needed marriage. I felt the commitment from the very first time Liebe and I slept together. That was real commitment. But I have been surprised at the difference it has made. I think our love for each other has really deepened. I also feel more confident in coming out to people since we got married.

Liebe: I also did not expect to feel different after getting married, but, surprisingly, I do. There is also a different level of respect that outsiders have for our relationship now that we are married.

Do you think marriages such as yours will help to change the way the Jewish community in South Africa feels about same-sex unions?

Margaret: I know that two women getting married in a religious Jewish ceremony must seem strange to some people. But a lot of new things feel strange at first. I think as time goes on people will accept it. My own family members have been very supportive.

Liebe: The Reform movement makes the point that Judaism is a living tradition – so there is space for traditions to change.

Index

African Christian Democratic Party (ACDP), 94, 138-9, picture pages
African National Congress (ANC), 6, 37, 92, 107-10, 134-139, 141-2, 144, 167, 280-2, 325, 327; ANC caucus, 107, 108, 110, 138
adoption, 163(n42), 238, 264, 276, 325-6; rights, 19, 23-4, 32, 34, 38, 44, 60, 91, 94; international rights, 193, 195, 290, 297(n35), 298(n44)
age of consent: for sex, 19, 26, 27(n15), 156; for marriage, 156, 304
anal sex, 223 (*see also* sodomy)
Anglican Church, 113, 127, 213, 253-245, 257(n4, n11), 274
ante-nuptial contract, 202-3
apartheid, 3-5, 34, 35, 37, 105, 170, 184, 187, 189, 194, 241, 243-4, 264, 268, 270; struggle against, 127, 186, 194, 223; post-apartheid as condition, 186, 190; biblical legitimation of, 243; demise of, 174; laws, 104, 184, 157, 165, 275
artificial insemination, 102, 195, 258-9, 264

Baehr v Lewin (USA), 286
Baehr v Miike (USA), 286
Baker v Nelson (USA), 285
Behind the Mask, 146(n5), 306(n1)
Bill of Rights, 5, 14(n5), 23, 42, 55, 60-2, 66, 69(n1), 92, 94, 103, 105, 117-8, 135, 137, 142, 166-8, 170(n6), 171, 187, 188, 200, 212, 217(n4), 243, 249, 258-9, 279 (*see also* equality clause; religion, freedom of)
Buddhism, 8, 235-245, 325, 241-344

Cameron, Edwin (Justice), 2, 60-3, 86(n8), 181(n19), 184-5, 191, 192(n9), 192(n12, n13, n19), 265, 300
Catholic Church, 40(n43), 119-120, 343
Centre for Applied Legal Studies (CALS), 91, 123-4
Christianity, 7-8, 13, 49, 50-2, 77-8, 83, 96(n8), 122, 145, 149, 156, 160, 173, 177, 194, 209-218, 221, 227(n19), 228-231, 232-245, 268-273, 318, 327-8 (*see also* Anglican Church; Catholic Church; religion)
Christian Lawyers Association, 122-3
civil partnership: definition in Civil Union Bill, 128, 132, 142-3, 150-3, 160(n4), 165-6; as opposed to marriage, 29, 37-8, 41(n52), 48, 115-6, 118, 123-4, 126, 142, 143, 145, 149-55, 159, 162(n27), 167, 202-5, 228, 271, 293, 296(n23), 343; Civil Partnership Act (UK), 161(n6), 162(n2), 180(n4), 291, 299(n60)
Civil Union Act: and African culture, 97-104, 171-81, 300-6; amends existing legislation, 37, 38; definition of unions under, 41(n52); designation of marriage officers, 12, 26, 29, 38-9, 54, 68, 95, 118, 128, 138, 141, 144, 157-8, 166, 203-6, 228-9, 230, 236, 241; as discriminatory, 26, 38, 271-2; as inclusive, 56, 153, 228, 249, 252; marriages and civil partnerships under, 14(n19), 225, 228-31, 232-4, 249-57, 317-347, picture pages; provisions, 37-9, 149-63, 202-6; conscientious-objection clause ('opt-out' clause, Section 6 of the Act), 6, 12, 26, 39, 109, 130, 144, 157, 158, 197; as Western-style pact, 255
Civil Union Bill: first draft of, 4, 29, 37, 44, 37, 39(n2), 54, 93, 108, 115, 127-8, 150-1, 153-4, 159, 161(n12), 270; debate on, 5, 107-8, 164-70, 187, 211-2, 238, 259, 308-10; in National Assembly, 134-42; in National Council of Provinces, 143-5; hearings on, 80, 92-5, 102-3, 115-46, 214-5, 224, 226, 227(n13) (*see also* Parliament); legislative process, 26, 29, 85, 115-46, 279, 308; minister meets activists on, 93, 153; vote on, 110, 134-45; unconstitutional, 29, 118, 146(n7), 122, 130, 138, 150-1; referred to Contralesa, 131-2 (*see also* Congress of Traditional Leaders of South Africa); as 'separate but equal', 4, 29, 35-7, 54, 67, 116, 118, 128, 142, 165, 196, 343
Commission on Gender Equality, 21, 91, 96(n6)
commitment ceremonies, 4, 11, 49-50, 163(n46), 232-3, 237, 324-6, 329, 339

349

Constitution, 1-3, 5-6, 13, 14(n8), 43-47, 52, 108-9, 115, 117, 123-7, 130, 132-5, 137, 139, 141-2, 144-5, 149, 151, 153, 157, 161(n15), 163(n36, n42), 164, 166-170, 170(n8), 173, 183-191, 192(n12, n18), 193-6, 199, 200, 212-4, 219, 227(n9), 238, 240, 249, 257(n1), 258-9, 266(n1), 273, 275, 279-80, 293, 327, 344; interim Constitution, 2, 17, 18, 26(n2), 27(n3)
constitutional amendment, calls for, 5, 116, 126, 129-30, 132, 135, 149, 191
Constitutional Court, 2-4, 6, 7, 50, 51, 52, 55, 58-9, 63-9, 73, 85(n5), 89, 96(n2), 104, 108-110, 115, 117, 120, 121-2, 124-32, 135-9, 141-2, 145(n1, n2), 146(n6), 149-52, 159, 164-9, 175, 182, 185, 188-91, 195, 197, 200, 213-4, 217(n4), 249, 258, 275, 277, 281, 327, 341; judgment in *Fourie*, *see* Sachs judgment
Congress of Traditional Leaders of South Africa (Contralesa), 8, 80, 82, 85(n2), 94, 102-4, 260, 265, 266(n6), 277, 277(n7); parliamentary submission, 131-2, 163(n41)
customary marriages, 46, 101-2, 155, 158-9, 172-4; Recognition of Customary Marriages Act, 41(n53, n54), 47, 101, 103, 158, 163(n40), 172-3, 178, 180(n8), 204, 158

'decriminalization case' (*National Coalition for Gay and Lesbian Equality and the South African Human Rights Commission v Minister of Justice and Others*, also referred to as 'sodomy case'), 3, 18, 20-1, 26(n2), 27(n6, n17), 28(n22), 31, 39(n12), 40(n16), 192(n11), 182, 185, 188-191, 195, 279
Defence of Marriage Act (USA), 287
democracy, 5, 10, 21, 52, 60, 64, 65, 77, 79, 81, 83, 90, 92, 94-6, 104-6, 108, 110, 116-8, 122-6, 131, 134-5, 164, 185, 213, 278, 280-3, 277, 303 (*see also* majoritarianism); constitutional, 36, 117, 165-70, 189, 195, 201, 214, 277; transition, to, 2, 10; democratic elections (1994), 325; democratic process, 86, 240, 293
Democratic Alliance, 136-7
divorce, 11, 32, 50, 74, 78, 101-104, 156, 194, 198-200, 204, 221, 242, 258, 264-265, 269, 299(n59, n61)

Doctors for Life, 116-7
domestic partnerships, 45, 119, 121-3, 126, 136, 142, 145, 155, 159, 290; Domestic Partnerships Bill, 14(n11), 26, 144; in draft Civil Union Bill, 116, 123, 136, 142, 144, 150; recognition of, 19
Du Plessis v Road Accident Fund, 23, 57
Durban Lesbian and Gay Community and Health Centre, 2, 28(n41), 59, 103, 146(n5), 206, 259
Dutch Reformed Church (Nederduits-Gereformeerde Kerk or NGK), 48, 235-45; submission to Parliament, 129
Du Toit and De Vos v Minister of Welfare and Population Development and Others, 23-4, 32, 41(n56), 57, 258, 326

equality clause (Bill of Rights), 2-3, 14(n5), 19, 43, 55, 83, 94, 101, 137, 141, 183, 185, 187, 227(n9), 249, 257(n1), 258, 273, 279, 300
Equality Project: *see* Lesbian and Gay Equality Project

family law, 3, 7, 10, 63, 69(n1), 88, 90, 95, 123, 149, 155, 160, 161(n16), 179, 265, 293-5; in Canada and USA, 288
Farr v Mutual & Federal Insurance Co Ltd, 23
feminism, 10, 12, 38, 237, 260, 258-65, 276, 307-13, 331, 345; lesbian-feminism, 194, 259
Forum for the Empowerment of Women (FEW), 2, 28(n41), 59, 146(n5), 259, 307, picture pages
Fourie case, 4, 14(n4), 58-69; in High Court, 2, 58-9, 63, 167, 170(n10); in Supreme Court of Appeal (SCA), 2, 61-3, 167, 170(n10), 184, 188-9, 192(n10); in Constitutional Court (*Minister of Home Affairs and Another v Fourie and Another*), 2, 4, 59, 60, 63-9, 89, 97(n2), 103, 115, 117, 125-7, 145(n1, n2), 146(n6), 149-51, 160(n1, n5), 164, 167, 169, 170(n1, n12), 182-92(n5), 192(n17), 195-6, 200-1, 217(n6), 259, picture pages
Freedom Front (FF), 138

Gay and Lesbian Organization of the Witwatersrand (GLOW), 4, 42, 319
gender, 5, 10, 11, 30, 139, 153, 172-3, 179, 199, 216, 221, 237, 240, 241 (*see also*

INDEX

transgender people); gender equality, 13, 78, 81, 170, 171, 216; gendered construction of institutions, relationships, 10, 152, 156, 176, 177, 153, 163 (n42, n44), 262-3, 276; de-gendering, 10, 266-275; gender norms, 161 (*see also* norms/normativity); gender-neutral definition (of rape), 26; gender-neutral language and definitions (of marriage), 54 119, 120, 122, 150-1, 156, 202, 271-2; gender-specific language, institutions, 32, 131, 221; gender roles, 5, 6, 12, 73-86, 163, (n41, n42), 178, 261-3, 276
Gender DynamiX, 146 (n5), 206, 331
Goodridge v Department of Public Health (USA), 151, 161 (n7), 200, 288
Gory v Kolver NO, 39, 41 (n56, 57), 57
Greyling v Minister of Welfare, 258, 266 (n2)

hairstyling, 76-7, 84
hate crimes, 11, 212-3, 302 (*see also* homophobia; rape; murder)
hate speech, 5, 13, 95, 113, 114, 121, 127, 164, 196, 239, 278
heteronormativity, 4, 13, 31, 195, 260-5, 268-70, 274, 310 (*see also* norms/normativity)
heterosexuality: disappearance of, 261; as dominant, normative, 30-1, 265, 311; rape as 'conversion' to, 191, 259, 302 (*see also* marriage)
Hinduism, 8, 172, 235-45, 268, 325
HIV/AIDS, 78, 79, 112, 210, 234, 282, 317
Home Affairs, Department of, 24, 50-1, 108, 125, 127, 145, 150, 161 (n12), 203, 228; Director-General, 21; lobbied, 92; marriages at, 10, 11, 45, 49, 205, 230, 251, 319-20, 321-2, 326-7, 329-30, 339; Minister of, 93, 128, 134-4, 142, 153, 158, 197, 229; Parliamentary Portfolio Committee on, 32, 37, 85 (n2), 90, 92-5, 115, 121, 127, 129, 131-3, 135, 137, 165-6, 214, 217
homophobia, 8, 9, 12, 13, 94, 125, 134, 136, 145, 170, 190, 191, 196, 212-7, 226, 231, 240, 243, 277, 282-3, 301-3, 306, 310-3; in parliamentary hearings, 164, 167, 249; state homophobia in Africa, 306 (n1); as Western import, 9 (*see also* hate crimes; hate speech)
homosexuality (male and female): acts versus persons, 119, 122; and African culture, 8, 9, 31, 73-86, 131-2, 163 (n43), 171-81 180 (n12), 249-57, 274, 277, 278, 300-306; African terms for, 176, 81, 82, 84, 177-8, 317, 321; as 'unAfrican', 47, 83, 91, 94, 274-5, 302, 303; decriminalization campaigns, 42, 44, 17-28, 55-7 (*see also* 'decriminalization case'); as deviant or inferior, 31, 275, 301; as 'lightning rod', 9; normalization of, 13; religion and, 53, 65, 91, 103, 113, 119, 209-18, 219-27, 228-31, 232-4, 235-45, 226-73, 274, 300-306; and struggle against apartheid, 70, 186-7, 192 (n16); as Western, 84, 172, 177, 179, 213, 239, 242, 299 (n64), 306 (*see also* gender; sexualities)
Horizon Community Association (Rwanda), 300

identity/identities, 47, 60, 104, 256, 265, 274-5, 289, 317, 331, 333; African, 9-11, 105, 159, 172, 177, 179, 256; gender identities, 11, 88, 125, 176-7, 206; heterosexual, 79; national, 172, 185; identity politics, 249; multiple, 47; same-sex/gay/lesbian, 103, 105, 159, 161 (n18), 172, 175, 226, 249, 260, 262, 274-5, 275, 291, 312, 324; as 'Western', 84, 172, 177, 179, 213, 299 (n64), 306; sexual, 47, 112, 125, 244; transgender, 331, 333, 337; versus behaviour, 276 (*see also* sexualities)
'immigration case' (see *National Coalition for Gay and Lesbian Equality and Others v Minister of Home Affairs and Others*)
immigration rights, 38
Independent Democrats (ID), 137
inheritance rights: 19, 23, 35, 39, 41 (n56, n57), 57, 213, 250, 253, 255, 265, 281
Inkatha Freedom Party (IFP), 137
Inner Circle, The, 219, 223-7; submission to Parliament, 121-2
Integrity (Uganda), 300
in vitro fertilization, 23, 57, 269
Ishtar MSM (Kenya), 300
Islam, 8, 11, 121-2, 139, 155, 171-3, 219-27, 235, 243, 268, 338-40

J and Another v Director General, Department of Home Affairs and Others, 23, 40 (n22, n56), 57

351

Jewish OutLook, 146 (n5), 345
Joint Working Group (JWG), 88-92, 94, 96 (n2), 146 (n5), 182, 206, 279; submission to Parliament, 124-5; statement in NCOP, 143-5
Judaism, 12, 235-4, 325, 345-7

Karner v Austria (EU), 291
Lekota, Mosiuoa (Minister of Defence), 127-8
Langemaat v Minister of Safety and Security and Others (also known as 'Polmed'), 22, 27 (n10), 28 (n27), 55, 192 (n6, n18), 182-3, 187
Lesbian and Gay Equality Project, 2-4, 14 (n3), 24-6, 28 (n42), 44-6, 49, 52, 55, 58-60, 67, 79-80, 87-9, 93, 145 (n2), 162, 206, 233; as *amicus curiae* in *Fourie* cases, 24, 28 (n38, n42), 57-60, 170; as *amicus curiae* in *Du Toit*, 41 (n46); direct application to Constitutional Court (*Lesbian and Gay Equality Project and Others v Minister of Home Affairs and Others*), 2, 14, 20, 25, 26 (n1), 52, 55-9, 145, 161 (n1); same-sex marriage case in High Court, 25, 59; submission to Parliament, 120-1
Lesbian and Gay Equality Project and the South African Human Rights Commission v Minister of Justice and Others: see 'decriminalization case'
Lesbian and Gay Equality Project and Others v the Minister of Finance, 56
life partnerships, 61, 123, 159; recognition in law, 38, 56; Life Partnership Act, Germany, 290
Little Sisters of Rwanda, 300-1
lobola, 47, 97-102, 105 (n1), 163 (n44), 249, 251-257 (n3), 318, 322

majoritarianism, 65, 118, 168, 189-90, 293, 309, 325
marriage: common-law definition of 274; as companionate, 63, 173, 268-70, 272, 304; as contract, 101, 121-2, 199-200, 205, 221, 241, 264, 346; decentring of, 155, 160; definitions of, 220-1, 225, 238, 254, 260, 263, 273, 275, 291, 297 (n26); designation in Civil Union Act, 41 (n54), 101, 109, 271, 343; heterosexual marriages, 2-5, 12, 29, 37-8, 46, 109, 176, 212, 261, 263, 268, 270, 290, 312; as exclusively heterosexual, 2-5, 12, 14 (n13), 31, 33, 38, 47, 64, 117, 122-3, 126, 128, 149, 156-7, 220, 252, 260-3, 265, 286, 288, 297 (n26), 334; and family, 230, 250, 252-253, 256, 258, 264, 276, 298 (n64), 319-320, 322, 325-327, 332; and female husbands, 163 (n43), 174, 180 (n12), 253-4, 298 (n50); institution of, 272, 281, 287, 332; interracial, 34, 130, 157, 168; legal consequences of, 255, 264, 268, 270-3, 275, 281, 286, 289, 290-2; meaning of, 219, 229, 230, 233, 237, 249, 250, 251, 268, 274-6, 304, 328, 334, 342-4; mine marriages, 174, 176; Muslim marriages, 172; as oppressive, 38, 259-263, 276, 307-313, 325, 347; and procreation, 9, 36, 79-80, 84, 119, 122, 131, 140, 216, 220-1, 268, 272, 275, 311; religious marriages, 69, 111, 318-20, 325, 327, 345-7; social significance of, 221, 245, 250-1, 255, 256, 264, 276, 319-20, 332; status of, 5, 7, 24, 29, 37, 38, 116, 117, 143, 149, 151, 155, 160, 290-1; woman-to-woman marriages, 163 (n40, n42), 174-5, 180 (n8), 253-6 (*see also* civil partnership)
Marriage Act (1961), 51, 66, 144, 172, 204, 333; age of consent under, 156; in Bible, 268-70; challenges to, 2, 5, 59; as Christian, 145, 173; as civil not religious, 168, 334; and Recognition of Customary Marriages Act, 41, (n53, n54), 143, 204, 271 (*see also* customary marriages); designation of marriage officers under, 38-39, 229; as discriminatory or unconstitutional, 4, 5, 25, 26 (n1), 68, 156, 164, 228, 271; marriage formula in, 33, 37, 58, 88, 120; amendment to, 3-4, 54, 68-9, (n1), 109, 119, 126, 128-9, 131, 137, 149-53, 160, 164, 214, 228, 236; as redundant, 130, 137, 141, 156, 334
Marriage Alliance, 40 (n43) 146 (n46) 129-30
Martin v Beka Provident Fund, 28 (n30), 56
Metropolitan Community Church (MCC): Glorious Light MCC, 146 (n5) 228; Good Hope MCC, 52, 113, 146 (n5); Hope and Unity MCC, 146 (n5), 232, 318; House of Rainbow MCC (Nigeria), 300

Minister of Home Affairs and Another v Fourie and Another: see *Fourie* in Constitutional Court
Mohapi v Mohapi, 258, 266 (n2)
murder, 215; of gay men, 113; of lesbian women, 113, 127, 182, 191, 196, 209, 217, 259-60
Muslim Judicial Council (MJC), 122-3, 223, 225

National AIDS Control Council, 302
National Coalition for Gay and Lesbian Equality, 2, 17, 18-22, 27 (n14), 28 (n20), 44, 49, 55, 87, 278-9, 300
National Coalition for Gay and Lesbian Equality and Another v Minister of Justice and Others: see 'decriminalization case'
National Coalition for Gay and Lesbian Equality and Others v Minister of Home Affairs and Others ('immigration case'), 21-2, 27 (n4, n12), 28 (n23), 31, 195, 258
National House of Traditional Leaders (NHTL), 5, 73, 78, 81-4, 94, 129, 159
Nigerian Same-Sex Marriage (Prevention) Bill, 277, 303, 306
norms/normativity, 13, 30, 31, 35, 44, 47, 49, 66, 73, 76-86, 91, 111, 129, 131-2, 161 (n14, n18), 175, 178, 188-90, 195, 210, 293, 299 (n58, n64), 309, 312, 327; human-rights, 289; legally normative, 31, 188; normalization, of homosexuality and homosexual relationships, 13, 127, 236-8, 244, 276; and values, 98 (*see also* heteronormativity)

O'Regan, Kate (Justice), 13; dissenting judgment in *Fourie* in Constitutional Court, 3, 68-9, 120, 170 (n2), 190, 199
OUT LGBT Well-being, 2, 28 (n41), 59, 87-93, 125, 146 (n5), 161 (n11), 206

Paganism, 8, 128-9, 235-45 (*see also* South African Pagan Rights Alliance)
Pan African Congress (PAC), 140-1
Parliament, 3-6, 51, 55-8, 62, 66-8, 80-1, 89-96 (n7), 102-3, 107-10, 112, 114, 115-46, 149, 150, 152-3, 159, 161 (n11), 162 (n20), 164-90, 196-9, 279-81; parliamentary hearings (on Civil Union Bill), 7, 8, 52-3, 115-46, 151, 164-8, 170 (n11), 190-8, 209, 215, 224, 265, 280; parliamentary submissions (on Civil Union Bill), 6, 90, 108, 112, 115-46, 149, 153, 165
pension benefits, 23, 38, 40 (n22), 44, 56-7, 60, 175, 195, 197, 258, 280-1, 341
Pietermaritzburg Gay and Lesbian Network, 103, 145 (n5), 321
'Polmed': see *Langemaat v Minister of Safety and Security and Others*
procreation: in LGBTI unions, 264; sex limited to, 176 (*see also* marriage and procreation); in woman-to-woman marriages, 253-4

Rainbow Project (Namibia), 300
rape, 209, 215, 217 (n2), 262-4; of lesbian women, 13, 127, 259-60; 'corrective', 191, 302; intramarital, 209
religion: and Constitution, 65, 68, 95, 126, 171, 184, 188, 189; freedom of, 139, 144, 158, 163 (n36); condemnation of homosexuality, 49-50, 113, 132, 274-5, 282; and rights, 95, 184, 300-6; and same-sex marriage, 7, 10, 11, 36, 38, 144, 166, 204, 209-45, 257, 260, 317, 338-40, 341-4; sanction of slavery, colonialism, male domination, 168 (*see also* Buddhism; Christianity; Hinduism; Islam; Paganism; sangomas)
Reforming Church, 48

Sachs, Albie (Justice), as supporter of LGBTI rights, 189
Sachs judgment in *Fourie* (Constitutional Court), 3, 4, 7, 21, 27 (n9), 31-2, 37-9 (n9, n12), 63-9, 117, 121, 137, 141, 164, 168-9, 182, 185, 186-90, 193, 195-8, 214-5, 218 (n6)
same-sex marriage campaign, 87-96, 228, 233, 279-282, 319, 339
same-sex marriage, opposition to, 5, 6, 14 (n13), 32, 93-4, 102-4, 110-3, 114, 118, 126, 131-2, 137-8, 159, 165, 167, 171-3, 184, 223, 239, 242-3, 249, 265, 276, 282-4
sangomas, 84, 174, 177, 235-45, 254-7
Satchwell v President of Republic of South Africa and Another, 22, 32, 36, 40 (n22), 41 (n56), 195, 258

353

sexuality/sexualities, 6, 11, 12, 13 (n2), 31, 81, 83, 84, 87, 91, 122, 176, 177, 182, 222-3, 226, 232, 234, 239, 240, 255, 260, 263, 265, 275-7, 279, 287, 341; asexuality, 272; bisexuality, 244; as continuum, 324; and human rights, 301; and marriage, 9, 249, 261, 277; and religion, 8, 235-45; and rights, 7; Tantric, 238 (*see also* heterosexuality, homosexuality)

Sexual Minorities Uganda, 300, 302

sodomy: as common-law crime, 17-20, 26 (n17, n18); in Criminal Procedures Act, 30, 39 (n11); decriminalization of, 3, 18, 55, 56, 60, 27 (n6), 269 (*see also* 'decriminalization case')

South African Catholic Bishop's Conference, 119-120

South African Council of Churches (SACC), 91, 138, 209, 214, 217 (n1); submission to Parliament, 129-31

South African Human Rights Commission (SAHRC), 91, 96 (n6), 164-7, 270-2; submission to Parliament, 117-9

South African Law Reform Commission, 45, 49, 62, 69 (n1), 120, 135

South African Pagan Rights Alliance, 128-9

Special Pensions Act, 27 (n3)

State v Kampher, 17-8, 20, 26 (n1, n2), 55

S v Makwanyane, 188, 192 (n4)

Supreme Court of Appeal (SCA), 2-4, 25, 27 (n1, n4, n9), 28 (n29), 58-9, 73, 78, 184, 167, 192 (n17), 265; judgment in *Fourie*, 2, 61-3, 167, 170 (n10), 184, 188-9, 192 (n10)

transgender, 156, 211, 224, 245, 330-5
transsexuality, 177, 206, 304, 331, 335-6
Triangle Project, 2, 6, 28 (n41), 52, 59, 111-4, 146 (n5), 206; submission to Parliament, 127-8

ubuntu, 103, 125, 191, 213, 274; justiciability, 217 (n4)

United Christian Democratic Party, 192 (n15)
United Democratic Front (UDF), 280

Women's Legal Centre (WLC), 116